SO-ATL-843

1817

HARPER & ROW, PUBLISHERS, New York

Cambridge, Philadelphia, San Francisco, London, Mexico City, São Paulo, Sydney

SCAVULLO

WOMEN

by Francesco Scavullo with Sean Byrnes

Also by Francesco Scavullo
Scavullo on Beauty
Scavullo Men

Copyright © 1982
by Francesco Scavullo

All rights reserved. Printed in the United States
of America. No part of this book may be used or
reproduced in any manner whatsoever without
written permission except in the case of brief
quotations embodied in critical articles and re-
views. For information address Harper & Row,
Publishers, Inc., 10 East 53rd Street, New York,
N.Y. 10022. Published simultaneously in Canada
by Fitzhenry & Whiteside Limited, Toronto.

FIRST EDITION

Designers:
Rochelle Udell, Doug Turshen

Library of Congress Cataloging in Publication
Data

Scavullo, Francesco
  Scavullo women.

  1. Beauty, Personal. 2. Woman—Interviews.
3. Women—Portraits. I. Title.
RA778.S274   646.7'042   81–48326
ISBN 0–06–014838–1   AACR2

82 83 84 85 10 9 8 7 6 5 4 3 2 1

PICTURE OF FARRAH FAWCETT REPRINTED
COURTESY OF *COSMOPOLITAN* COPYRIGHT ©
1975, THE HEARST CORPORATION. PICTURE OF
MIRELLA PETTENI REPRINTED COURTESY OF
HARPER'S BAZAAR © 1964, THE HEARST COR-
PORATION. PICTURES OF ADELLE LUTZ AND
TINA CHOW REPRINTED COURTESY OF
HARPER'S BAZAAR COPYRIGHT © 1979, THE
HEARST CORPORATION. PICTURES OF PRINCESS
CAROLINE AND ORNELLA MUTI REPRINTED
COURTESY OF *HARPER'S BAZAAR* © 1980, THE
HEARST CORPORATION. PICTURE OF LENA
HORNE REPRINTED COURTESY OF *HARPER'S BA-
ZAAR* COPYRIGHT © 1981, THE HEARST CORPO-
RATION. PICTURES OF ORIANA FALLACI, PRIN-
CESS ELIZABETH AND CATHERINE OXENBERG,
AND KIM ALEXIS REPRINTED COURTESY OF
VOGUE COPYRIGHT © 1980, CONDÉ NAST PUB-
LICATIONS, INC.

Hairstylists:
Michael Anthony
Phyllis Della
Andre Douglas
Bob Fink
Garren
Pamela Geiger
Maury Hopson
Harry King
Suga
Deborah Tomasino
Harie Von Wijnberg
Michael Weeks

Makeup Artists
Way Bandy
Sophie Levy
Sandy Linter
Joey Mills
John Richardson
Harie Von Wijnberg

Photo Editor: Sean Byrnes
Fashion and Beauty Editor: Sean Byrnes

My Thanks To:
Connie Clausen, my agent
Nancy Crawford and Elizabeth Perle, my editors
Doug Turshen and Rochelle Udell who designed the book
Jim Reiher, my studio manager
Frank Tartaro and Bob Bishop for work on the color photographs
Dick Cole for work on black-and-white photographs
Edith Loew Gross
Anne Rostaing
Kit Hawkins
Steve De Canio

Contents

The Women

Color

Black and White

nterviewers frequently ask me whom I have most enjoyed photographing and seem surprised when I don't instantly come up with the name of a famous fashion model. In the first place, I don't just work for *Vogue* and *Harper's Bazaar;* I also work for *Cosmopolitan* and for *Time* and *Newsweek* and I do album covers and a tremendous number of private portraits. I adore photographing women. Every time a woman walks into the studio, into the dressing room, and we begin the process of hair, makeup, accessories, I become really excited as slowly we bring out the best in that woman. When we go into the studio and I start photographing, the excitement comes all over again. It mounts and mounts and mounts until the final fabulous photograph of a woman looking the best she's ever looked in her life.

And that's what this book is all about.

The forty-six women in this book are a cross-section of that variety. Less than half are models; the rest are novelists, journalists, housewives, princesses, singers, schoolgirls, fashion editors, designers, businesswomen, movie stars, theater stars, television personalities. And—to lay to rest the myth that youth is an occupational obsession—more than a dozen are over forty.

The truth of the matter is, I am that most fortunate of human beings in that what I do for a living is what I love most in this world to do, which is to photograph women—all women. People who think it must get boring "just taking pictures" year after year, day after day, are way off base. Every day is different; every woman—every face, every personality—is a new, marvelous experience. Something in my head gets turned on by seeing a woman's looks really come together with the right makeup, the right hair style, the right

clothes: the whole pre-camera dressing-room ritual. I like to be right in there, along with the makeup artist and the hairdresser, getting the transitions on film, step by step as they happen; it's exciting to see a woman metamorphosed into something extraordinary, and I've included some of these transitional stages in the pages ahead.

But what gives me the biggest kick of all is to see a woman come out of that dressing room not just looking her best but *knowing* she looks her best. She doesn't have to say a word; the pleasure she feels in herself radiates like an aura. For me, that's the ultimate thrill of taking pictures: the look of someone who knows she's at her best. I don't know how you define glamorous, but to me that's it—not Movie Star, but simply any woman at her best.

Now, obviously, to be at your best you've got to know what's best for you. In other words, you've got to know yourself—know what you really look like. You have got to learn to look in the mirror objectively, which isn't the same as looking ruthlessly. Too many women get so hung up on a single imperfect feature—a too-prominent nose or too-small eyes or too-square jaw or too-thin mouth—that they never see themselves whole, and therefore they never discover their good points and how to make the most of them (which is often the secret of a so-called "great beauty": not flawless features but knowing how to accentuate the positive and eliminate the negative).

Another trap that women fall into in front of a mirror is that they look at themselves with a mind's-eye vision of some other person—someone they've seen in a film or in a magazine—and this is the image they take with them when they go shopping or go to the hairdresser. And this way disaster lies; it's why we see so many little tiny

women walking around in ridiculously oversized layers of clothes that looked terrific on a six-foot model in a magazine, and why we see so many Farrah Fawcett hairdos on women who would look stunning if their hair had something to do with their own looks instead of some other woman's.

I'm not saying that you should turn your back on fashion and go off in a totally opposite direction (though there are a lot of women who do, and a lot more who could learn from them; it's riskier being a rugged individualist but so much more interesting than being a sheep). What I am saying is this: A fashion magazine is a guide, not a bible. It tells you what's new and available. Some of those things are going to be good for you. Others could be, if you make some adjustments in the basic premise—I mean, if oversized clothes and voluminous layers are in and you love them and you're barely five-feet-five, you don't have to deprive yourself, but you do want to think in scale: fewer layers, a little less volume.

Still other things are to forget about. The most sensational-sounding diet is anything but, if it omits a food that your system may require—the way to find out is to consult your doctor or nutritionist. (This goes for all diets, by the way, including the ones you'll read about here: Judy Collins, for instance, thrives on a diet that cuts out red meat except for liver once a week; you may need more—know your needs.) Or you read that bright-red lipstick is hot stuff. Not if your lips aren't perfectly smooth and full and symmetrical, it isn't— again, know yourself. That's the key that's going to open all the doors for you, as it did for the women in this book. . . . Granted, they had the help of top makeup artists and hairdressers, but anyone, I think, can learn—and profit—by their experience.

Any Woman Can Be a Beautiful Woman

On Being a Beautiful Woman

To me, the word woman is synonymous with beauty, because I believe *every* woman has some natural beauty and has the potential to become even more beautiful than she thought possible.

What's the secret? It starts with being aware that as a woman you are a very special human being, endowed with physical features, characteristics, a personality, and a spirit that are uniquely yours. And it grows as you realize that it's up to you to make the absolute most of your special qualities and individual potential. Being a woman today means you have a tremendous number of options available, more so than at any other time in history. Whatever your personal goals are —whether it's to be a loving wife and mother, a good companion, a friend with whom to have fun and to share experiences, a confident professional who can achieve success in any arena and still retain her femininity and allure, or all these things and more— with the unprecedented freedom and opportunity available to women today, you can realize them . . . gloriously. With the joy and vitality of this kind of full, active involvement in your own life and the lives of those around you, also comes beauty.

''Beauty means intelligence and vitality.''

Beauty is . . .

Over the course of the nearly thirty-three years I've been photographing women, perceptions of beauty have changed dramatically. Perhaps the biggest change is that beauty today means *courage, intelligence,* and *vitality.* You no longer hear people talking about a woman who's beautiful but dumb; the two simply don't go together. It takes a courageous woman, an intelligent and aware woman, to carry the banner of beauty. In the forties, for example, the concept of feminine beauty hadn't evolved to the point it's reached today; the revolution where women were no longer relegated primarily to the home or placed on a pedestal was just beginning. The Victorian notion of the woman who dutifully raised her children and tended to the needs of her husband and home but had no real outside occupation or interests was already disappearing, and, for the most part, it's been a steady growth since then. The one exception, however, was in the late sixties and early seventies, when women seemed to feel they had to compete with men and this feeling was reflected in how they dressed and how they looked and acted. Things got very uniform looking—all the same suit, the same kind of makeup—it was too restrained. Women just didn't want to be bothered with their appearance and that part of their femininity. But women *must* be bothered with that part because that's what makes them female! No matter what a woman wants to be—even if it's president of the United States or the chief executive of an oil company—she's a woman and she must never forget it. And, really, after all, why should she want to?

Just as women search for certain desirable characteristics like intelligence, a sense of humor, breadth of interest (and, let's be honest, money and power never hurt!) in the men they're attracted to, so too do men seek out special qualities in a woman. A woman who's interested and curious and has many different facets to her personality is automatically a woman who's interesting; and if she's got a healthy body and a healthy mind, she's going to feel secure and happy with herself as a woman. She's going to be beautiful, too, because when you feel good about what's inside, you also want to make sure that the outside, which reflects the inner you, is as attractive as possible. Feminine beauty is an incredible kind of treasure, and instead of hiding or subduing it, women—all women— should use it to maximum advantage.

One of the first things I discovered when I began photographing women (and it's been a constant source of surprise ever since) is that your face is just like a screen, a blank canvas on which all the many aspects of your being alive are portrayed for others to view. I've seen women who started out as attractive young ladies become breathtakingly beautiful over the years because their attitude about themselves and their outlook on life had improved. The opposite is true, too, of course, and there's nothing sadder than to see a beautiful woman lose the fresh, alive quality of her looks because she's unhappy and doesn't keep up her appearance. So, then, what a woman should do to keep beautiful is quite simply to *be happy with herself.* Barbara Walters is a good example of this. I first photographed her in 1966, and I think with each year that has passed she has become more beautiful. In today's world when women are out doing exciting new things and have unlimited options, it's easier than ever to have a positive outlook.

Being young at any age

What about youth? Well, youth is just fabulous, but it's a *feeling* about yourself and about life that has nothing to do with your age. Physical youth is one thing; a 100-year-old tree, no matter what condition it's in, is still a 100-year-old tree. Youth, like beauty, is a spiritual quality; that's why you have fabulous people like Katharine Hepburn, Georgia O'Keeffe, Louise Nevelson, Gloria Swanson, Greta Garbo, Valentina—all these women have a glorious free spirit. Diana Vreeland has it too; so do Lena Horne and Ruth Ford. These women

"You've got to experiment a little."

are the real beauties. If you worry about age, how many years you have lived, or dwell on your birthdays, it makes you unhappy—and that's terribly aging. So why worry? Besides, as Lauren Bacall said, your only other alternative is to slit your throat!

What's fresh and new and youthful is how a woman looks and feels when her mind and her body are in great shape and she's got the right hair, the right makeup, the right clothes and accessories to go with them. Women who have it all together can't help but feel young, just as they can't help looking youthful.

Making the right decisions for you

Being beautiful involves making some personal decisions, starting with the makeup and wardrobe that are right for you. The first thing to understand is that there are no hard and fast rules. What's right is what works best for you and feels comfortable. So you've got to try different things, experiment a little, use the fashion magazines as guides for getting new ideas. Young girls, for instance, should have some throwaway clothes—try short skirts, tight skirts, pantaloons, whatever you want. You can use a certain part of your wardrobe to have fun. But nothing's worse than a woman who becomes a fashion victim, who tries everything she sees in a magazine. I know a woman, for instance, who wears a tricorn hat, probably because she saw it presented in a magazine and so went out and bought it. But when I see her walking down the street, I think, Here comes the lady with the tricorn hat. I don't see the woman as she really is because the hat dominates her, and the hat is a mistake. Magazines are only there to show you, to give you ideas; it's like window shopping. When you purchase something and adopt it for yourself, on the other hand, it should be suited specifically to you and to your personality.

Once you know what works for you, stick with it. Just because fashions change seasonally doesn't mean you should throw out everything you've got. Add slowly and gradually to your

wardrobe, especially as you grow older. As a woman matures, she's changing all the time—the way she feels, her makeup, the way she dresses. If a woman is unhappy with herself and feels she wants to change her looks to improve them, I approve most heartily. But simply changing for the sake of change is wrong. Look at women like Gloria Vanderbilt and Diana Vreeland, who have kept their look for a long time. Classic beauties, they've found what's right for them and shouldn't change. Actresses, of course, have to change their looks for different parts, but in life you're not an actress, you're *you,* and who you are is very important. Once you've found the style you like and that works for you, keep it.

Staying beautiful

I've photographed many of the same women again and again over the course of years and so I'm always asked, What should a woman do at the different stages of her life—twenties, thirties, forties, fifties—to stay beautiful? The answer is this: You must always keep up healthy skin and healthy hair and a healthy body. And your mind, your psyche, has to be healthy, too. These are the most important things. You can't be beautiful if you don't feel healthy and if you haven't worked at maintaining your body and mind. You have to take care of yourself as a whole; think of it as adopting a holistic approach to beauty. Beauty includes your outlook, your optimism about life, your enthusiasm, your intelligence, and so on, every bit as much as what you do with your physical features. A great example of this is Rose Kennedy, who's known so many tragedies and had so many things in her life that would send other women around the bend, but there she is. And it's because she's simply got indomitable courage, faith, and spirit. Where it comes from doesn't matter. Courage and spirit are what give you the strength and conviction to lead your life in the best way possible. These qualities are also what keep you beautiful and young looking; the important thing is to find them from whatever source is right for you.

The beauty basics

When a woman walks into my studio to be photographed, the first thing I notice about her is the general picture she presents, whether she looks good or not. I don't focus on details immediately because I'm trying to get an overall impression of who and what this woman is, just as anyone would do upon meeting a person for the first time. Once I have this overall sense, I start to analyze the details—eyebrows, makeup, hair, skin, and so on—until every feature has been catalogued in my mind and I know exactly what improvements have to be made before we begin to photograph.

Every woman should go through this same procedure for critically evaluating herself at *least* once in her lifetime, and probably periodically over the years. To do it, stand in front of a full-length mirror with light that's not too harsh or bright. Do this twice—the first time *fully dressed, with your usual hairstyle and makeup;* the second time *without clothes and without makeup.* Be objective about what you see in the reflection. Concentrate initially on getting a general impression of yourself, and then start to analyze specific features. Use a magnifying or double-sided mirror for a close-up inspection of your face.

The basic beauty guidelines that follow will help you begin the process of refining and improving to maximize your beauty potential.

Eyebrows—Most women make a terrible mistake when they tweeze, pluck, and shape their eyebrows. The thing to remember is that eyebrows balance your face and frame your eyes, and you can change them to enhance your looks. You can't change your eyes too much except for the subtle addition of some color to bring out their natural beauty, so if you change your eyebrows and make a mistake, it sticks out like a sore thumb. There's nothing worse than a woman whose eyebrows have been plucked or penciled to a thin, straight, ugly line or to end halfway across her brow or extend too far down, distorting her whole face. Your eyebrows should always follow the natural curve of your eyes, beginning at about the point formed if you hold a pencil vertically next to the base of your nose. As for thickness, often the brow's natural fullness is the ideal texture. If you think you need to make adjustments, it's a wise idea to consult a professional makeup artist before doing any significant plucking or tweezing.

Skin—A woman with beautiful skin is a truly beautiful woman. Carmen, for instance, has absolutely exquisite skin, which she takes care of by using moisturizers and mineral oil and by observing a strict regimen of cleansing, proper exercise, and nutrition. Every woman has to find her own balance of the right creams and conditioners, moisturizers, foods, vitamins, water intake, exercise, and sleep, as well as the type of cleansing routine that will bring out the best in her skin.

Clean skin is a must, and the first step in proper skin care is to learn how best to clean it. Everyone's skin is different, and for this reason it's a good idea to make an appointment with a good skin-care specialist or dermatologist to help you analyze your skin and then formulate a cleansing routine. Some women can use almost any kind of soap to cleanse their faces; others have such delicate skin that soap is too abrasive and milky cleansers are best. Some women can have facials as often as once a week or as infrequently as once a month to keep their skin glowing; others should never have facials at all. It all depends upon your skin. The same holds true for squeezing, using astringents, scrubbing with a washcloth or loofah. The same procedure that is perfect for some skin types simply cannot be tolerated by other types of skin. Cosmetic products, too, include ingredients that have different effects on different skin types.

In general, creams and moisturizers specially selected for your skin type and age are good for keeping the skin soft and supple and preventing it from aging prematurely from too much exposure to sun, dry heat, and other factors that damage and dry skin. There are only two absolute rules about skin care that every woman should observe: (1) good hygiene (cleansing) is imperative and (2) never, never wear makeup to bed. Makeup that's worn all the time clogs the pores so they never breathe and dries and ages the skin.

Makeup—Common sense, basic good taste, and a sure instinct about what works for you are your best allies in applying makeup that looks and feels right. Not every woman needs to wear foundation, for example. If your skin is in good condition to begin with, it's a mistake to cover it up with makeup that's not necessary. Even if you live in an area like New York or Los Angeles where smog and pollution are a problem, you don't necessarily need a foundation. A light cream or moisturizer and careful cleansing twice a day to maintain the skin's clear, healthy look are sufficient. If you do use foundation, make sure it's specially selected for your skin type, and always wear it as lightly as possible. Also, when applying foundation, the sponge or other applicator you use should be perfectly clean.

In general, makeup should be worn lightly, and this is especially true in the daytime. Sunlight and the fluorescent lighting in offices are just not good on makeup. And a lot of makeup for daytime is inappropriate. If you've ever seen a woman walk down the street in bright daylight wearing too much makeup or a harsh eye shadow or a too-brightly-colored lipstick you've seen how it jars the eye. Office lighting magnifies this even more. During the daytime, lip gloss, a little blush for a touch of color, and a light application of black or brown eyeliner or mascara are plenty for most women.

Nighttime makeup can be much more exciting and daring; this is the time for heavier colors, eye shadow, and for really playing up a distinctive feature, such as a beautiful mouth or beautiful eyes (just be sure you don't play up every feature, or you'll cancel them all out).

If you wear eye shadow, *flat, matte* colors like *taupes, grays,* and *browns* are best. They give a smoky, sexy, subtle look that is great on any woman. Too much color around the eyes, on the other hand, takes away from the natural beauty of your eye color. Blue shadows, in particular, are disastrous for most women. Of course there's always the exception—like Elizabeth Taylor, who uses violet shadow, and on this rare beauty it looks stunning. To add more color around the eyes, try combinations, like a purple with a brown or taupe to give a little life. Blending different colors together with

a brush or accenting with a subtle touch of highlight like peach or beige can be great as long as the result looks natural and there are no lines. If you use pencil liners, again, blacks and browns or even a little blue mixed with a gray or brown are best, depending upon the color of your eyes. Never use iridescent shadows; they look gaudy and dry out the delicate skin tissue on the eyelids, thus aging it.

Even at night, you don't need much makeup to look glamorous. Oriana Fallaci and Florinda Balkan, for example, both look best with a minimal makeup that doesn't detract from their strong, distinctive features. Brooke Shields, a young girl, looks great either with a lot of makeup or none at all. And if you're lucky enough to be like Janis Savitt, who's so knock-out glamorous she can get away with a lot of makeup even on the beach, pulling out all the stops with a lot of makeup tastefully applied can be simply magnificent.

Hair—Your hair can make or break your face. It doesn't really matter what you do with your hair provided that you do it well and it works for your face and your personality. There are two major sins women often commit with their hair. These involve *shape* and *color*—and they can be corrected.

Shape is something you have to work out with your hairdresser. You should have a general idea of what shape and length of hair is good for you, but ask yourself some questions: Is the cut too blunt? Too long or too short for your face? Is it all one length, too many lengths? Younger women can look sensational in all different cuts and lengths of hair; most women in their forties and fifties, I find, tend to look better with shorter hair rather than longer hair. If an older woman wants to have long hair, then usually it looks best if it's pulled back or in a chignon. A glamour bob, for example, is not the best look for a woman who's over fifty. Just look at the photograph of Polly Mellen, who

leaves her hair gray and gets a marvelous straight blunt cut that looks perfectly smashing on her.

Hair color is also crucial, and for this you absolutely must see a good specialist. Robert Renn, for example, is a very good hair colorist, probably the best in New York, because he doesn't dye hair one color—he streaks it. If he streaks in a lot of gray salt-and-pepper, as he did recently for my sister, he doesn't change anything; rather, he improves on the natural and makes the hair look the way it did ten years ago. If you dye or frost your hair instead of streaking, you really take a chance because it's a major change, and if you dye it a bad color or frost it so that it looks artificial and terrible, you're going to be stuck with it during an awkward transition period. Plus, if you dye your hair, you have to have it done every ten days or so as the natural color starts to grow out. Streaking or highlighting, on the other hand, need be done only about every four months.

What to do about graying hair is definitely a matter of individual preference. On some women, gray looks distinctive and elegant; others just can't abide it under any circumstances. If a woman in her twenties or thirties starts to go gray, especially a brunette, it adds a bit of light that picks up the face and can look marvelous; this should be left alone. In general, as the skin starts to age and have lines, lighter hair colors soften the face. A shorter, softer cut and a lighter hair color minimize the harsh look that darker hair tends to create. A wonderful thing you can do when your hair begins to go gray is to keep streaking in a million highlight colors. Sometimes you see a woman and you don't know exactly if she's blond, beige, gray, or what—just that she looks terrific. If you decide you want this look for your hair, be sure to go to an expert instead of trying to do it yourself.

All these rules about hair color apply in general, but there's always an exception to the rule or a rule that you break.

Ruth Ford, for instance, in her earlier picture ten years ago had short, dark hair; in the picture I took of her ten years later her hair is long and blond and looks much better on her. Ruth, of course, has a real sense of style; I think she had her hair done blond for a play she was in and realized that she really looked better. So you break rules, too. A lot of brunettes, for example, choose to keep their hair dark instead of lightening it as they get older. Gloria Vanderbilt and Diana Vreeland both color their hair to keep it dark, and on them it looks perfect and amazingly youthful. It depends on the woman.

Of course, you have to take care of your hair as well as having the right shape and color for it to look its best. If you blow your hair dry, color it, use heat or hair spray on it, or do anything that's going to damage it or dry it, you must be careful to condition it. A good trichologist, like Philip Kingsley, will tell you what shampoo to use, what conditioner, and all the things you need to know to maintain the texture and quality of your hair.

Nutrition—You've got to be as healthy as can be, which means eating the right foods in the right amounts. Many attractive women who are impeccably groomed miss being truly beautiful because they get lazy when it comes to using a little self-discipline to control their eating habits. Nutrition, like any other aspect of body maintenance, has to be keyed to the individual—you're the one who knows best if you aren't eating enough of the proper foods, to keep your energy level high or are abusing your body with too much sugar or too many of the non-nutritious temptations it's so easy to succumb to.

A balanced, nutritious eating regimen supplemented by vitamins is the basis of proper nutrition. And it's essential, I think, for every woman to consult a diet specialist or nutritionist to plan a diet that is tailored specifically to her body's individual needs. Some women, for instance, can do very

well without breakfast; others, with low blood sugar, need as many as six small meals a day to keep up maximum energy level. Different blood types also have different nutritional requirements: type A blood, for instance, may require lower-grade food and less protein for the system to operate optimally; other blood types, like O, may need higher-grade food, higher in protein. B and AB blood types often require the best of both kingdoms in moderation. Remember, protein and starch eaten together are more difficult to digest; I find it better to combine protein with a vegetable or starch with a vegetable. And always wait one to two hours before eating fruits or desserts.

Everything you take into your system is going to have an effect on it, either positive or negative, and so it's important to be aware of what your body's needs are. This applies especially to smoking and drinking. I'm totally against cigarettes because they pollute your body and pollute the environment, and smoking them is the single worst thing you can do to harm your system. I've never done cigarette advertising; it's geared to young girls and young women and I don't want to encourage this destructive habit. Drinking, on the other hand, when done with moderation and intelligence, is fine, depending, of course, upon your body's tolerance. As a child I was brought up with my grandfather from Italy, whose attitude was that everybody needs red wine to digest their food, so as kids we drank water with a splash of wine. That's stayed with me through the years, and I enjoy a glass of red wine with dinner (never white, which gives me a headache and has a high acid content). Some people have no tolerance for drinking alcoholic beverages, though; a good nutritionist can advise you on this. For daytime, plenty of water, fruit juices (apple juice is especially tasty), and herb teas are a healthy substitute for coffee and alcohol.

Proper diet is especially important for women who work in offices during the day where there's a lot of tension. In this kind of environment it's easy to slip into the coffee-and-Danish habit during the morning and sending out for whatever's quick and inexpensive for lunch. Don't do this to your body! It's just the worst, and the sugar actually adds to your feeling of stress. If you work in an office, try bringing your own herbal teas and fruit juices and plenty of bottled water to drink during the day. If you have a luncheon appointment at a restaurant, choose one that serves healthy food in sensible portions and is located several blocks away—walk over and back for the exercise. Try to avoid drinking alcohol at lunch; it's a depressant and makes you sleepy, despite the immediate high the sugar provides. Bottled water, fruit juices, and herb teas are much healthier for you and if you drink them in lieu of a cocktail or wine you'll find you've got more energy for the rest of the day.

One final note about diet: if you need to go on a weight-reduction program, be sure it's one that's approved by your doctor. Fad diets and crash diets are dangerous to your health, and the pleasure you get from losing a few pounds in a hurry is going to be wiped out by the negative physiological effects rapid weight loss has on your system. Plus, weight that's lost rapidly never stays off permanently.

Exercise—Everybody should exercise daily, and with enjoyable exercise programs available by merely turning on the television, there's no reason even the busiest executive can't devote fifteen minutes a day to this important part of your beauty routine. You can buy an exercise mat for a few dollars and lay it on the bedroom floor for calisthenic routines. Tennis, jogging, jazz dancing, and aerobic exercises, especially swimming, are also excellent ways of keeping in shape, particularly for women with sedentary jobs. If you've got the time and money, try using the facilities at a health club. Walk as much as you possibly can—if you're staying in the office for lunch, make a point to reserve ten or fifteen minutes for a brisk, invigorating walk to help clear your mind. The point is that exercise gets your circulation going, helps minimize stress, and elevates your spirits. Just try worrying about a contract or an unfinished memo after a half hour of vigorous movement! The physical and psychological feeling that comes from having a healthy, beautiful body cannot be measured in dollars and cents. What are you waiting for?

Environment—I'm a firm believer that there can never be too much beauty in the world. Oriana Fallaci says that beauty is something that our eyes caress and that it's very important to us as human beings and to our lives to

Attitude—Your attitude about life is the finishing touch on the beautiful canvas that's you. Even the most magnificent oil painting doesn't look as good as it could if the frame isn't right. So it's important to envelop yourself with a positive, optimistic attitude about everything and everyone you come into contact with. Spend a few minutes in the quiet hours of the morning in meditation or contemplation, refusing to let any worrisome or negative thoughts enter your mind. Throughout the day, congratulate yourself on the things you do well, the compliments you get. Once you develop this kind of rewards system, you won't want to give it up! In addition, try giving yourself a treat whenever you can. It mitigates stress like nothing else. At the end of the day, lull yourself to sleep with happy thoughts about yourself and those you love. The inner peace these kind of thoughts and feelings bring also brings exterior beauty.

Your ideal beauty regimen

1. Understand yourself. Take the time to get to know yourself. Study yourself, your habits and features, and evaluate each of them realistically. Which are best? Which have areas for improvement?

2. Consult an expert for advice. Every woman's features are different, and to be truly beautiful, your makeup, hair, skin, and wardrobe should be suited specifically to you. Let an expert teach you how to maximize your own beauty potential.

3. Develop a style of your own. What you're trying to achieve is a look that enhances your features as much as possible and at the same time lets your natural beauty shine through.

4. Allow yourself enough time to be beautiful. Give yourself enough time to improve those areas that need it and to maintain a balanced beautiful look.

5. Be open to new ideas. Be flexible and experiment with new ways to accessorize, apply makeup, and so on. Freshness only adds to basic beauty.

"Always maintain an attitude of respect for yourself . . . a positive attitude is the best incentive to beauty."

---

surround ourselves with beauty. I think she's definitely right about that. The small ways in which a woman pampers herself—like wearing a clean, fresh white terry-cloth robe after taking a bath, using soft, subtle lighting in an office instead of harsh fluorescents, spraying a little Evian water on your face for instant refreshment—all add to this immediate sense of beauty, as, of course, do the bigger ways, like always wearing the most attractive makeup and clothes you can to bring out the best in you. We must see the beauty in life and strive to make life as beautiful as we possibly can.

Discipline—Montaigne said it all in the sixteenth century: Moderation is the key to life. Being moderate—knowing what's best for you in every area and sticking with it—brings harmony and beauty, and that takes discipline. Take the time to figure out what your best beauty regimens are, including makeup, hair, diet, and exercise, and then use just a little self-discipline to keep with them. Once you've determined what's right for you, it takes only thirty minutes a day to maintain your body and mind in the proper, healthy balance you need to be a totally beautiful you.

6. Keep your body healthy. Always get enough sleep and exercise, eat properly, and maintain good nutritional habits.

7. Be disciplined. Once you've found what works for you, stick with it. Being beautiful is a kind of positive addiction, and once you've developed the habit you won't want to give it up.

8. Have respect for yourself. Always maintain an attitude of tremendous respect for yourself and for the people you come in contact with, so that you always try to look your best. A positive mental attitude is the best incentive to beauty; if you love yourself and you love life, you can't help being naturally beautiful!

Every woman — every face, every personality — is a new, marvelous experience. The forty-six women in this book are a cross section. . . . Less than half are models; the rest are novelists, journalists, housewives, princesses, singers, schoolgirls, fashion editors, designers, businesswomen, movie stars, theater stars, television personalities. And — to lay to rest the myth that youth is an occupational obsession — more than a dozen are over forty.

Something in my head gets turned on by seeing a woman's looks really come together with the right makeup, the right hair style, the right clothes . . . it's exciting to see a woman metamorphosed into something extraordinary. . . . But what gives me the biggest kick of all is to see a woman . . . not just looking her best but *knowing* she looks her best. . . .

Elizabeth Taylor

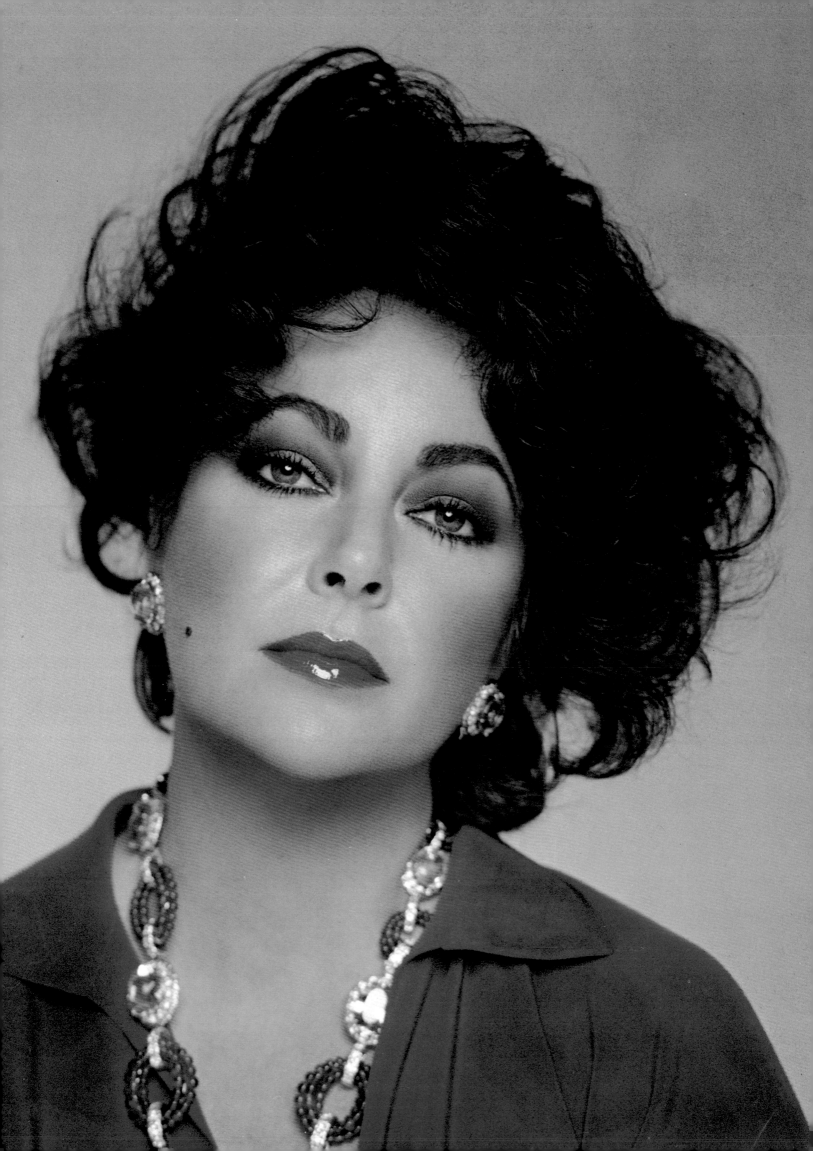

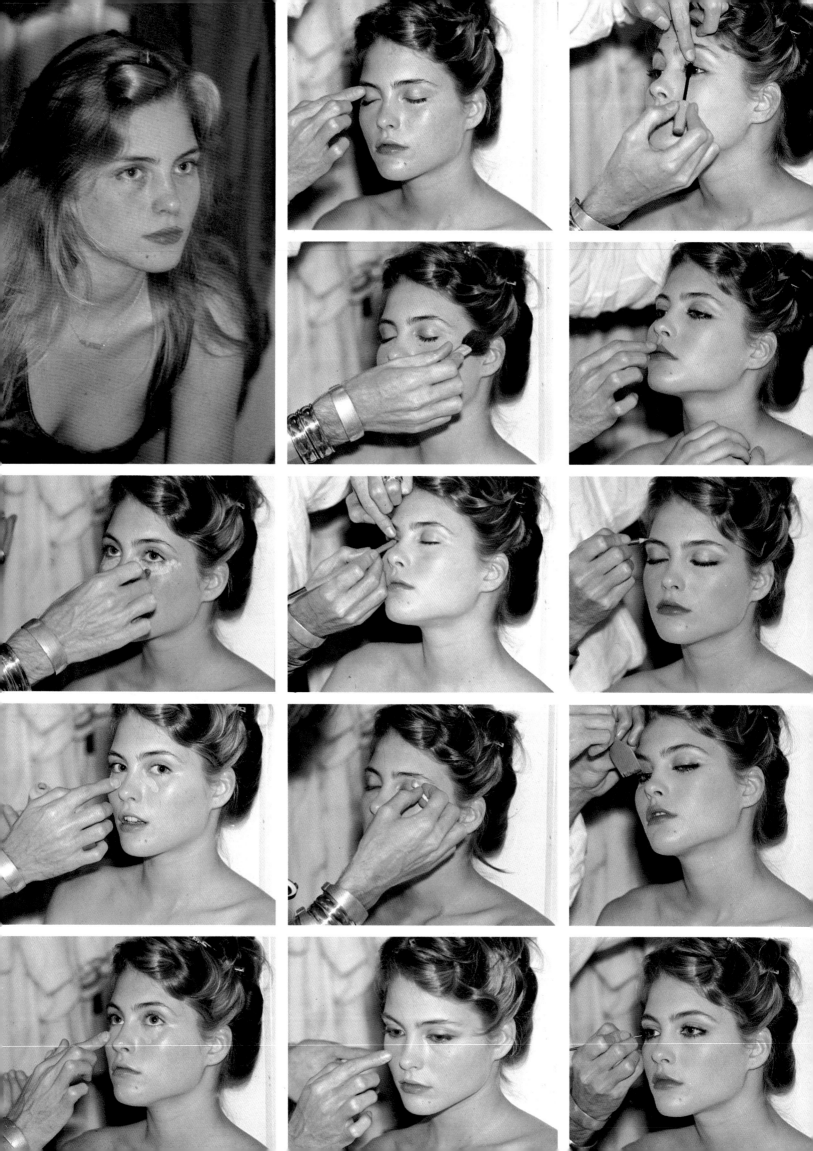

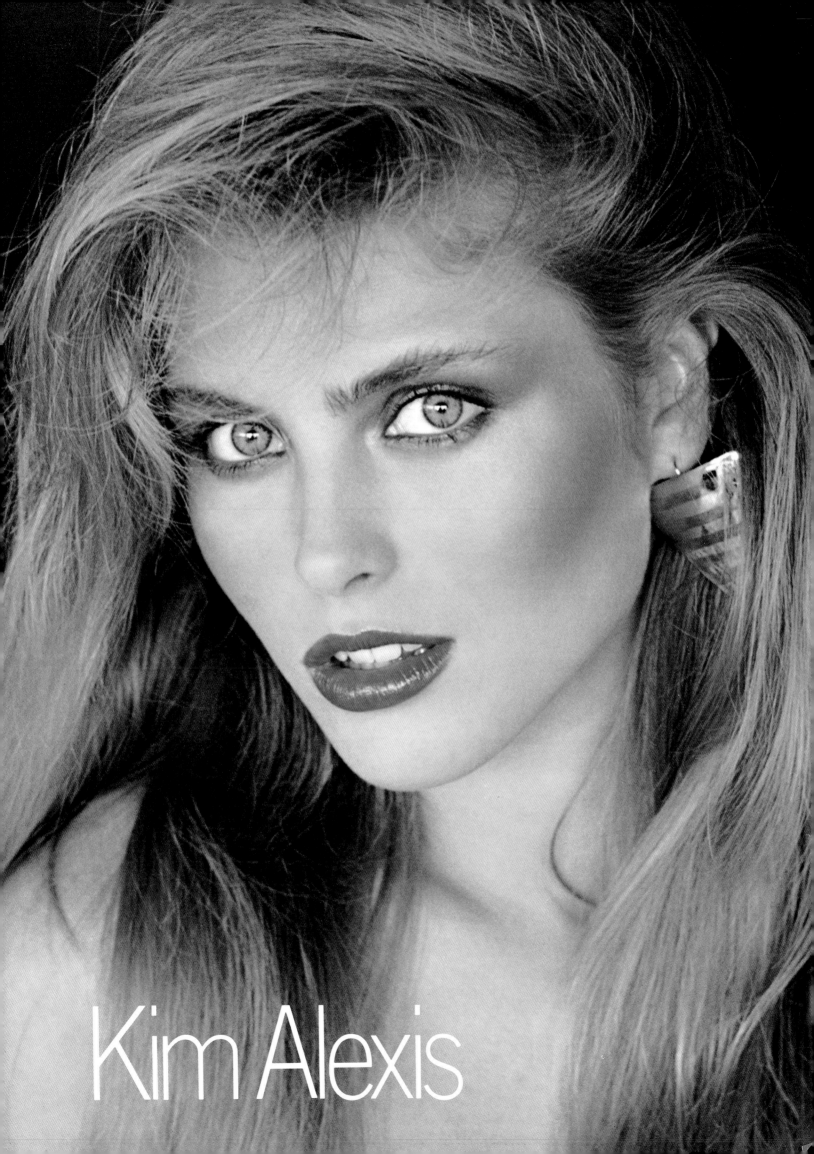

Kim Alexis

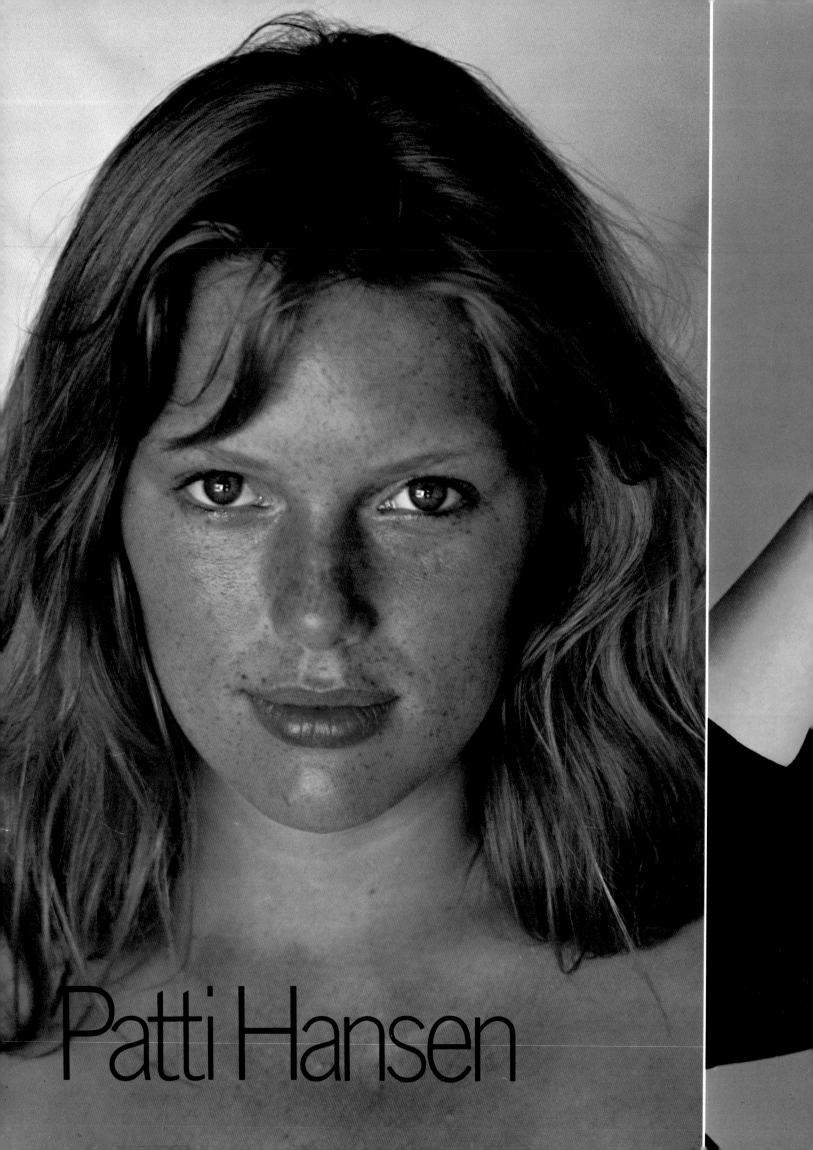

Patti Hansen

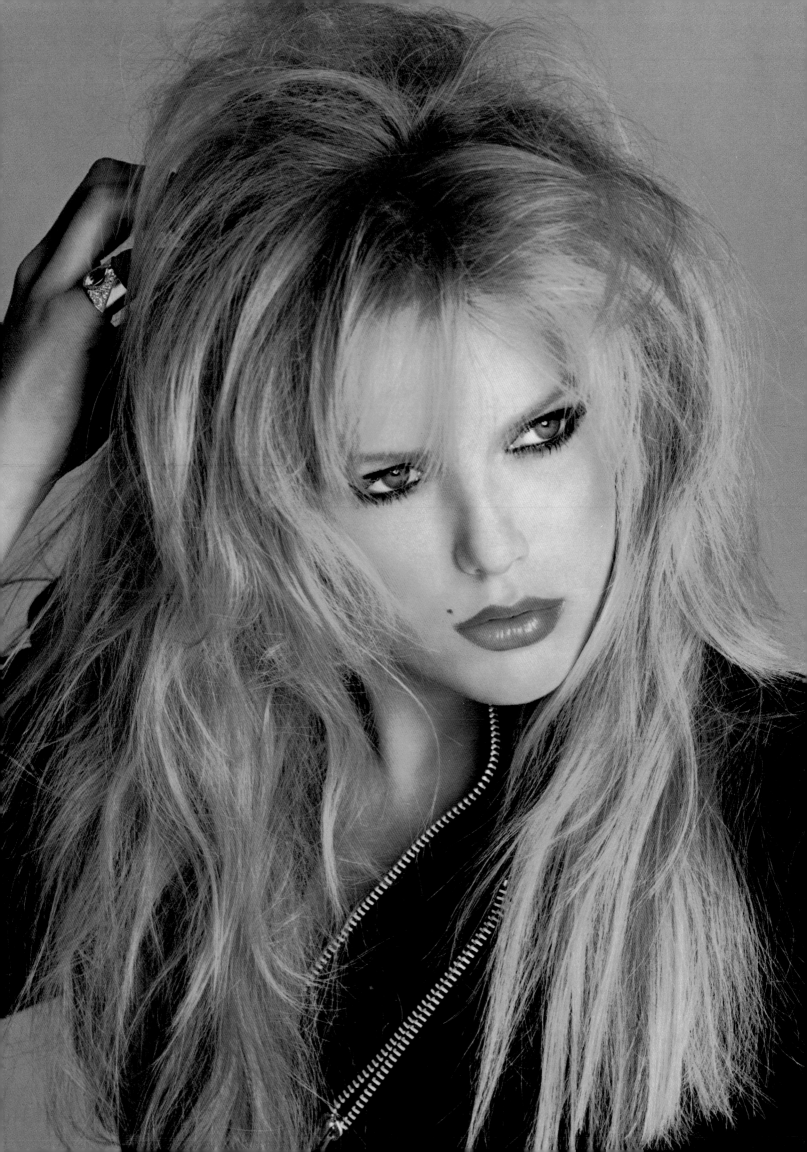

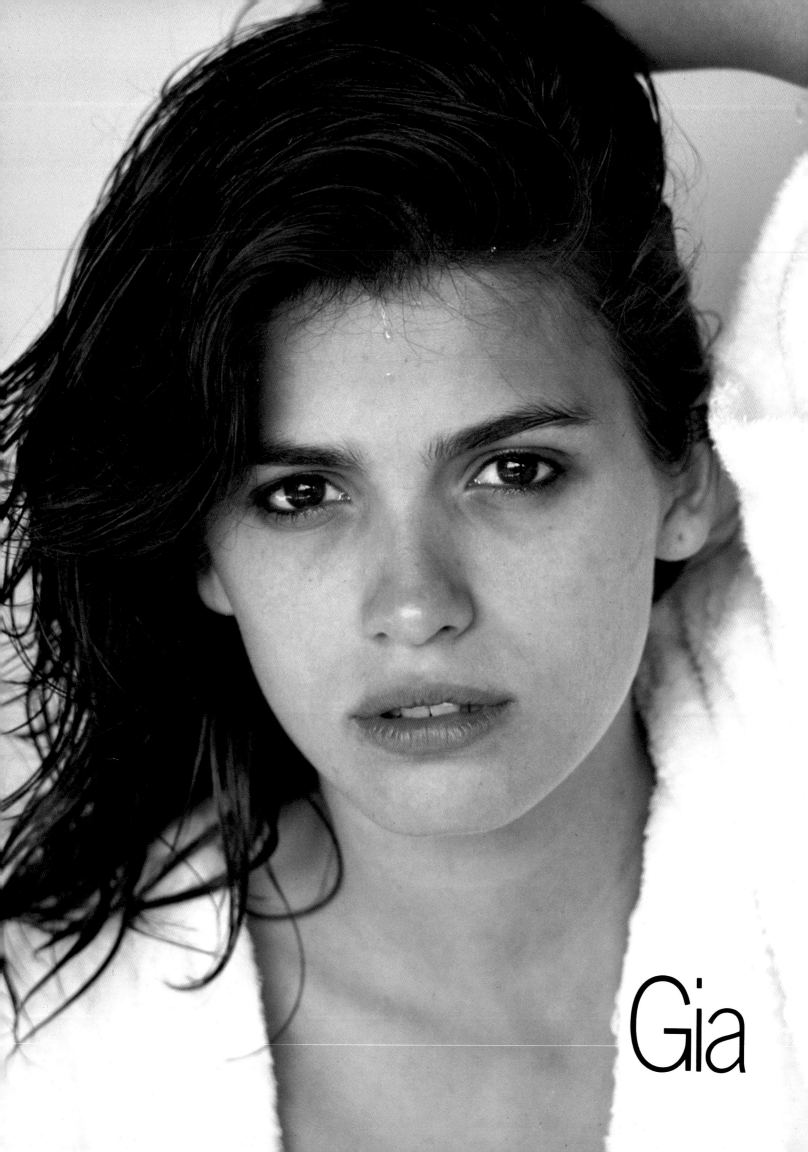

Gia

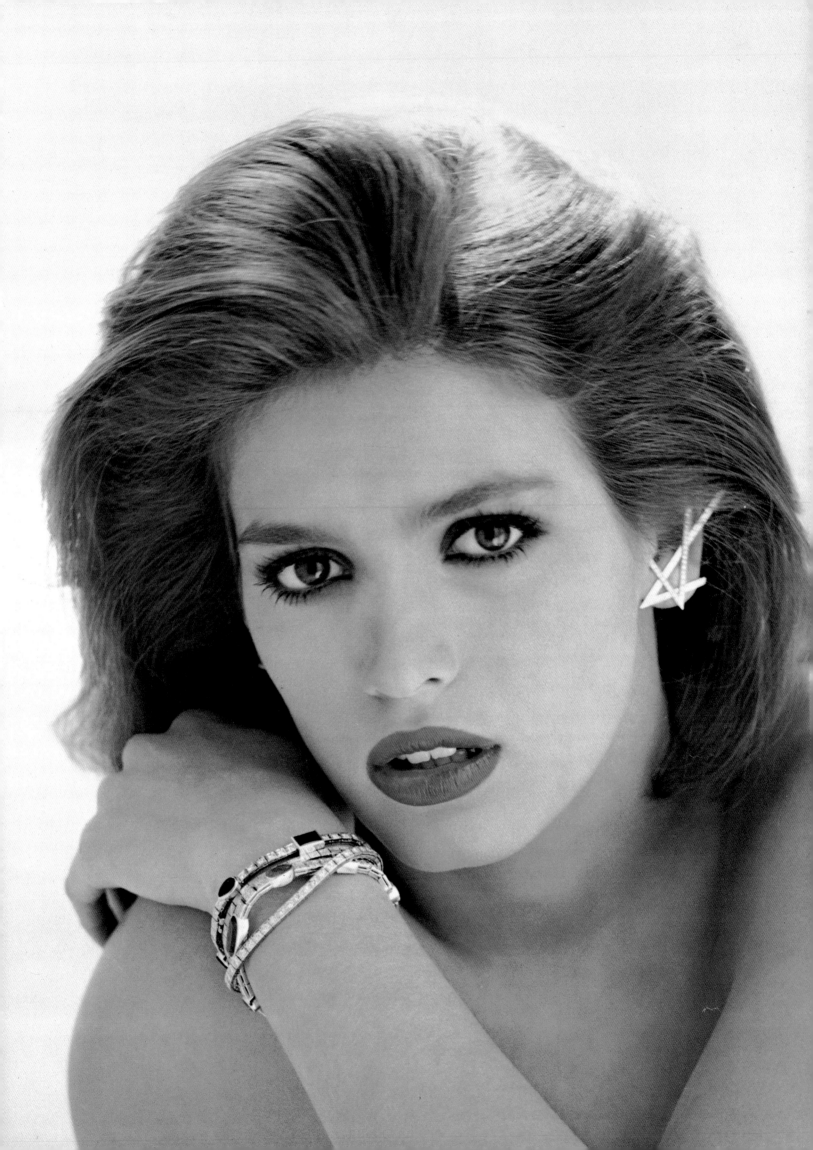

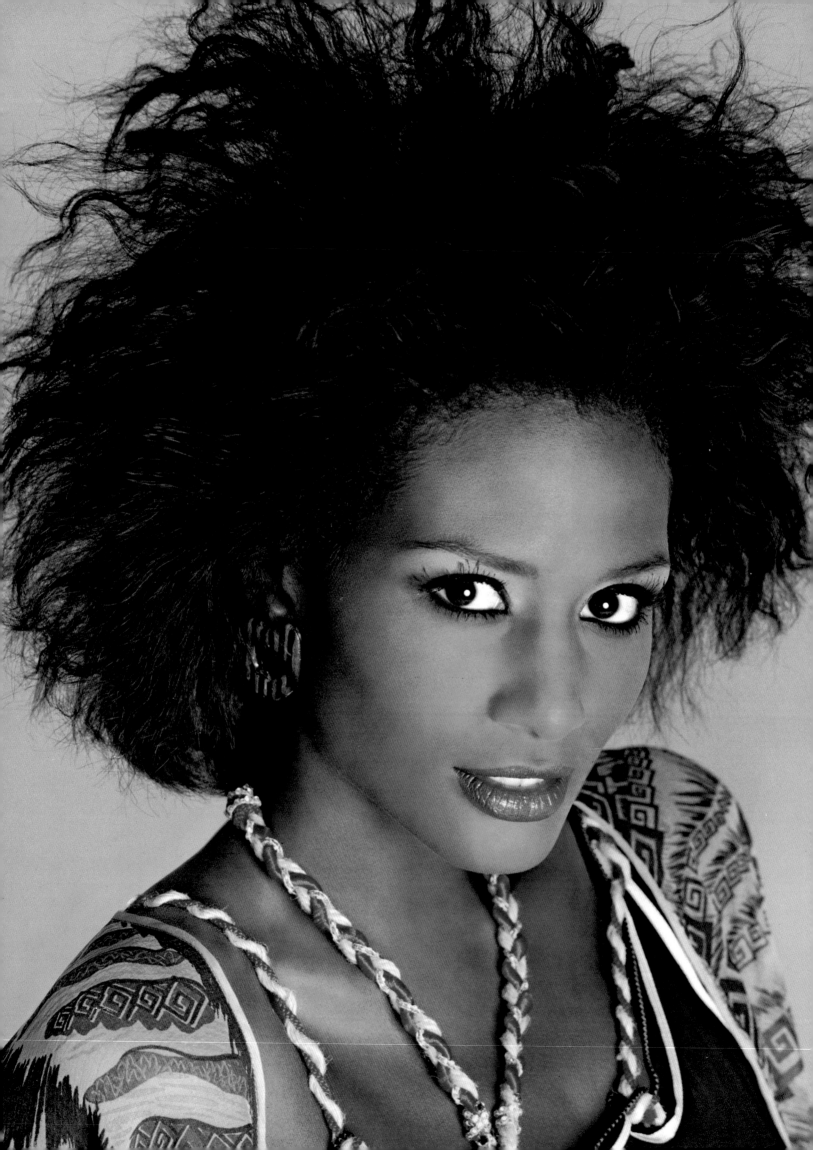

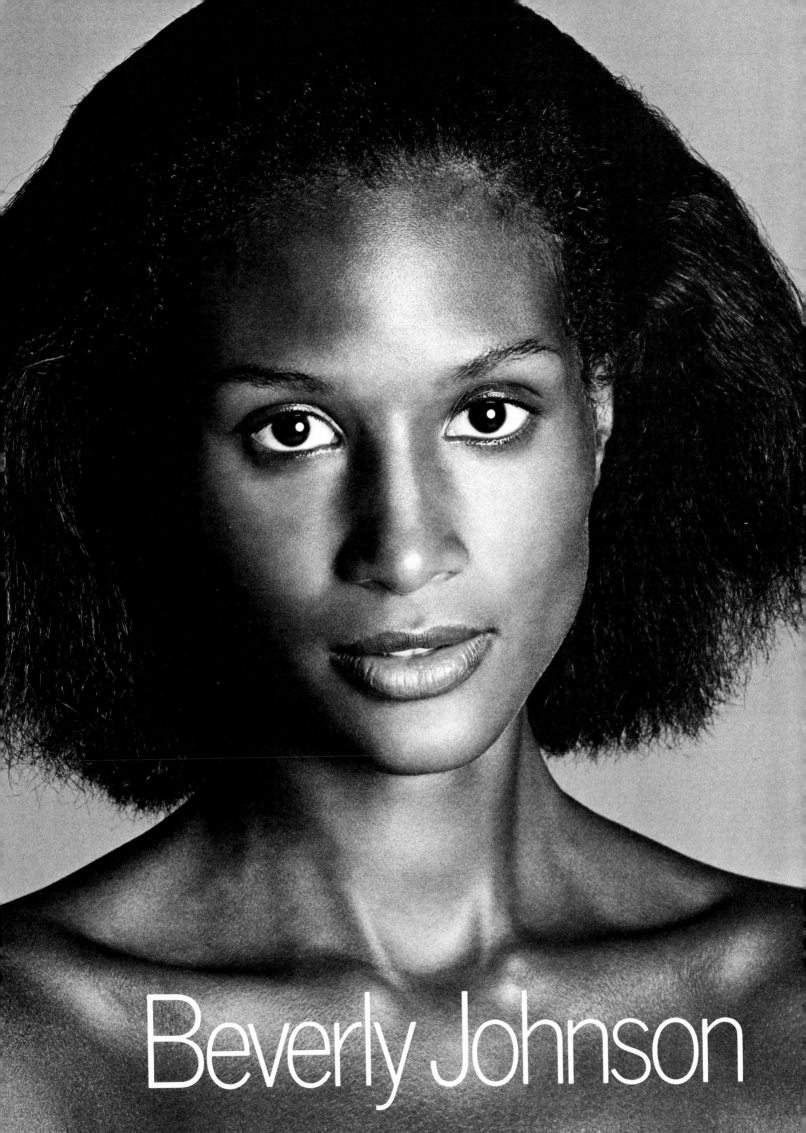

Beverly Johnson

Elizabeth Taylor

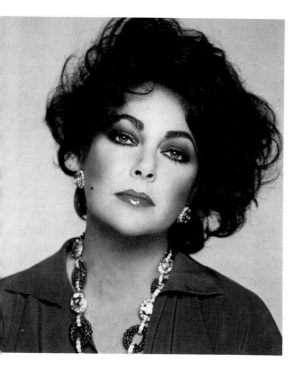

The truth about Elizabeth Taylor is that she is an earthy, intelligent, bubbly, amusing woman, almost entirely without vanity and more casual about how she cares for her looks than women with considerably less at stake. She washes her face—that still fabulous face—with ordinary soap. In a hotel, she'll use the soap the hotel provides; if she happens to be laid up in the hospital, she uses their brand. And afterwards she puts on a hand lotion that she has used since the age of ten ("Don't say the name; it grotzes me to give them free plugs when all they've ever given me is a case of the lotion").

Elizabeth has often been overweight ("I didn't start having a weight problem until after having my children"). I have a fantasy in which I run away with her to a health spa for six months, and when we get back, she has the figure she had at sixteen. As a matter of fact, she has been to a couple of spas for a couple of weeks, "to exercise, tone up. I like the discipline and the regime. I think it's healthy for you. I could have had more pampering, more facials and hair treatments and fingernail treatments and all that stuff. I chose not to get it. I chose to have more exercise. For the first three days, I could barely walk." Between the exercise and the diet she lost five pounds—it is definitely *not* true that she lost thirty pounds, as she was rumored to have done, in a single all-out weekend at the Golden Door.

All sorts of myths attend Elizabeth, one of the most enduring being the myth of the violet eyes. She has astonishingly beautiful eyes—hauntingly expressive eyes. She can break your heart with those eyes, or she can break you in two with them. But they are not violet eyes; they are *blue* eyes, which on an Irish girl, with thick black lashes and black hair and white skin, isn't anything you'd want to take back to the store for a refund. On the other hand, if it's violet eyes you crave, Elizabeth knows the trick; she wears purple a lot, she wears sapphires a lot, and as long as I've known her she's worn violet-blue eyeshadow. On her, I go for it. Everything she does with makeup is brilliant for her; she puts her finger into the paintbox and pulls out . . . Elizabeth Taylor!

Way Bandy does her differently from the way she does herself: the softly smudged eye versus the boldly outlined eye. "I couldn't stand it the first time Way made me up, mostly because I don't like people putzing around my eyes. I always feel they're going to stick a pencil in. He was the first person I'd let make me up, and I was very, very happy that I did. But he had to fight me to do it. I'm just so used to doing my own. Of course, there's always a makeup man on the set to help. But the actual application—I've been doing that for years. I even did it in *Cleopatra.* I didn't start out to, but after about a month and a half, the makeup man developed disc problems in his back,

"Even three years ago, I wouldn't have said that I might ever, under any circumstances have a face lift, because I'm of the grow-old-gracefully school, and every wrinkle I've got is a wrinkle I've earned. But it's wrong to discount any possibility."

and I did the rest of the film—designed the eye makeups and everything. I had a *ball!*"

She is reputed to be one of the great jewel collectors of the Western world. She is. "I like pretty things. You could also say I collect trees. And art." Her collection of French Impressionists, Art Nouveau, and Art Deco is "scattered around" in various houses, which she might also be said to collect—in the U.S., in Mexico, in Switzerland. And each is sufficiently staffed and outfitted so that, should she choose to, she could pop into any one at any time, without having to pick up even a toothbrush en route.

■

"I have two Oscars, and I am not at all unhappy about that; I wouldn't trade them for anything, but they are not my life."

■

As practically everyone knows, Elizabeth came to Hollywood from London at the age of seven, with her mother, a former actress, her father, an art dealer, and her older brother, Howard. Although putting Elizabeth into films was her mother's dream (and her father's nightmare), it wasn't the standard stage-mother obsession but something that "sort of dawned on her, because strangers kept coming up to her and suggesting it. They were doing *Gone with the Wind* at the time, and people would say, 'she resembles Vivien Leigh so much, you should put her up for the role of Scarlett's little girl.' " She didn't get the part—though it still pleases her enormously to be told she looks like Vivien Leigh—but she did eventually get a contract with Universal.

"You won't believe how I got that contract: it was because I sang!" Not, evidently, as well as Deanna Durbin, and six months later, ten-year-old Elizabeth was out of Universal—"the casting director said, 'She'll never do in films. She's got a very old, very sad face. That face won't sell' "—and into *Lassie, Come Home* at MGM. At twelve, she landed the title role in *National Velvet,* having worked out for four months in order to gain the three extra inches of height the role required —which may be the first recorded example of the famous Taylor grit and determination.

The equally well-advertised high temper and salty tongue appeared first at the age of fifteen. The object of her wrath was Louis B. Mayer, emperor of MGM, also known as "one of the biggest bastards that ever lived" and a man given to fits of rage: "I saw him actually foam at the mouth." It happened in his office. "My mother had asked him a very simple question, and he started to get *extremely* cross, really out of control. I blew up—it was the first time I had ever sworn—I told him that he and his studio could both go to hell, but he could not talk to my mother that way. And I went flying out of the office. The vice-president, a sweet man named Benny Thaw, ordered me to go back in and apologize. I refused. I never did go back."

Although she has allegiances within the industry ("Roddy McDowall has been my oldest, most consistent friend. . . . I had a great empathy with Judy Garland, and Liza [Minelli] and I are very close. I was surrogate mother at her wedding"), and she treasures the recognition the industry has given her ("I have two Oscars, and I am not at all unhappy about that; I wouldn't trade them for anything, but they are not my life"), she has no nostalgia for the Hollywood years: "Hollywood is a little tiny town. It is—or was—a narrow, gossipy community that talked about who is going to bed with whom, who is making how much money, and who could beat whom. It was a very ungenerous atmosphere. . . .

"It wouldn't be fair to mention the lady's name, because she's dead and can't defend herself. But this lady— this actress did a film with somebody very close to me, who didn't go to the rushes. And she said to him, 'Why don't you go to see the rushes?' He said, 'Because I don't like to see myself on the screen; I really cringe.' She said, 'Well, I go to the rushes every night, and I see them three times: The first time is exclusively to see myself; the second time to watch the entire scene, myself and the other players; the third time I go to see whom I have to defeat!' "

Elizabeth doesn't go to rushes. She sees the final product, and that's it— except once, when her children were very young, and *Jane Eyre* was playing on television: "I propped them in front of the set, feeling all puffed up about it. They were going to see their mommy on the screen when she was a little girl. And there I am, waiting. And I wait. And there's Peggy Ann Garner, Jane as a little girl. And all of a sudden, there's Joan Fontaine, Jane all grown up. But I keep the poor kids there—the oldest was only five; none of them understood what was going on. And I keep saying, 'Now wait just a minute, Mommy will be coming on soon.' Well, Mommy never did. Mommy had been cut out of the whole picture!"

The children, now grown, are Michael, twenty-seven, a musician, her first son by the late Michael Wilding; his brother, Christopher, twenty-five, a photographer-cum-mining student; Liza, twenty-three, a sculptor, whose father, Mike Todd, died when she was an infant; and Maria, nineteen, a model, Elizabeth's adopted daughter with Richard Burton. She is close to her children, proud of them . . . she likes the way they live their lives. Which is what she might say about her own life. "I've had the highest highs, the lowest lows. And lots of gray. But gray is when you use your gray matter, your little gray cells. You had better, because our lives are fundamentally based on gray, not the huge ups and downs. And what it's all about, I think, is coming to terms with the gray and making it not only acceptable but exciting."

Elizabeth is one of the very few stars for whom getting older has not been a problem, possibly because she has been doing—insisting on!—character parts throughout her career. She hasn't had a face lift, though she wouldn't hesitate if she thought it necessary—"Why not? Everybody has them now. I definitely would if I felt my eyes needed lifting, or anything else." This is a new attitude: "Even three years ago, I wouldn't have said that I might ever, possibly, conceivably, under any circumstances have a face lift, because I'm of the grow-old-gracefully school, and every wrinkle I've got is a wrinkle I've earned. But it's wrong to discount any possibility. I don't think you should ever put yourself in the position of saying, No, never; you just don't know how you're going to feel in ten years. So the option is open, but at the moment, I don't feel the need. I feel that my experience has shaped my face. And you know," she said, smiling that delectable pussycat smile of hers, "there's nothing to be ashamed of in the way I look."

Kim Alexis

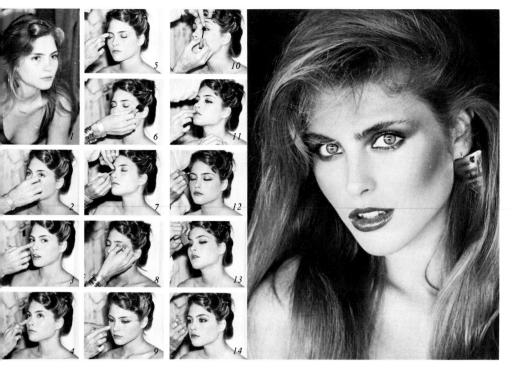

"For breakfast, I'll have half a V-8 juice, a little plain yogurt with wheat germ, bran, and a few raw almonds on top. I do twenty leg-ups each—on my back, my stomach, and my side."

1. Kim as she entered
2. Flesh-color pencil to conceal darkness
3. Darker foundation over light pencil
4. Blend to avoid light and dark rings
5. Dark shadow on outer half of lid for eye length
6. Loose base powder for matte finish
7. Rimming underneath top lashes with black
8. Bronze shadow to highlight under eyebrow
9. Rose rouge high on cheekbone to blush
10. Hold lid to apply black mascara cleanly
11. Sheer lip color to tint lips
12. Beige eyebrow pencil to fill in sparse brows
13. Use comb to separate lashes
14. Apply charcoal line inside lower lid for strong look

In my entire career as a photographer, I can think of no question I have been asked more often than "How do I get into modeling?" I could give the answer backwards, upside-down, and in my sleep: "Get yourself over to a reputable agency." If they think you have it—or with a little work could have it—they'll take you under the agency wing: advise you about clothes, makeup, diet; see that you get some decent test shots; and send you on go-sees (the model's equivalent of the actor's "making the rounds") to prospective clients. There is no secret, better way. I know that girls have been discovered on street corners, on buses, even at pizza parlors, but it's rare. Least likely of all is that a hot new model will be plucked from the student body of a modeling school.

And yet . . . in Buffalo, New York, there is a modeling school that has tripled its enrollment, because among its recent alumnae is Kim Alexis, who is, no question, one of the hottest young models ever to hit the business. How much the school had to do with this is debatable ("We had to learn this funny walk, where you tuck in your rear and slouch down a bit, keeping your back and shoulders straight and your head forward, and then sort of glide with your knees . . . when I got to New York, forget it!"). Still: "The school made me feel secure about myself." And even more to the point: A local photographer spotted her there, took some pictures, and sent them to agency owner Johnny Casablancas. The rest, as they say, is history.

Two days after her eighteenth birthday, Kim Alexis (her paternal grandfather, in his army days, simply got tired of being yet another Anderson in the Swedish military) came to New York. Two days after that, Italian *Bazaar* booked her for the fashion collections in Paris and Rome. By the age of nineteen, she was earning over $100,000 a year. She has a condominium in Florida, two fur coats, and "some liquidation stocks and things." For his birthday, she gave her boyfriend, a photographer, "a huge twenty-five-hundred-dollar lens." He gave her, for her birthday, a string of perfectly matched white pearls . . . she recently turned twenty.

Why? What's so special about Kim Alexis? Why this girl on every other

dressed me to a T—on Fridays, I could wear jeans to school; otherwise, forget it—you wouldn't believe my closets back home! My New York closet has nothing." Not nothing, exactly; it may be a sparely furnished closet, but the contents are chic. And there are plenty of jeans, which may be leather or suede, as well as blue denim. Jeans are pretty much her uniform, only now she wears them with "a nice silk shirt, a classy leather belt," and throws on her new, full-length, dark-green beaver coat.

She has dyed her pale-blond lashes navy/black ("so when I don't wear makeup, I don't have to worry about mascara"). She doesn't wear makeup often, but when she does it doesn't look like Buffalo. The difference is blending: "People I know who aren't in the business don't blend their makeup. They put the pencil on and leave it. And you don't want those harsh lines; you want it soft and pretty. You have to take your finger and blend it out. Or, after I've put on a liner in pencil, I put a shadow over it. Then I go over it with a powder brush, just to blend it a bit. Finally, after I've powdered my whole face with a brush, I take the brush again and go *whish, whish* over everything, which takes care of any little unblended residue."

Kim's eyebrows are thick and dark, and there is no way that anyone is going to pluck and/or bleach them: "It's the only thing Way Bandy and I ever fight about, so we compromise: he puts on a golden powder. . . . Then I go to the next booking, and they love it that my eyebrows are dark and bushy." As for the two tiny moles on her upper lip and chin: "Anyone who hates them can airbrush them out of the picture. They're part of me, and I'm not going to change myself for this business. . . . Besides, in full-length shots, it's how my mother can tell it's her daughter."

■

"People I know who aren't in the business don't blend their makeup. . . .
You don't want those harsh lines; you want it soft and pretty. You have to take your finger and blend it out."

■

cover of *Vogue?* What is there about this sweet little cupcake that editors and advertisers are falling all over each other to get her face on their product? Surely, there are girls more extraordinary-looking, sexier, more sophisticated—Lauren Hutton, for one; Janice Dickensen? Absolutely—but America had to get used to them. Nobody has to get used to Kim. That's the bottom line: She has a face that is instantly understood and instantly appealing, right across the board—rich, poor, young, old, male, female, everybody loves that face. It's part of our national mythology: The All-American Beautiful Blond Dream Girl. In the forties, when I was starting out, a model named Anita Colby had it. Grace Kelly had it for the fifties. Kim Alexis has it now.

She looks, in fact, the way she was brought up to look: "I was a country-club girl. My mother said, 'You're going to marry someone, and if he wants to go golfing you don't want to be embarrassed and not know how to golf.' So I used to take golf lessons and riding lessons and tennis; I water-skied, snow-skied, all that stuff—ping-pong—everything. . . . I already knew how to swim; I'd been swimming competitively for twelve years (I think I still hold the New York State record for the butterfly). . . . My mother used to take me shopping and spend a fortune. She

K im has changed her look in other ways: she is thinner and less muscular ("In Buffalo I was swimming three miles a day. I was an athlete and I ate like an athlete. I used to eat French toast and pancakes and eggs; now, for breakfast, I'll have half a V-8 juice, a little plain yogurt, with wheat germ, bran, and a few raw almonds on top. I do twenty leg-ups each on my back, my stomach, and my side. But I don't swim; I don't want to develop those muscles again"). She goes to a dermatologist once a month to have her skin cleaned. She goes in the sun more carefully than she used to; she doesn't "just lie there and listen to myself fry," and she uses a sun block around her eyes. She uses a hairdresser's trick in the sun: "Not just plain lemon juice, because it's drying, but you add some coconut oil, and a smidgen of peroxide, then mix it all up and put it in a spray bottle and spray it on your dry hair."

■

"I don't want to have to dream about things. I like to go after them."

■

Success is nice; she enjoys it, but she isn't awed by it. And she isn't surprised: "Ever since I was very young, I've had it in my mind that I was never going to have problems, that I'm a very lucky person. . . . People say I'll last another ten years in modeling; by that time, I'll be thirty and I'd like to be on my way to L.A. I can see myself in the movies then. It's going to happen. . . . I'm not saying that I want everything at thirty. But I want to know that I'm going to get there. I don't want to have to dream about things. I like to go after them."

Patti
Hansen

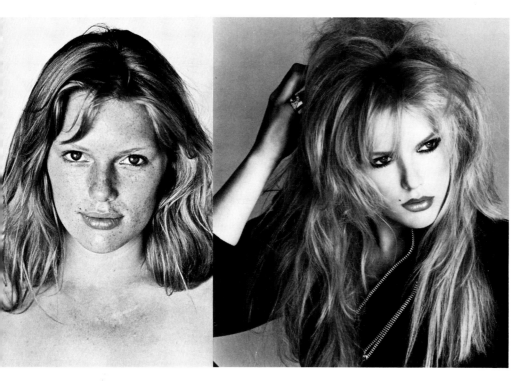

"I don't take very good care of my skin. But I'm better than I was . . . I use a moisturizer. And I wipe the makeup off with baby oil. Then when I'm in the shower, I wash my face with soap and water—a Neutrogena-type soap, without fragrance."

T he big cliché about high-fashion models used to be that they were nothing but skin and bones and remote as the Himalayas. And then came Patti Hansen, the country girl from Staten Island. Big-boned, rounded, full-bosomed, and full of life, she knocked the old high-fashion stereotype into a cocked hat. Suddenly, in *Vogue* and *Harper's Bazaar,* the haughty-looking, cavernous-chested models of the past were replaced by a different race of women. These girls were flesh and blood: healthy, outgoing, and real. And Patti was first—the first modern sexy girl.

Nowadays, a Patti Hansen type would be high fashion from the start. But in the early seventies, when Patti was discovered—selling hot dogs at her father's van—an energetic sixteen-year-old, with shagged strawberry-blond hair and freckles popping out all over was automatically a junior. For three years, you could hardly open an issue of *Glamour* that didn't have Patti running, jumping, horsing around on the beach; she never stopped moving, never stopped smiling, and never ever wore makeup; every freckle was like an ounce of pure gold.

At nineteen, Patti busted loose. "I went to Europe and did some pictures for Italian *Vogue*. They were into severe makeup and straight, severe hair. And I looked real tough . . . you know, you squint your eyes. But when I came back and American *Vogue* saw the pictures, they went, 'Oooohhh, my God! The baby's grown up.' " Two minutes later, Alexander Liberman, Editorial Director of Condé Nast, which includes *Vogue,* is on the phone. "She's gorgeous," he says, "shoot a cover." She was. I did. And Patti took off.

That sitting is memorable for several reasons. One, we got rid of the "tough look," which has nothing to do with Patti. She had acquired it, I think, because she wasn't used to looking directly at the camera. Her "thing" was action; she ran and the camera followed. But a cover shot is another story —all face and eyes, and you go right for the camera. So here was Patti trying on an expression that didn't come naturally but maybe the camera would love anyway. It never works that way. As Patti recalls, I coaxed her out of it: "Don't look so mad; don't look at me so angrily." Gradually, she says, "I started feeling at ease with myself. I realized I didn't have to *do* anything; I could just sit there. And I didn't have to smile; I could pout. Once I began to feel that way, I just relaxed into my own face. . . . And the eyes: All of a sudden I understood what you do with your eyes: you love. Let's say I'm in love with someone, I think of that person; I sort of say to myself, 'This one is for you, doll.' "

Vogue says if you don't lose fifteen pounds, forget it.' And I looked at the photograph, and I was really *plump*—I mean, it was like no neck. It was terrible. I did some fasting, went on a diet. I'm always going on and off. But most of the time, I eat anything I want. I've never worried about my weight."

She doesn't worry about many things that one might expect would drive a superstar model into deep depression. Getting older, for instance. Patti has been at the top for nearly a decade; she is now twenty-five. "I love getting older. It's amazing how quickly it's happening, but I love it. It's lovely seeing other people grow up, and seeing

came an excuse not to continue with the class. But it was good."

The film is Peter Bogdanovich's *They All Laughed,* in which Audrey Hepburn and Ben Gazzara star, and Patti plays a Patti Hansen–type New York taxi driver. In the film, someone suggests to Patti that she go into modeling. To which she replies, "I did a little bit of that once upon a time, and it's a pain in the ass . . . that's not for me." Which is hardly a case of art imitating life. While she would like to get more into films, she isn't quite ready to close the book on one of the highest-paid long-run careers in the business. Not that she has amassed a fortune; she isn't the type.

She is this type: "I have no idea how much money I've made. I haven't had good management. I have different accountants every year. I go with one because someone I know is going to him, then the person I know leaves and I don't get around to it, and the guy turns out to be a real creep. But it's OK, because I've enjoyed every single penny. For nine years, I've really played around. I've spent my money and had a good time. I don't buy clothes or things like that. But I like to buy caviar and champagne. I like to visit Europe and stay in hotels. I love hotels. I love living out of suitcases. On my last vacation, with my boyfriend at his place in England, I pretty much kept everything in suitcases; you never know when you're going to pick up and go."

"I like to buy caviar and champagne. I like to visit Europe and stay in hotels. I love living out of suitcases . . . you never know when you're going to pick up and go."

This was also the first time we did a real makeup on Patti, and the change was extraordinary. There are some girls whom the camera will always perceive as full-grown women, with or without makeup, no matter what their age. Brooke Shields is one. Patti isn't. For her, makeup is the difference between cute kid and all-out sexpot. Not that she has to pile it on. It's just a question of darkening the eyes, emphasizing the ripe, pouty mouth, and paling down the freckles with a light base. Also—because Patti is one of those rare models who photographs better when her weight is up rather than down—we usually put dark contour rouge under her chin. That's OK; I'd rather go through pots of contour rouge than have her lose a pound. In Patti's case, thin is gaunt; healthy is sexy.

On the other hand, there is a point beyond the powers of contouring. Patti nearly reached it a couple of years ago. "I had gone to Spain to do a film—a spaghetti Western—that never happened. It turned out to be a fiasco, and the people were a real disaster; at one point they threatened to throw the cameraman out the window because the camera wasn't working. For three months, we just sat and waited—and waited and waited. And I put on so much weight! . . . The week I came back I worked for *Vogue*. I put on the clothes, and this thing went *rrrrrip!* And the bra went shooting across the room. The next day, the agency calls me up: 'What happened yesterday?

all the changes you go through yourself, and how you deal with life. . . . I used to be so nervous I wasn't able to go out to dinner parties; I couldn't hold a conversation at the table. I can do it now, though I actually am very nervous and shy. I smoke; I bite my nails. In spite of it, I think I've become much more sure of myself.

"I don't take very good care of my skin. But I'm better than I was. I used to say in interviews that I didn't wash my face at all, just kept putting my makeup on over and over again. But it does start to show, you know—plus flying so much and wearing makeup all the time—your skin really dries out. As much as I like getting older, I don't want my face to droop later on. So I use a moisturizer. And I wipe the makeup off with baby oil. Then, when I'm in the shower, I wash my face with soap and water—a Neutrogena-type soap, without fragrance."

Patti exercises "when I'm in the mood; then I do sit-ups and leg raises and just bending." In a recent "fat period," she noticed the beginnings of "saddlebags . . . these awful things that women get on their thighs. So I started going to a great exercise class—the Lotte Berk Method. I looked around at all the little fatties in the class, and I thought, Oh, wow, this is going to be great; no contest! Well, by the end of the first class, I couldn't lift my leg. And these tubby little bowls had their legs wrapped around their waists. I was so embarrassed! This was just before I started to work in a film, so that be-

In her less transient moments, Patti lives in New York's Greenwich Village, in "a lovely apartment, with a fireplace and beautiful wooden floors and high ceilings," and a couple downstairs who apparently hate most what Patti likes best: "Music makes them crazy. I love music. I love musicians. My ex-boyfriend was a musician. And now I'm madly in love with this guy who's a great musician. So the music is constantly going in my apartment. And they come banging on the door—in the middle of the afternoon; on a Saturday morning—'Don't play your music!' So it's time to start looking. . . . I think I'd like to buy a place of my own."

She could probably pay for it in cash; Patti may not know what she has in the bank at the end of the year, but she knows what goes on the voucher at the end of the day: "My price is twenty-five hundred a day. Negotiable." And just in case you're thinking of booking Patti Hansen on the cheap, she adds, "It could go higher, depending." But don't despair; as Patti would be first to tell you—and everyone in the business will verify—"I have just never been pushy about prices." Or about anything else . . . a *good* girl.

Gia

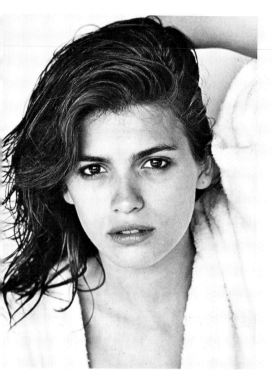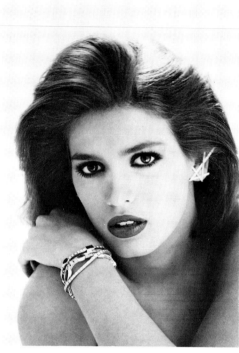

"There's a lot more to being good-looking than makeup and prettiness . . . there's a lot more to being a woman than that. When I look in the mirror, I just want to like myself . . . And if I like myself, then I look good."

Gia is my darling—old, young, decadent, innocent, volatile, vulnerable, and more tough-spirited than she looks. She is all nuance and suggestion, like a series of images by Bertolucci. . . . I never think of her as a model, though she's one of the best. It's that she doesn't behave like a model; she doesn't give you the Hot Look, the Cool Look, the Cute Look; she strikes sparks, not poses. Out of doors, especially, I have never known anyone so excitingly free and spontaneous, constantly changing, moving (which drove me crazy until I got smart and learned to focus the camera faster)—she's like photographing a stream of consciousness.

Gia—her last name is Carangi—is twenty-one ("going on eighty-four"). She came to New York three years ago from a small town in Bucks County, Pennsylvania, and landed like the Marines. Everyone was nuts about her— editors, photographers. "It was fun. A lot of models have a rough time, but things started happening pretty quickly for me." Maybe too quickly: By the end of her first year, she'd been to Europe "at least ten times" and could say matter-of-factly, "I'm able to buy whatever I want . . . if I see something, I can buy it." Well, why not? She was booked to the eyeballs. Only it wasn't always so much fun. "When you're in demand, and people are saying, 'I want you, I want you,' it isn't easy to say no. I don't like to disappoint people; I'm basically a satisfier. So you find yourself working a lot—a *lot*. And if you want to take a day off, because you need a day to rest or to get yourself together so you can be there and together and have your energy for the next day, it's hard. Models are never supposed to be down or be tired or have a headache. They've got to be up all the time."

Gia wasn't. And sometimes she

turned up late, or she didn't show at all, or she showed and then vanished from the set. The talk was, Gia was into drugs. And the truth is, she was. The more important truth is that she isn't; as I said, there's more toughness here than meets the eye: "It wasn't just a matter of stopping. It was a matter of wanting to live in the world that I live in, and making it work for me instead of against me.

"The world seems to be based on money and sex . . . I'm looking for better things than that, like happiness and love and caring."

"I think the reason someone gets into something like that is because—for me, anyway—there were a lot of unanswered questions in my mind about work and about life. Money didn't interest me. I got to a point where I had all this money. I had everything I ever wanted in life—or thought that I wanted—and I said, What the hell is this all for? I mean, you need money to survive. But I think people value it too much; the world seems to be based on money and sex. And I'm looking for better things than that, like happiness and love and caring. . . . I was really down on society, but then I found that I was part of society too. And for me to be doing drugs made me just as bad as I thought society was. I think maybe society is kind of what I make myself. And that makes me happy, happier than being high.

"If anything, I'm high on being straight because now I can feel my body, I can feel my head. Before, I was like numb. It's really just selfish. I don't care if you're on Quaaludes or you're a nice housewife hooked on diet pills and Valium, it is just a selfish way to live. . . . I learned a lot from my experience, so I don't regret it. It was good for me, like a slap in the face. . . . I'm an extremist, you know; I had to go all the way."

Now she has come all the way back; she's taking control of her life. "I'm

disciplining myself. If I have a booking, I plan for it the day before. I have to; if I didn't, and if I were late or didn't show up or something, they'd think I was goofing off, so the thing is to make sure that I'm together and that I get enough sleep. I'm basically a night person, so it's hard for me to go to bed at a normal hour. Then, in the morning, I just want to keep sleeping. I don't want to get out of that bed because I'm

hiding in that bed; it's so nice and warm. I've had this problem all my life; it's why I was always late. . . . I was really spoiled, you know. I was a brat. And that stays with you. It's a hard thing to change. But once you know these things about yourself, you have to try to discipline yourself, because after a certain age nobody else is going to do it for you."

Some things — happily — haven't changed. The way she dresses, for instance, which is thrift-shop chic and pure Gia: flat boots, tuxedo pants, and an oversize man's jacket. She looks marvelous. "I just like to be comfortable. I don't do it purposely, but I have my own style of dressing, and it just comes out kind of different. I don't like to dress like anybody else, and I'm not into designer clothes . . . I'm not into anything. I just pick up pieces here and there and throw them together. Sometimes I go shopping in the nicer stores, too; I buy a shirt or a belt or shoes. But

I like the things they have in the thrift shops even if they are old; they're cut a lot better than the newer things."

She thinks she is shapelier now than when she started modeling. She's right; it's the difference between a fabulous body and a more-fabulous body. Exercise isn't the secret. "I get my exercise from walking or running or riding a bike or swimming. I don't go home at night and pump iron or something." And for sure diet has nothing to do with it. "I eat a lot. I eat everything—except, I don't go for mixed salads. I eat pizza and hamburgers, and I eat pheasant and Jell-O and steak and spaghetti. Home cooking. I hate going out to eat. I think it's a bore, sitting there and drooling over your food for hours and hours."

Her skin-care regime wouldn't tax a very small child. "I wash it with soap and water and a washrag, and once in a while I put on a little vitamin E. I try to keep my face very clean. I never leave makeup on—no, no, no, no matter what. I couldn't go to sleep without washing my face. All that makeup! I like makeup—just in photography, though. I like the creativeness of it, what it can do, how it can transform you. But when I'm finished working, I run for the soap and water.

"You have to try to discipline yourself, because after a certain age nobody else is going to do it for you."

"You know, I thank God that I'm good-looking, or that people think I'm good-looking. But there's a lot more to it than makeup and prettiness and all that stuff . . . there's a lot more to being a woman than that. When I look in the mirror, I just want to like myself, that's all. And if I like myself, then I look good." . . . Gia has got to be liking herself a lot these days.

Beverly Johnson

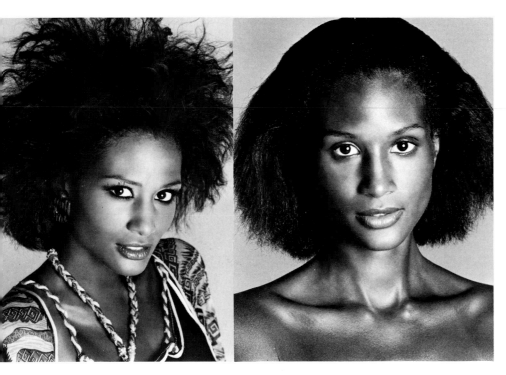

"When I am working I'm very conscious that I've got to go home and cleanse. I cleanse with yogurt and soap and water. I use a natural unscented moisturizer ... I like any kind of cream I can get from the health-food store."

Beverly Johnson is unique: A black woman at the very top of what is still very much a white woman's profession. A twenty-eight-year-old in a business that tends to assign senior-citizen status to anyone over twenty-four. A ten-year veteran of this business, which runs through pretty faces as though they were panty hose and craves new ones the way the lions in Rome craved Christians, Beverly endures.

Actually, she does better than that; she prevails. And I can think of at least one reason—I mean, beyond the obvious fact that she is more beautiful than she was at the beginning (in those days "they said I was 'cute' "): It's that she keeps growing. A lot of models don't.

But Beverly was more divine to photograph for this book than she was in 1973, when we started working together, or in 1974, when we did *Vogue's* first black cover—more exciting, with more style, more force, more vitality, more of everything to give to the camera.

You don't just luck into a great photograph. Beverly knows what she's doing out there; she has learned and polished and perfected. And it didn't happen overnight: "At first, I just sat around. I didn't know what to do, so I didn't do anything. Then the pictures come back, and you look at them, and you start looking at other magazines and other models. And then you try. One time you try putting your hand on your hip . . . or you try putting it in your pocket. You practice in front of the mirror at home, and you work at it.

"There are things you just learn about . . . space and composition and shape and line . . . how to make good lines with your body, how to position yourself. You don't hold your hand out toward the camera, or it's not going to be on the same plane as everything else; it'll be big or out of focus. You can't hold your head up too high, and you can't hold it down too low. Because sometimes a photographer shoots from a low position, and if your head is low it's going to be distorted. And if it's very high, you're not going to see anything. You have to learn to hold it up —not straight up, like a turtle pulling out of its shell, but a little sideways and up, so that you have a long neck and the whole face is there.

"You have to learn the angles each photographer shoots from. Some shoot low. Some shoot straight off. Some like to shoot down. And you have to learn what to do when they're shooting— and when it's good not to do anything, to be just sort of open and natural so that you can come up with these beautiful expressions that are really no-expressions, but more like the hint of a mood."

Beverly knows all the angles . . . and all the little tricks: "You put some lipstick on your cheeks and use it as a blush—Way Bandy does that a lot. It's fantastic, nice and fresh and glowy. Powder blush is too dull; it gives you too flat a finish. And I don't think they've really gotten out a good cream blush yet. . . . I think it's good business to have specialized markets, black markets. But the truth is, in our business, everybody uses everything—including Posner's, Fashion Fair, Revlon's Wine Polished Ambers, whoever's color is good. A lot of models—Lauren Hutton, for instance—wear this bronze foundation by Fashion Fair. It's great on white skin; it makes you look as if you have the most beautiful suntan. . . . A nice touch to point the lips: You take a brown eyebrow pencil, or a black one, and put it just in the corners of the mouth—not on the outside; you don't want to look like a clown.

"If I'm doing the best makeup I can ever do for myself, I would start with foundation—I use a liquid, and in summertime I cut it with a water-based foundation, because I need less oil then —and then the most important would be the contouring. I like to play up every last one of my features. I like to make my eyes really big and the lids really deep. I put black or dark-brown shading pencil in the crease of the eye and smudge it with my fingertip; that's your Greta Garbo line. Then I line the eye inside and out—top of the lid, under the lower lashes, and inside on the rim of the lower lid—and smudge, smudge, smudge. That is the whole secret of eye lines: *no* lines—you have to smudge like crazy.

"Most people don't know how to contour the nose, but it's like contouring any other part—chin, cheeks, or the bone in your forehead. The point is to accent good bones and give character to the face. You want your contouring rouge darker than your foundation, of course, but still relating to it—and to your skin tone. I usually use a light brown and blend it very, very well; it can't be noticeable or you'll look as if you've got a dirty nose. Then I put a highlighter down the tip to bring out the bone. . . . So basically, your makeup is foundation and contour. Then you add your colors very lightly, and powder. I like to use a lot of baby powder, which is translucent and gives you that really porcelain-doll finish."

"Basically, your makeup is foundation and contour."

Whether she does it herself or it's done for her (Way Bandy did it here), there is no question that for Beverly makeup is a tool to be used for art, the way an actress uses it, to project different moods, different emotions, different kinds of women: "You take on different personalities . . . depending on how you're made up, you're rich, you're elegant, you're sexy, you're fresh and young. When your makeup is on, you look at yourself in the mirror, and what you see there is what you think you are when you go on the set." There is also no question that without makeup—as she is in the photograph at right—she is just as gorgeous as with. Mostly she goes without. "When I'm not working, I try to use as little makeup as possible —meaning, none.

"And when I am working, I'm very conscious that I've got to go home and cleanse. I cleanse with yogurt and soap and water. I use a natural unscented moisturizer. Kiehl's makes the best, but I don't even know the name of it. Also, I like any kind of cream I can get from the health-food store—vitamin E, C creams, A and D, PABA. . . . If your diet is good and your skin is normal, I think massages and facials are great. I have facials maybe twice, three times a year, with Adriana at Suga. She cleans every single pore. Immediately after I've had a facial, you see all these little tiny sort of bumps, but they go away quickly and my skin is perfection. And if I stay good on my diet, it will be that way for months.

"I eat fresh vegetables, nuts, fruits, seeds, grains; I take vitamin supplements; and I exercise—I run and I bicycle, and in the summertime I swim. All these things generate good skin. I can always tell the difference in summer, because then I sometimes slip and sneak in a lot of ice cream. That sugar tears your skin up. It gives you whiteheads and pimples . . . if you find your skin breaking out, just cut down on your sugar and you'll see; it will clear up.

"Three years ago I changed my way of eating. I became a real vegetarian and a health fanatic. And my skin has been fantastic, and my energy is up, and I haven't had a weight problem . . . if anything, I have to worry about going under. I don't like to be too thin; everybody says, 'Oh, you're so *skinny!*' It shows everywhere—my face, my body. I mean, I become a skeleton. It just doesn't look very good."

Beverly has a two-year-old daughter, Anansa, named after the role Beverly plays in *Ashanti,* the movie she made with Michael Caine, Rex Harrison, William Holden, and Peter Ustinov. "I was pregnant during the filming . . . and I modeled the entire time." In addition, she has done one record album, is rehearsing for another, has written two health-and-beauty books, and is working now on a book about modeling. . . . What makes Beverly run? Easy: "I *want* to do it.

"It was a decision and a commitment that I made when I started modeling, because when I started I was going to college—at Northeastern in Boston, where I grew up—and I wanted to be a lawyer, to be a professional. We're a professional family: My sister is a teacher and my brother is a lawyer. I was the first one to spring off into a world that I never even knew existed. But once I did, I knew I wanted to be an artist, total and complete." Beverly was eighteen when a photographer talked her into doing some pictures; she wasn't overly impressed. "I said, 'To hell with this, I'm going back to school.' And I did. Then the check came, and I said, 'Well, wait a minute, you know, let's be realistic. . . . I can handle this *and* college.' So I came to New York, got married to my first husband, transferred to Brooklyn College. I was going to school at night, modeling during the day, and working part time at a boutique. And then I said, 'Forget it, I'm an artist, not a professional,' and I started acting classes at Lee Strasberg's Workshop. . . . I knew that modeling wasn't going to be enough."

But it has been a lot—enough to put a lock on the gold-dust twins, fame and fortune. From her modeling career alone each year, Beverly earns "a hundred-thousand plus, and that's working kind of nice, not really killing yourself. . . . I love the business. I love it now more than ever."

Which doesn't mean she would kill to stay on top; her attitude toward her profession is loving but objective; she sees the traps. "Modeling is a very physical world, and it can come to a point where the only stimulation you get is from looking in the mirror and looking at your pictures. It becomes your whole life. You think a man likes you because you're pretty and you have a sexy body. It has nothing to do with your personality, your intelligence, what you know; it has to do only with the physical being. And if that's all there is, then at the end, when you age, as we all do, it can be very frightening and very destructive. You have to have a mind, and you have to nurture your mind as well as your body. I think everything I've done—having the baby, writing books, making the movie, the record—has helped me to grow mentally.

"Also, mistakes—you can learn your best lessons from your mistakes. But the key is not to keep making the same goddamn mistakes over and over and over again; then it becomes a detriment." Or a wrinkle. Or a line. "I never give it a chance to develop. I'm very open about emotional things I'm going through. I don't want to hold it in, because that leads to bad health and all other kinds of complications. I get it out and get it over with. I keep going, and I don't look back."

If that's her secret, then treat it like the beauty tip of a lifetime. Because I promise you—Beverly Johnson, pushing thirty, has never looked so breathtaking and fresh as she did for this sitting, although she says, "If you want to photograph me at my most beautiful, photograph me at midnight; that's when I wake up. I'm not awake at nine in the morning. Nobody notices . . . but when you see me at a party at night, you go, 'Damn!' . . . I *feel* more beautiful at night. It's a creative time, a bewitching time . . . a much higher energy. I love the night life . . . the lights. If I could stay out all night long, I'd do it. But I love the mornings, and I love the days . . . I wish I could do everything all the time!" Why not? She's already more than halfway there.

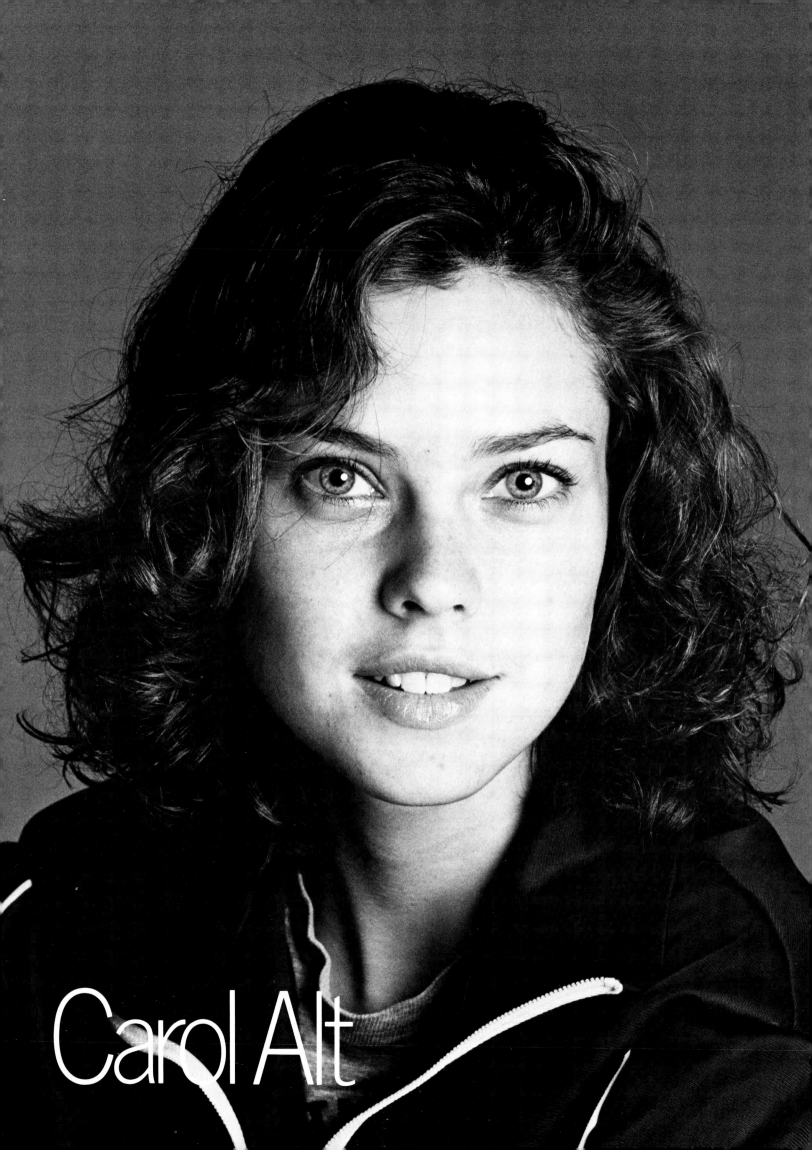

Carol Alt

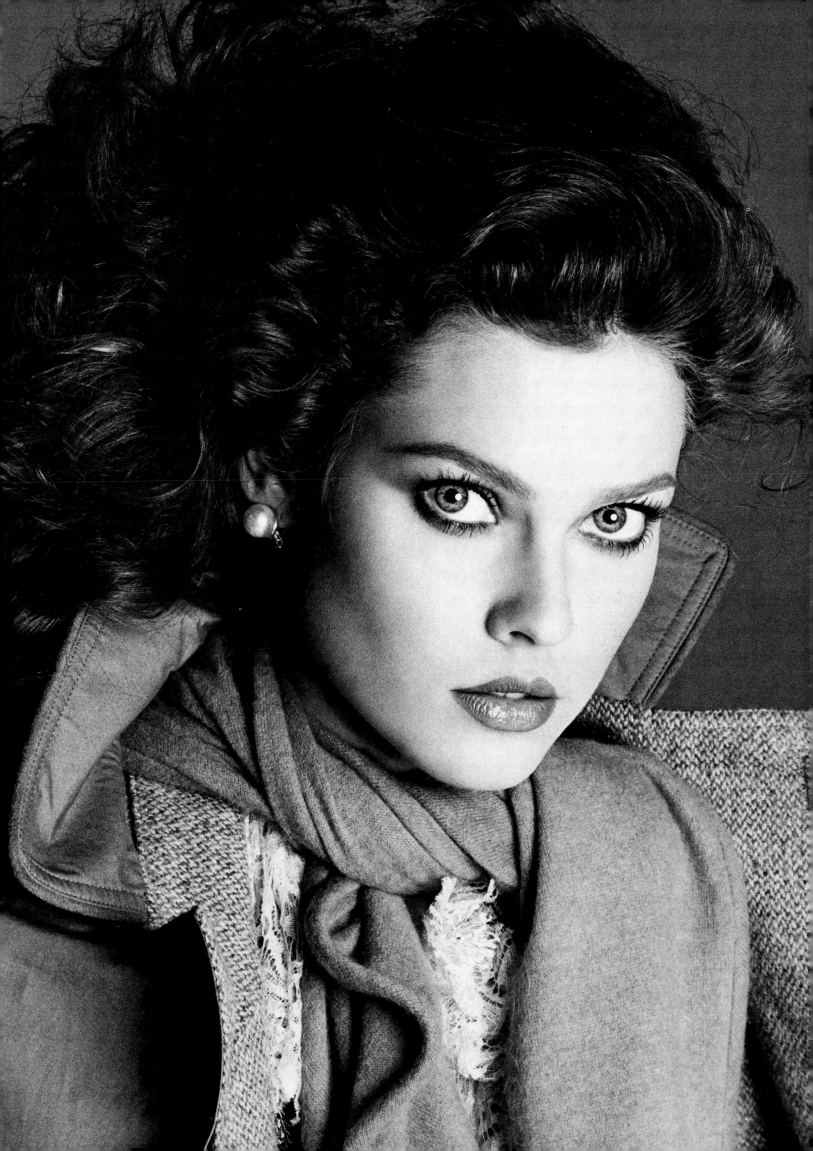

Carol
Alt

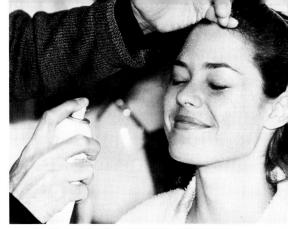

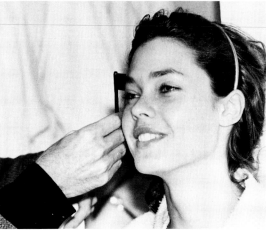

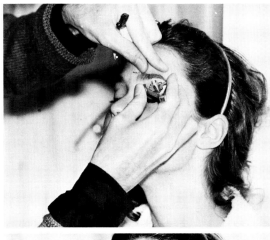

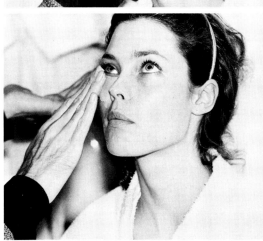

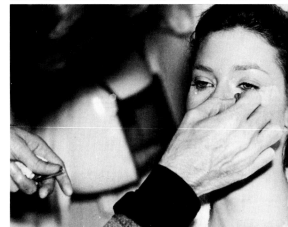

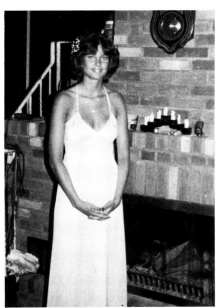

1978

The first time I saw Carol was at the airport. We were on our way to Paris to photograph the collections for *Vogue,* and Carol was one of two models the magazine had booked for the trip. When she walked in, I had one sinking moment; she was so young. This was only two years ago, and she was barely eighteen. Her hair was just washed, and her face clean—no makeup at all, as in the small photograph above. Then, as I kept looking at her, I thought, She's got lots of animation—lots of sparkle in her eyes and tons of expression. Plus she has a beautiful body and a very contemporary look. I was struck by her freshness and vitality.

I was also aware that Carol had—has—dark shadows under her eyes, which could make her look tired in photographs. Carol's shadows had nothing to do with tiredness; they're just a physical thing that she has. I'm sure she had them when she was six—a lot of women do. And I wasn't concerned; I knew we could get rid of them with makeup.

Carol's eyebrows are naturally very dark. People tend to forget that eyebrows are the most emphatic lines on the face. When they're too dark, they dominate every other feature; in photography, they can overwhelm the picture. Again, no big deal—nothing that couldn't be handled with a little bleach. And a tweezer to clean up the scraggles.

All of this—the erasing of Carol's under-eye shadows, the lightening and neatening of the eyebrows—was worked out by Way Bandy in the course of a regular makeup, which goes as follows:

1. First, the eyebrow cleanup, always tweezing in the direction the hair grows, always following the natural shape.

2. A touch of bleach on the eyebrows—just for a quick second.

3. Preparing the "canvas": moisturizer is smoothed in all over her face . . . sprayed with Evian water . . . blotted with tissue. Now Carol's face is ready for makeup.

4. Way mixes several foundations to get the color he wants . . . then thins it out with a little Evian water to make it moister. A dry makeup can make you look older; moister is younger and more natural-looking. The whole point is that Carol (anybody!) should look as if she isn't wearing any makeup on her skin—it's fine to see makeup on the eyes and mouth, but you don't want to feel that your skin has a pancake mask on it. So the foundation is always thinned out . . . blotted with tissue if it gets too moist.

5. Now, with a soft off-white pencil, he goes after all the places that need to be lightened: under her eyes . . . along the sides of her nose . . . on her chin, where it goes in a bit . . . blending, blending. (This is one of

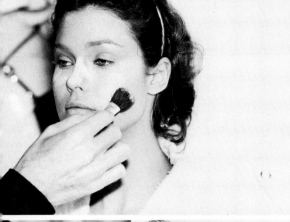

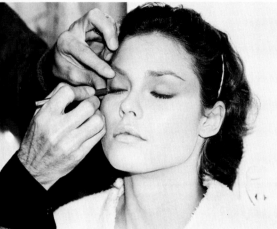

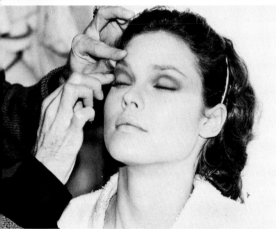

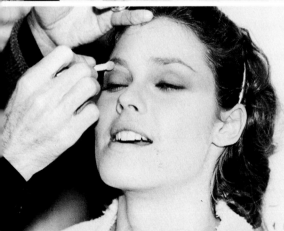

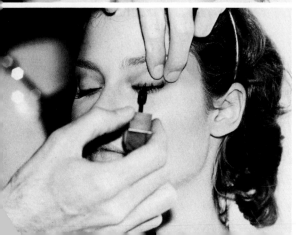

1. *Evian spray to freshen and moisturize*
2. *Groom brows prior to tweezing*
3. *Tweeze brows to follow eye shape*
4. *Foundation to even skin color*
5. *Light shade pencil to cover shadows*
6. *Dark powder to contour under cheekbone*
7. *Eye pencil to elongate eye*
8. *Dark shade to recess lid/deepen eye*
9. *Light shadow on brow bone to set off eye and brow*
10. *Mascara applied side to side for thick, even color*

the basic makeup tricks: light areas come forward, so when some part of your face needs to be pulled out of the shadows, add white!)

6. To seal the makeup and give a lovely sheen to the skin, he baby-powders with a brush.

7. Eyes next. Way uses a pencil to start drawing the lines, first in the crease between the lid and the brow . . . a stick to apply shadow . . . a tiny sponge applicator for highlights on the brow bone . . . always blending and smudging. That's Way's trip, the constant blending and smudging, and the absence of any hard lines

"I'm a jock."

(inspired, he says, by Vivien Leigh's makeup in *Gone with the Wind*). I love it too—that soft, misty look. It goes with the illusion I like to create in a picture. (Tip to the blue-eyed: Way never uses blue shadow on blue-eyed girls like Carol; it would take away from the color of her eyes.)

8. Way applies the first layer of mascara—upper and lower lashes, both sides—and combs them out.

9. Powdering again . . . and again . . . and again.

10. For the mouth, Way uses an old trick of mine that goes back to the fifties, when I used to do the makeup too: After outlining the lips and before filling in with color, a little bit of white right in the center makes the mouth "roll." A nice sexy touch.

11. Final mascara-ing, and . . .

12. Hairdresser Maury Hopson takes over: sprays her hair with water and then, because Carol's hair is very curly, puts on setting lotion (with straight hair, he'd use hair spray instead), and combs and back-combs. This gives hair the body I like in a picture and also helps hold the shape.

Once Carol is made up and her hair is done, that's it. I never get the feeling that she's worried about how she looks. In front of the camera, she is totally free and easy and marvelously animated. There isn't anything I have to be careful about—her eyes are beautiful, her mouth is beautiful. I just go with her, and she gives and gives. She is fabulous, a real performer!

When she isn't working, Carol turns off the glamour completely—the simplest hair and not a smidge of makeup. Most of the time, she's in jeans or jogging shorts—in her words: "I'm a jock. I've played everything from lacrosse to basketball. I jog. I run to bookings. I bicycle-ride. I love to dance. I've taken up tennis. And I've started to roller-skate." She burns up a lot of energy and she eats healthily. Now.

The old Carol was a pizza-pasta-Milky Way freak, who had one summer job at a bakery, another at a restaurant, and ate "everything in sight, any time I felt like it—a whole pizza, a whole box of candy." What turned her around was modeling.

Carol came into modeling at the beginning of June 1979, in classic movie-star style: She had just finished her first year as a pre-law student at Hofstra when she was "discovered" waitressing at a restaurant on Long Island. And the Big Break came right off the bat— a chance to go to Rome for Italian *Bazaar* on the nineteenth of July—provided she lost fifteen pounds. In case you're counting, that comes to one pound every three days for less than two months. But, as she says, "I had a goal. In the beginning, I was dumb; for the first two days, I fasted. I went totally without food and lost four pounds." After that, it was fruit juice and yogurt for breakfast, and salad all the way: chef's salad, Caesar salad, spinach salad. The punch line is, she didn't lose fifteen pounds; she lost twenty-five: "I just kept going till I reached a weight I felt comfortable at, about 120." Which is where she is now —and, at five-nine-and-a-half, in terrific shape.

P.S.: Carol got to Rome on schedule.

Dark shadow and a very light base
for a face with strong features

Florinda Balkan

"I think there is only one thing that is good for people's looks. And that is happiness. Anything else is silly. A face that is happy is beautiful. Your organs react differently when you are happy. And oh, they go so crazy when you are unhappy.... People complicate happiness, and I don't think it is complicated. It is knowing what we like and having it."

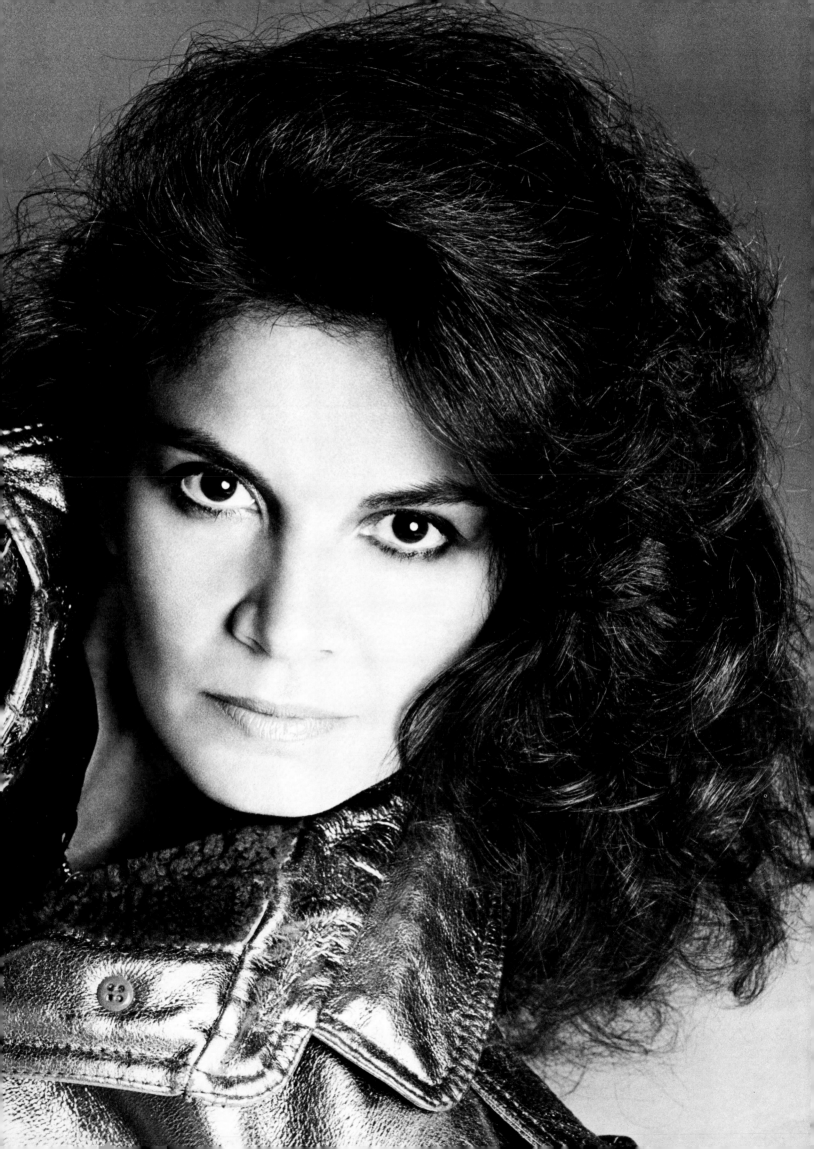

Florinda
Balkan

To me, Florinda Balkan, the Brazilian star of some thirty Italian movies—among them, *The Damned* and *A Brief Vacation*—is one of the most fascinating-looking women in films. There's an animal quality about her that just knocks me out; like a panther, she's all sinuous, long-bodied, restless grace. And I love the strength of that face—the intensity of the gaze and a certain world-weariness that I think of as being a particularly Latin kind of sexiness. Then you get this nice contradiction of girl-scout freckles and a perpetual suntan.

It isn't a face a makeup artist does a big number on; Harie von Wijnberg did the minimum: dark shadow around the outer corner of the eye, plus a very, very light base, and only on certain areas that needed to be pulled out of the shadows—around the eyes, mouth, nostrils, and a tiny bit on the forehead. Otherwise he went for totally natural skin, let the freckles come up and the outdoors come through. This side of her—and it's the dominant side—surprises me. Somehow, I tend to think of her prowling around some magnificently decadent palazzo at an hour when everyone else has turned into a pumpkin. Which just goes to show you. . . .

"I hate the night—I *hate* it. I don't know why. I go to nightclubs, I see people, I go out to dinner—I have to, because it's part of everything, and you cannot cut yourself off. But I don't like! I like to go home and go to bed. I'm a bed person; the bed is the best. I do everything in bed. I read in bed. I talk to my friends in bed. I could even have lunches and dinners in my bed. It feels cozier and more comfortable than any other place . . . on the ark of Noah, if I could take just one object with me, I would take my bed.

"I know what is good for me. I know what food I should eat. I know what people I should see. I know how many hours I should sleep. I have to sleep eight hours, and I don't like to go to bed late—midnight the latest. I could go to bed at seven o'clock and get up at five. I love mornings. I love the beginning of the day. When I read books of the seventeenth century—the period when people had a supper at three o'clock and then went to bed—I think, I could have lived then. That was my time.

"When I am in New York, I go running in the park at eight o'clock. I need a lot of exercise. I need a lot of physical, fresh, outside air. When I'm in Rome I go riding, in California I play tennis . . . it depends on what is close. I take flying lessons. I sail—I don't mean the big boat with three sailors who ask, Would you like to drink this? That I am not interested in. I'm interested in being one of the sailors who pulls up the sails, and the boat goes. And you can go anywhere; you are free in your mind. Obviously, I'm not going to take a boat and go to Australia all alone. But I could; I have the skills. I'm a good swimmer. I ski pretty well—and I'm not afraid, which is a good thing. I like everything where you have to stretch yourself against nature.

"But I don't exercise for the looks. I do it because I feel sick otherwise. I don't do anything especially for the looks. . . . I'm a mess if I put makeup on; it makes me strange, like a chorus girl. I do wear it, but very little. I use all Janet Sartin, and they are very simple things, very easy, like nothing on the face." Her hair, once almost black, is now a sort of very dark red: "It's henna, natural henna. But twelve years I am using it, and if you wear for a long time, the reddish comes—slowly, slowly. . . . One day I'm going to be like those girls from Morocco, you know, that the hair is *orange*. If I have to be blond for a film I wear wigs, because it's not worth it to bleach; the bleaching is very bad.

"I think there is only one thing that is good for people's looks. And that is happiness. Anything else is silly. A face that is happy is beautiful. Your organs react differently when you are happy. And oh, they go so crazy when you are unhappy. I have my problems—my liver, my this, my that—and I realize I'm unhappy. Then I do *everything* to be happy. I don't think there is a pill that one takes to be happy, but there is a way to avoid being unhappy. It's a discipline. For example: You're in love with somebody who is not in love with you. What do you do? You don't *see* the person. You avoid. You *kill* the person . . . in your mind. The person is dead . . . he went to Vietnam . . . a bomb. And that's it. ¡*Basta*!

"Of course it's hard. Everything is hard in life. To stop seeing the person you love is as difficult as to stop smoking—maybe easier for some people—or to stop eating chocolates, if you really like them. It's all the same, and the cure is the same: You just kill. There is no other way. There is no such a thing as soothing and trying to make easier—you know, Maybe if I see him three times a week, or at least once. No good. Unless we are masochists—then see all the time; it's no problem if it makes you happy. So it's important to know what brings us happiness, and we know . . . we know.

"I'm a bed person. . . . It feels cozier and more comfortable than any other place . . . on the ark of Noah, if I could take just one object with me, I would take my bed."

"People complicate happiness, and I don't think it is complicated. It is knowing what we like and having it. For me, it can be a meal. A Brazilian meal. Beans. I'm crazy about Brazilian *feijoada,* which is beans, and I don't have it every day. It can be so many things: It can be a person . . . a dress that is silly . . . a pair of jeans. It all has to do with the measures we make. If I dream of a castle in Ireland I'm going to be unhappy, because the castle is never going to be mine, probably. So I don't think about that. I think about things that I *can* have. Small, so that if they come big—ah! what a big, big happiness.

"Unhappiness is like birds when you cut their wings or people when you cut their legs; it makes them unbalanced. And there are so many unhappy people, especially in America. I think among men in this country there is a

---

"I know what is good for me. I know what food I should eat.
I know what people I should see.
I know how many hours I should sleep."

---

great confusion in accepting what they are, what their likes are, because there is a very strong *matriacado*. Men become like children to women here. The men one sees in New York, absolutely —children. They are afraid of so many things, are afraid of their sex—they don't even know what sex they like— and I think that is greatly the influence of women. Women are too *important* for them, too strong, wanting to prove too much. I don't think it's Women's Lib; it was always like that. Women here had somehow five husbands, and men died of heart attacks at the age of forty-five—that's unique, no?"

As Florinda sees it, there is one very basic difference between American women and women of more traditional cultures: "What they have together, the Italians or Latins or Brazilians, is the sense of family—of being embraced by a family, of being loved, of loving what they do. If they are housewives they adore that, and they are protected by their surroundings—the children, the household are very important. In America, people are born, they grow, and immediately they are out, out, out. They go to university, and they try to find in other people their mothers, their fathers, their sisters, their brothers. And those other people don't have to deal with them in the same way, because they don't have the same blood, they don't have the same patience. And they don't care."

Florinda is one of five: "Thank God I come from a large family—thank *God!* Anything but the need of that kind of love, because that kind of love

is something you carry with you. You have it and you give. It's a natural thing. If you don't have it you can't give. That's why American women somehow keep a distance, I think. They never had that easiness; they don't know how to approach people."

Like most actresses, Florinda lives where her work is: New York, Los Angeles, Rio, Rome. "I *think* I like living best in Europe, but I'm not so sure . . . it depends. I like the decadence of Europe, by which I mean there is a feeling of a long shadow: Things are not new, are not made yesterday, are not to be thrown out of the window; they are to be kept. . . . Love is a very complicated thing. It's not the man sees the woman, falls in love, gets married. No. It's *more* than that. There are other lovers. There are sisters that fall in love with their brothers, there are fathers who adore their sons or daughters. There are certain strange things in life that nobody talks about here. Everything is very clear and clean in America . . . a puritan outlook.

America is the country that has all the answers; people go crazy on numbers: 'How many orgasms?' 'One million five hundred.' Making love is more complex; it's a complete thing, like going to God. People should limit their sexual desires so that what they have is really good, not mediocre. Instead, today, a man likes a woman, he doesn't just take her to dinner and for a walk and to look at beautiful pictures in a museum . . . building to the big moment. Now they go to bed

right away. And the fantastic thing is to wait, to hope, to expect—that's the beauty of life, not to have right away. We are not animals; we have to have beauty, we have to have measurement. But people are wanting to have *all* right away. And the pity is, they can. So they become bored. . . . Boredom is the capital sin. Nothing is worse; it means you've had it . . . you have always to have a dream."

Florinda has many dreams, film projects among them. Her dreams are one of the very few subjects she is silent on. "I don't like to talk about these things, because then they never come. It's mainly that I'm Brazilian. Brazilians are superstitious. Italians are superstitious. Americans are less so. I'm very fascinated by the idea of people not having these hang-ups, because they limit a lot—the pleasure, for instance, of telling. But I feel it will not become a reality if I tell. So I tell very little. One day I'm not going to tell anything; I'm going to say hello and goodbye."

There is one other non-negotiable subject: "I'm at the point where I don't say my age, but I am not a baby. I am over thirty-five, and when I am seventy I will be 'over thirty-five'; from thirty-five up I am just 'over.' A funny thing that I always remember—Marie Bell, the French actress, used to travel, and wherever she went people would ask, '*Née?*' and she would say, '*Oui!*' . . . No group of women, I think, is more threatened by aging than actresses. You play the woman when she's young, then you play the thirty-five-year-old, then you play the mother. And nobody wants to play the mother. People resent—*I* resent—I *resent* the idea. I've already played the mother. I played Maria Schneider's mother two years ago, when she was eighteen. In fact, I won in Italy the Donatello prize. People didn't expect me to play a mother, and I played it quite well. Still, I don't think it's very flattering to be sent the script. . . ."

On the other hand, she has no inclination to recapture her "under thirty-five" image. "I don't even think about it, because I don't believe there is any way to go back. From now on it's going to be this to worse. There is no other way to be looking. Of course there are a lot of things one can do, but I don't think I will. . . . The most important thing is to think that one day one is going to have the face that one has." I can think of a lot of women who would kill for that face . . . and I wouldn't blame them one little bit.

Carina and
Yasmine Bleeth

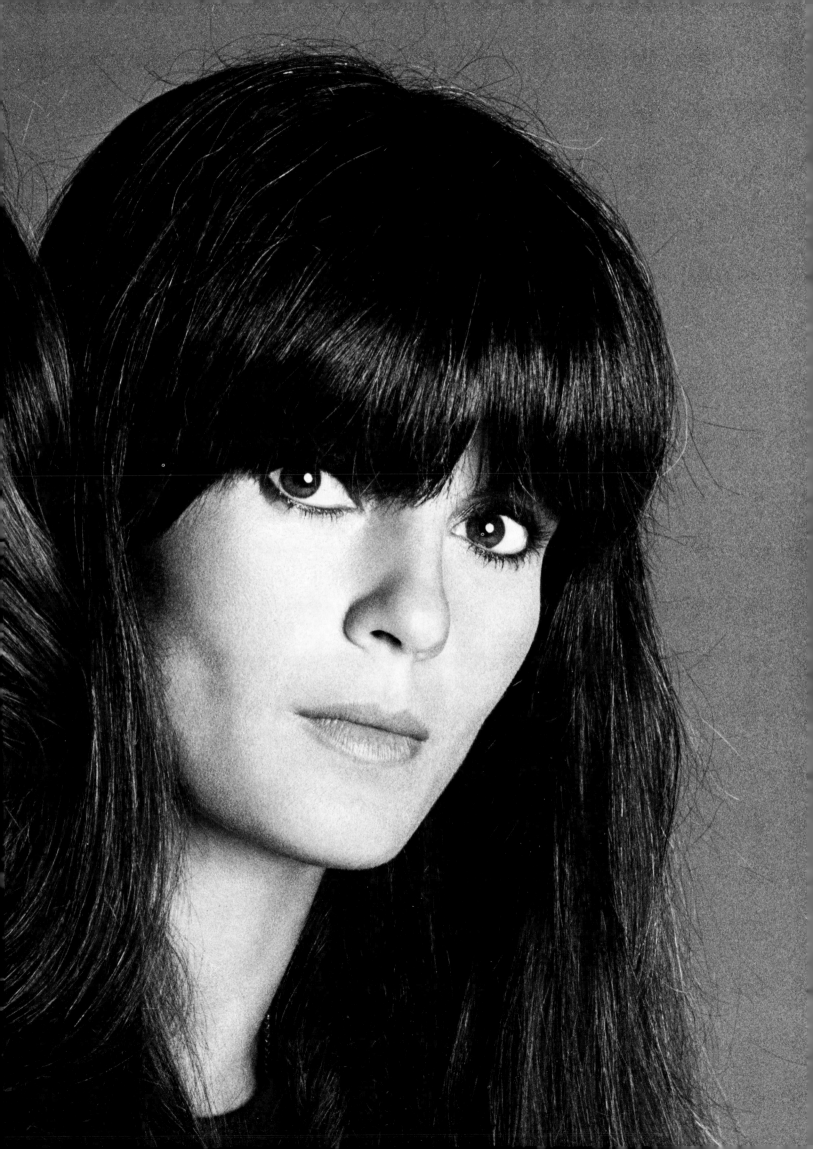

Yasmine Bleeth

Everybody should have a daughter like Yasmine Bleeth. She's bright, beautiful, well-mannered ("except once, when I was six, I went up to this photographer . . . I go up to him, and I go to his nose, and I say, 'You know something, your nose is really big!' My mother reminded me of that; I was so embarrassed!"), level-headed. She does her homework, goes to bed when she's supposed to, does her own laundry. And she makes a lot of money.

I took this early photograph of Yasmine when she was seven; she's twelve now and has been modeling since she was six and a half months old. Nowadays, she's doing less print, more commercials. She has done a children's jeans commercial for Gloria Vanderbilt: "It was fun, but I don't like the idea of wearing other people's names on your pants. In middle one—that's what we call sixth grade [Yasmine attends the UN School, a bilingual private school in New York]—designer jeans were In, and everyone wore them. So I did too." But from the sobering heights of the eighth grade, "when you can get a pair of Levi's for fourteen dollars, and then you hear forty dollars for designer jeans—!"

Yasmine likes modeling—for the moment. It hasn't interfered with her schoolwork ("I'm not the most outstanding student in the entire world; average for me is usually good, or sometimes very good. Every once in a while, I'll get an excellent"), and it hasn't cost her friends ("They don't treat me like Miss Goddess; I'm just another friend. It's like some people take ballet or play the violin; modeling is just another thing that I can do"). But she doesn't plan on doing it forever. "I have no intention of being a model when I grow up. I just don't think you need anything to be a model except good looks and being able to pose. You don't have to have any intelligence. You don't have to study anything in college. I'm looking forward to going to college. I want to go to Colorado. Or Princeton. Or Yale, maybe. I want to be a doctor when I grow up. Or an interior decorator. . . . There are just so many things!"

There is also acting. Yasmine has made a movie, *Babe,* in which she plays a little girl, an orphan, who fantasizes that she is a star. Yasmine is the star. Buddy Hackett is the co-star. "He was fun to work with. He taught me a lot: about saying lines . . . how you should move your eyes in a certain way. . . . I'd never seen myself on a big screen before. It was like, Oh, my *God!* My voice sounded different. I looked different. Everything was different. But I guess it was all right. Still, I don't want to be an actress when I grow up, but it's sort of an interest now . . . maybe I will be. . . . "

She has her Junior Lifesaver's card in swimming, her own roller skates, a white Maltese terrier named Frankie-O ("because most people name little fragile dogs Champagne or Snowball"), almost all the Beatles' records, and no dresses—except one, for summer. She likes books about girls her own age and books by Judy Blume. But only the ones she wrote for children. "She wrote two adult books, which are very disgusting. The story was good, but every other page was, like, Oh, my *God!*—instead of just saying, 'They did this and they did that,' she describes *everything,* and you know, it's not bringing anything to the book."

The facts of life didn't come to Yasmine via the Book-of-the-Month Club. "My mother told me . . . and around school . . . the streets. But my mom never hid anything from me." There is a further reason for her sophistication: Having lived for a while in Brazil, where she skipped a full year in school, she is now by far the youngest child in her class. "All her friends," her mother, Carina, told me, "are older, and I am astonished by the conversations they have: about boys . . . sex. They make fun, they make a joke out of it. But there is an awareness. They are aware of homosexuality; they accept it. There is nothing they don't know."

Sexual conversation used to be more intense. "Mostly, we used to talk about boys, and it was like, 'Oh, I'm so in love with him. Ohhhh!' We don't talk about it so much anymore . . . actually, we got over that last year." A typical date is five girls and five boys on roller skates, although "I've gone out once to a movie at night. Afterwards we went to an ice-cream parlor. And then we just went home. It wasn't like, And then he dropped me off and we kissed good night. Nothing like that; it's not serious. Also, we paid our own way."

Yasmine gets an allowance of $6 a week: "three dollars from my mom and three dollars from my dad." That her parents are separated troubles her less than the tension of their living together. "That bothered me. It would be nice if they could live together, but I understand that they have problems. So I'd rather they live this way. Besides, they only live a block away from each other. And they're friends; they go away together on the weekends. . . . I see my dad three or four times a week, and I sleep over at least twice. Usually, I tell both of my parents everything, but I tell my father *everything* . . . sometimes things I don't tell my mom."

> "Some people take ballet or play the violin; modeling is just another thing that I can do."

She has a close, easygoing relationship with her mother. Still, Carina is the in-charge parent. "She doesn't tell me, Brush your teeth, wash your hands before dinner, do this, do that. But she, you know, takes care of me. I have to be home after school no later than five, because of homework. And sometimes she's not home, so I would get home at five thirty or a quarter to six. . . . There's a sort of hangout for the kids after school. We all stay there. I did a couple of times, but I don't anymore, because my mom calls home at five o'-clock. And if I'm not home, she knows. One day, she goes, 'Were you home on time?' And I go, 'Yes.' And then she gets really mad at me. . . . I don't usually lie to her."

What worries Carina a great deal more than homework is drugs. "My biggest concern is that someone will hand her something when she goes out from school. And that is the only thing I'm really afraid of for her: drugs." Yasmine says, "It goes around the older grades, and it went around the sixth and seventh grades this year. I don't do it at all. There's no point to doing it. Most of the people who are doing drugs just do it because they think they're being really cool. If they were, they wouldn't be doing it. That's how I feel." Pretty cool for a twelve-year-old—that's how I feel.

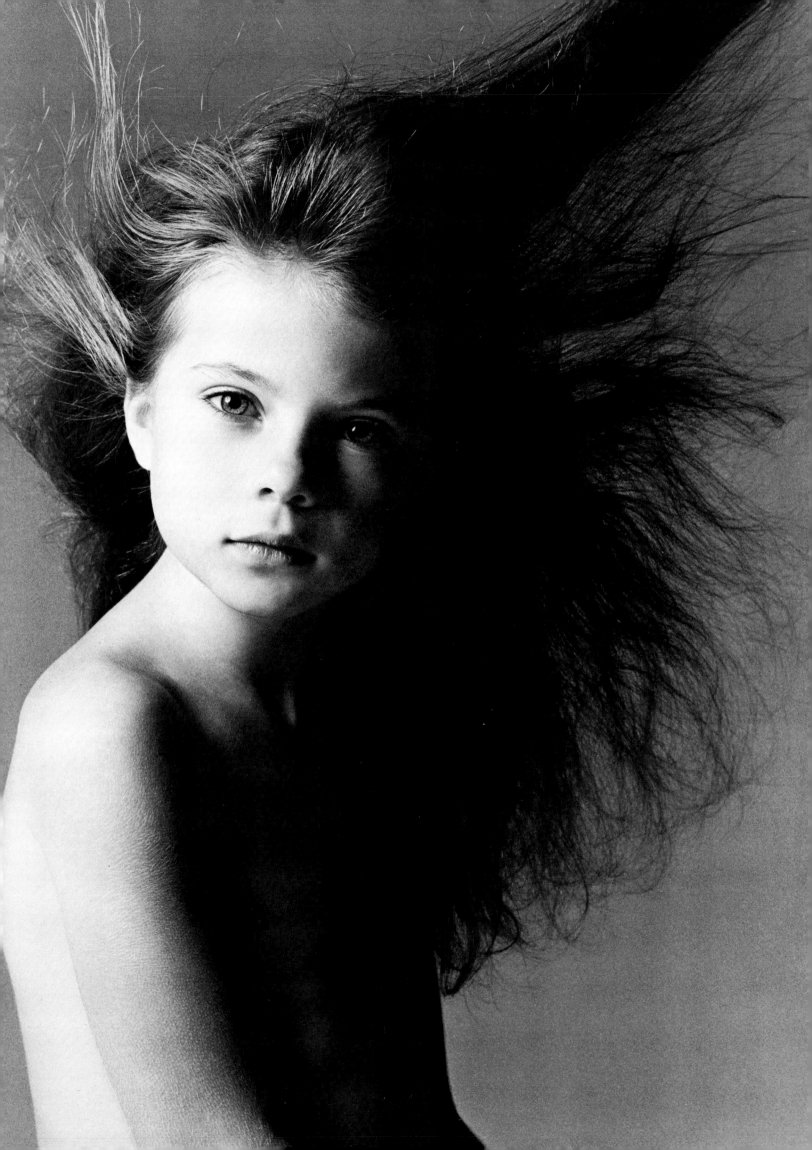

Carina Bleeth

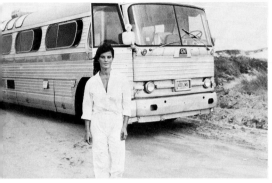

1975

I'd love to see Carina Bleeth go on one of those TV shows like *What's My Line?* where a panel of experts have to guess your profession. Model, they'd probably say—what else, with those sensational cheekbones and almond eyes? Of course a model. But that's only what she used to be. She gave it up a dozen years ago to become a wife, mother, and—are you ready for this?— a bus driver! And I don't mean some cute little minibus. This reed-slim slip of a woman, who looks about as tough as a piece of Lowestoft, drives a *major* bus, big enough to haul around the whole crew and all the paraphernalia of a fashion sitting when it's on location in and around New York.

It is one of two such operations in town; the other is owned by Carina's husband, from whom she is separated. It's an ambiguous relationship; they live a block away from each other in the city and often spend weekends together in the country. "I love him. No question about it. Liking is something else. It doesn't have to do with the fact that he is my business competitor; I don't always like him as a person. I don't like that he is irresponsible as a husband and as a father. As a lover, he is not. I have to give him that credit— a very important credit."

Carina was born in Algiers and went to Paris with her family on the eve of Algeria's independence from France.

She was nineteen. Her long, straight black hair was wrapped on top of her head. Then, as now, she had bangs— "big, puff-puff bangs, and big eyelashes, and lots of black liquid eyeliner. People would stop me on the street and ask, Are you a model? I guess for the way I was dressing, or maybe it had to do with my youth. I didn't know about the profession; I never heard it when I was in Algiers. So, I'm going to check out the modeling. There was a school—a Madame Claude, who was teaching how to walk, how to pass the clothes. I picked up a job in a bank to be able to pay for my courses, and after a month a client picked me for fashion shows."

A girl can do well on the runway, but she can do better in front of a camera. . . . In the Paris of the sixties, the empress of photographic-model agents was the onetime American supermodel Dorian Leigh, who knew a good thing when she saw it. She grabbed Carina. "She said I was *très typée*. It is an expression that means you are not black, you are not white. You can pass for Eurasian, Spanish, Italian. It means you have a strong type. That was a must in fashion shows, because a fashion show is composed of girls who each has her own style. And I had one. It was the *très typée* style. I did very, very well. Then, in 1967, I had to run away from Paris."

Cherchez l'homme. "I was in love and the man was married. I was living, with him for three and a half years, and he would not get the divorce. He didn't want to go for the legality; he was afraid of it. At that time, I was very into getting marriage extremely clear. So I knew what I had to do. I knew that I had to put a distance between him and me. And—ah, well, the opportunity came along." The opportunity was Expo '67, in Montreal. With three other models (one of whom, "my best friend, was in a similar situation. So here we were, two broken-hearted girls . . . though she eventually succeeded better in the personal thing"), Carina went to Montreal to represent the Paris ready-to-wear. And from there, New York.

Two standout memories of her first day: a taxi driver who drove around for

blocks, shooting the meter to the sky. And model agent Eileen Ford, who loved Carina on sight but didn't feel New York was quite ready for *très typée*. Instead, she would turn five-foot-six-and-a-half-inch Carina into a junior model. First, "she picked up her own tweezers and plucked my eyebrows." Then she set out to get her a whole new portfolio. Now, when a new girl looks promising, photographers will often do test shots on her. What the girl gets out of this is a free photograph by a top fashion photographer. Eventually, when she collects enough of them, she has a book—a portfolio— to show to prospective clients. It takes time, and she doesn't get paid. And a girl gets impatient, especially if she's been one of the busiest models in Paris. Carina quit Eileen. "I made a mistake. She knew exactly what she wanted to do with me, but I didn't understand— at that time, I was not understanding very well English. So I went to another agent, and she sent me to people who were looking for my type, and who gave me work. And it went on.

"Then I met my husband, and a few months later I got pregnant with my daughter Yasmine. And that was the end of the career. There was no heart anymore to go to interviews; my personal life was taking too much of me. My relationship with my husband was such a stormy one—up and down, up

"You shouldn't worry about which angle; just be aware of the expression you are projecting to the camera. It is a matter of fantasizing."

and down." In 1971—on a big up—the Bleeths went into the fashion-busing business.

Even though I'd known Carina for years—through the bus, and having photographed Yasmine when she was seven—this was our first real sitting together. I loved it. So did Carina, even though, she says, "I had to drink a little wine to get in front of the camera again. But then it was nice." It was perfect; she wasn't nervous about how she looked or what angle I was catching. "You know, years ago, we were not aware that the model had this angle better than the other; that was the photographer's job. I still think you shouldn't worry about which angle; you should just be aware of the expression that you are projecting to the camera. It is a matter of fantasizing. As you are fantasizing, your face gets alive and that's what you project. You can fantasize anything. Fantasize that the photographer is your lover—I feel there is at the particular time of the shooting a very, very sexual relationship for the photographer and the model. I feel it is why photographers prefer to shoot with certain girls—and also vice versa—because they believe they have a contact with that person, a physical contact. And you definitely keep eye contact. This time is different, because it was a dual. My contact was with my daughter. Even if I was not looking at her, there was a physical contact with her sideways."

Carina gets to see a lot of makeup artists in the line of duty. "A lot of times they play with my face, and I was never satisfied." Until she worked with Sandy Linter on this sitting. "Sandy respected my suggestion not to put any foundation. She focused only on my eyes and my lips . . . just put some natural lip color and some gloss . . . maybe a little blush. She kept it really natural. As well as for Yasmine. Many makeup artists put foundation on her; she has a lot of freckles, you know. She has a very pretty pigmentation, and if you cover it, what's the sense?"

"At the particular time of the shooting there is a very, very sexual relationship for the photographer and the model."

The only difference between Carina's own eye makeup and this one is that "Sandy put a dark crayon underneath the lashes to make my eyes look bigger; over the lashes—that is to say, inside, on the rim of the eyelid—has the tendency to make the eyes smaller. So, if you put it there, you have to have already the pretty big eyes." Big-eyed Carina puts it there. And she uses pure kohl, as it comes from the souks of Morocco. "It has a beautiful shape of container, and they put the powder in that—kohl is a burned stone, ground into powder. With it, there is a wooden stick that is

shaved very pointy. So you have to be careful. . . . It goes on the lower lid and the upper lid at the same time. You do it by putting the stick inside, between the lashes; close the eyes, and just make the movement forward and backward. And that's it."

She rarely uses any other makeup. "I always look cheap when I put on makeup. So I never put foundation. Never. I don't wear eye shadow; it doesn't do anything for me; I have dark skin. I don't look good with mascara; on me, it is just a pasty thing." Her skin is so good—and her skin-care routine so simple—you could die. "When I take a shower I use soap, and I don't believe in using it every day on the face; it's too rough. I have a tendency to have dry skin, and I use a lotion that I buy at Kiehl's Pharmacy. It's all I use on my face. It has no fragrance, just natural oils from almonds and apricots. There is also a version for the body that

I tried to use for my face because it's cheaper. It didn't work. And baby oil and Vaseline don't work; they're too thick. The lotion is the only thing that works for me. . . . It's very popular; all the models use it."

Carina is thirty-eight. She has a theory; "A woman above thirty has only one direction to be aware of—that it's all going downhill from thirty on. Physically. And we are in a society where the physical projection you give is very, very important. It is related to the mind, as well; if you feel good physically about yourself, the mind goes with it. I've seen many times where I gain weight, and I get depressed. I will not go out, I will not go to buy clothes, because I know that I will not look good. . . . My husband is a very physical person, always involved with physical activities—thank God. That is the one positive thing—one of several things, actually—that he influenced me on. He really turned me on to it. Six months ago, I believed that lifting weights would be good for me;

the doctor has told me that I need strenuous exercise, because I have a slow blood circulation. So I joined the New York Health and Racquet Club, which is fantastic.

"Three times a week I go. I have a routine. I get there around ten o'clock. I run on a running machine for fifteen minutes, quite fast. Then I do the Nautilus weight-lift machines; you cannot exercise with these every day; you could actually destroy fibers. At eleven thirty, there is a yoga class. I always end up with that—in case I've done something wrong during my Nautilus routine, I know yoga will compensate. I even take belly-dancing once a week; I'm from an Arabic country, you know."

Carina has not much tolerance for orthodox medicine since the time, a few years ago, when she slipped a disc in her bus (not driving it; straightening out a mat on the floor), and a team of doctors told her that unless she underwent immensely costly surgery she would never walk upright again. Having neither perfect faith in the doctors nor insurance to cover their fees, she opted instead for bed rest and a chiropractor . . . and recovered. Her nutritionist is the only doctor who has her absolute confidence. "When I went to see him, I was losing my hair." The trouble, as he diagnosed it, was that Carina, an O-positive blood type, was trying to be a vegetarian, and the O's of this world want big-time protein. "It is not such a good blood; it's a low-grade blood. So you need high-grade protein food. He believes in all protein except red meat—fish, veal, lamb, chicken, and eggs—but no more than four a week. His diet is difficult in that he asks you to drink water and lemon when you wake up, which is fine. But then he asks you to wait a half hour before you drink your juice, and another half hour before you have your breakfast; who has the time in the morning?

"I'm very careful. I drink only raw milk. I eat a lot of fruit and nuts. I try to have a balanced meal. I always start with a salad—that means the big hunger goes toward the salad, and you don't stuff yourself. My weakness is sweets, no question about it. And I do cheat; it's why I exercise, to be able to cheat. It is the biggest pleasure remaining in life—food and love. Or love and food. Sometimes I don't know which goes first . . . they go together, yes?" *Oui*.

Maria Burton

"People expect much more when your mother is very beautiful. They're disappointed when they look at you and they say, 'Ah . . . er . . . um . . .' It sort of takes them aback. . . . It would be so much nicer if instead of saying, 'That's Elizabeth Taylor and Richard Burton's daughter,' they'd say, 'That's Maria Burton!' "

There are various family stories of how Maria Burton came to be adopted by Elizabeth Taylor and Richard Burton, ranging from the businesslike (an advertisement in a German newspaper placed by an anonymous "wealthy foreign couple") to the absurd ("they climbed up a ladder and sneaked into the hospital"). Maria says she hasn't the faintest idea what the truth is, but in the version she likes best, "Maria Schell, a very good friend of my mom's who lives in Germany, and for whom I'm named, helped in the adoption.

"She found six babies, and I was the ugliest. I was eight months old and I was bald, and my leg—it was only a dislocated hip, and afterward they operated and put a cast on it, and it was fine. But then . . . I mean, I was *ugly*. So Maria Schell put me out of sight; she didn't want Elizabeth Taylor to see this ugly baby. But when Mom came, she heard me screaming and carrying on, and she said, 'What's that noise in the other room?' 'Oh, that's nothing, just other babies.' But Mom insisted, and she saw me and picked me up, and she said, 'That's my baby!' "

All Maria knows of her natural parents is that they were German and poor. She has never tried to find out more. "There is a little bit of curiosity,

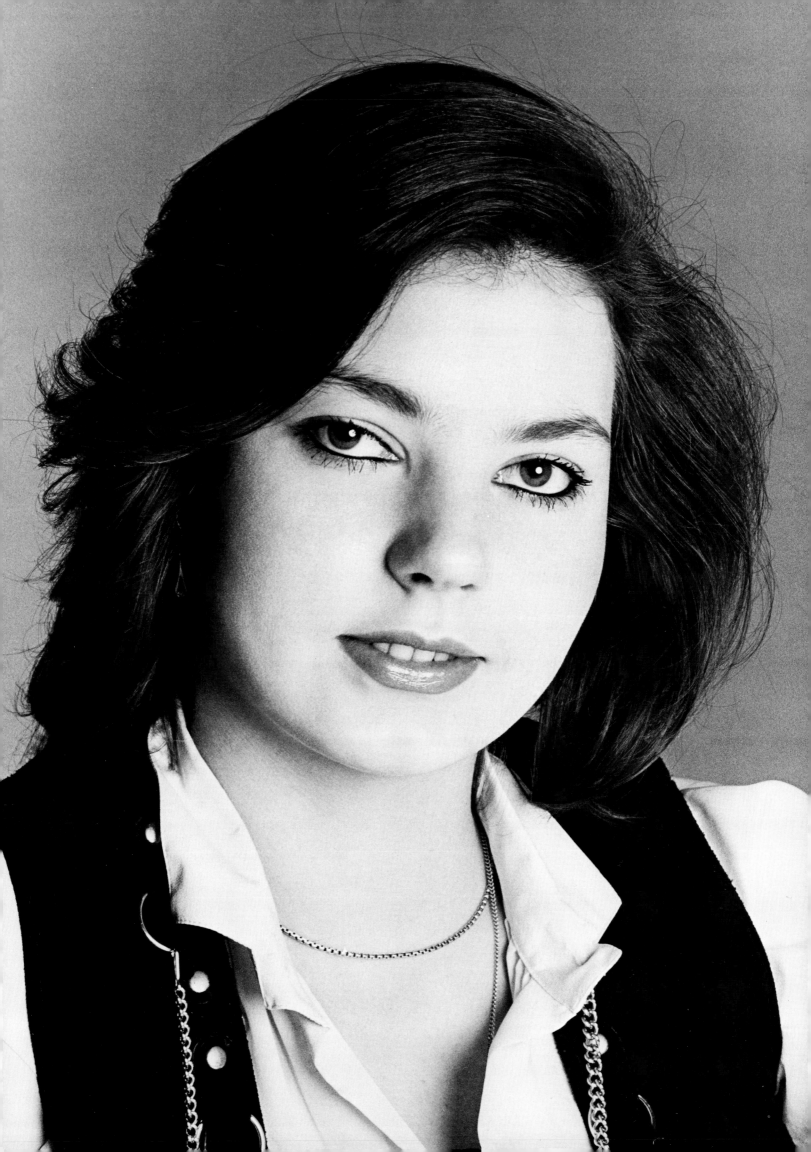

Maria
Burton

but then . . . I don't even speak the language." Being the adopted child of two extravagantly glamorous people has never troubled her—on either count. She can't remember ever not knowing she was adopted. "Dad and Mom always told me that I was. It wasn't sort of sprung on me; I was brought up with it." And while she could hardly have been unaware of her parents' celebrity, they have always been "just my parents, my father and my mother . . . just normal." Her relationship with her assorted siblings is equally normal. "We're a very close family. Usually you get half-brothers and half-sisters, and they're such a distance from each other, each completely different from the body of the family. Whereas us, we're all the same—we laugh at the same things, we joke a lot —even though we have our own lives and live somewhere else."

when, through a family friend, she began to model. "I like modeling. I feel I'm fulfilling something, doing something that's enjoyable . . . but I'm not very good at posing." Nevertheless, within a year she was successful enough to make New York worth a try.

So here she is, a lovely young woman, tall, slender, shy, and excessively modest. Apart from her eyes, which are large, hazel, and

---

"When the makeup is on, then I think I look good. . . . If I don't have eyeliner, I look like the pits. *Dreadful.* It's a trademark, my eyeliner—my lifesaver."

After ten years at Swiss boarding schools, Maria moved to London. "I wasn't sure what I wanted to do, so I went to secretarial college for a year. Mom thought it was a good idea. They all did, especially my dad; he said, 'That's great!' At least I know that if I don't make it in anything else, I can always fall back on my typing." So far, she hasn't had to. She had barely got started as an "office temp"

slanted like a cat's, she doesn't think she is pretty. "If people tell me that I am, I ignore it because I know I'm not. . . . When the makeup is on, then I think I look good. But without it, I look as if I've been dragged through the hedge backwards. And the makeup has to be right. I did my own makeup in London once, and I looked like God-knows-what. When those photographs came out, I said never again am I going to do my own makeup. I didn't put enough dark shadow to cut down my cheeks—my cheeks have always been too big; I've got to go on *such* a diet— and I didn't have any eyeliner, which was a very big mistake. If I don't have that, I look like the pits. *Dreadful.* It's a trademark, my eyeliner—my life-saver.

"Way Bandy told me that I ought to pluck my eyebrows. But I have a hor-

ror of doing it; it's agony! . . . Mom's eyebrows are absolutely fantastic—the shape and all—and I have never ever seen her pluck them. They fascinate me. And her eyes are so beautiful, as well; they really are." In general, I think, "Mom's" looks have a lot to do with the way Maria feels about her own. "People expect much more when your mother is very beautiful. They're disappointed when they look at you, and they say, 'Ah . . . er . . . um. . . .' It sort of takes them aback."

Elizabeth Taylor is her daughter's staunchest champion. She gives skin-care advice; at one recent middle-of-the-night session, "She was teaching me how to wash my face. She said, 'Take the cream—the hand lotion— and put it on your face. Then splash warm water on. And then take your facecloth and just go pat around your eyes to get rid of the makeup. If you don't get it all off, take a bit of soap and do the eyes. Take the facecloth and pat it around your eyes. Use a clear soap, like Pear's soap, the kind that has no perfume or any other stuff in it. You use that, and your skin won't get dry and cracked.' "

Her mother also says, "You'll make it." She pushes Maria on, which is not the same as mere pushing. "She doesn't push me; I push myself. My family encourages me a little bit here and there —challenges me a little bit—and then

---

"My cheeks have always been too big."

I'll go all the way on my own. . . . It helps that they're my parents. But I don't want to use that for the rest of my life. I don't want people to pinpoint me forever as their daughter. Then you don't have an identity of your own; it's all just your parents. It would be so much nicer if instead of saying, 'That's Elizabeth Taylor and Richard Burton's daughter,' they'd say, 'That's Maria Burton!' " . . . That's Maria Burton. It sounds good to me.

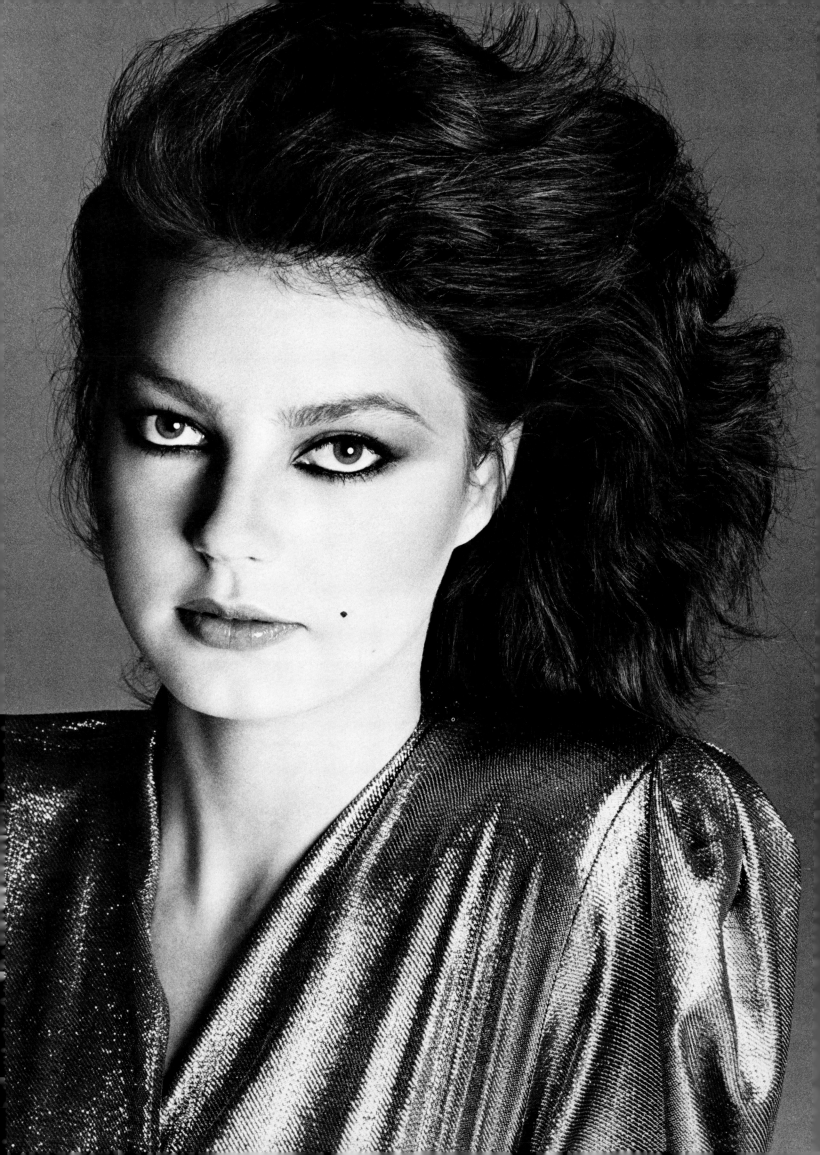

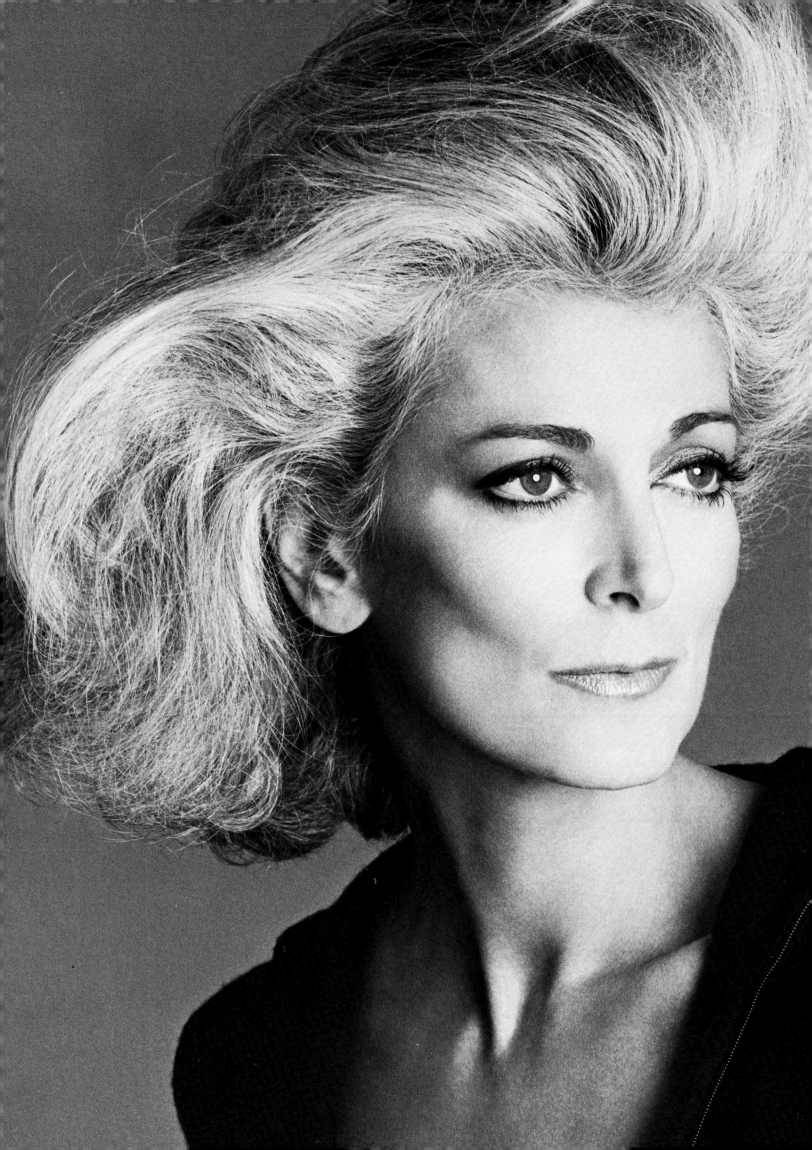

Fine skin and elegant looks start with self-knowledge and are maintained by discipline.

Carmen

"It's a pleasure to keep myself happy, which means keeping in shape. Women: Look in the mirror, a front mirror and a back mirror. See yourself the way other people see you. It's so shocking. It's so funny. The important thing is to be open, re-examine, redo. The process is fun."

Carmen

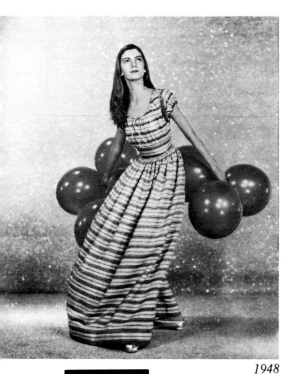

1948

The first time I photographed Carmen, in 1948, for *Seventeen,* they told me she was too old for the magazine. She was sixteen. But nothing about her look was childlike. It was high fashion, sophisticated, soignée—a woman's look. At sixteen, five feet nine inches tall, she was a *femme du monde* who didn't even have a bosom yet.

I tried to make her a little girl. I did Alice in Wonderland hair; I had her stand very demurely. And we got a good picture, but they were right: Carmen never did belong in *Seventeen.* But at *Vogue!* They'd put those Mainbocher clothes on this infant and she'd look as though she'd been born in them. She was phenomenal—she *is* phenomenal. Carmen at fifty is as exciting to photograph as she was at sixteen or twenty or thirty-three. And believe me, that's rare. Usually when I photograph someone at fifty whom I've photographed as a girl, it's depressing. I look through the lens and my heart sinks. With Carmen, it flies. She gives off sparks; there's so much spirit and such an elegance of line. And she needs very little retouching; she's marvelous

as is, with that fine skin and those wide, long-lashed, cool green eyes and the gray hair she wears like a banner.

Carmen has always had a good deal of gray in her hair, which she covered up until a few years ago. "My last husband turned over in bed one morning—I thought he was reaching over to caress my face—and he pulled out a gray hair. That's about as close as I've ever come to feeling offended. So I let the gray grow in: my rebellion."

Carmen Dell'Orefice Miles Heimann Kaplan ("Being a well-brought-up Catholic girl, I hadn't heard that I didn't have to marry every man I fell in love with"), sometimes known by her maiden name ("it's one of the few things a man has given me and not taken back"), but sufficiently celebrated to get along on just Carmen, was discovered in 1945 by Carol Philips, now president of Clinique, then a *Vogue* editor. The dramatic version is that Carol spotted Carmen on the 57th Street crosstown bus. The truth is, they met at Carmen's godparents. Who discovered Carmen on the bus was the wife of a *Harper's Bazaar* photographer. He was underwhelmed. "You have a charming child," he wrote to Mrs. Dell'Orefice, who framed the letter and hung it in the bathroom, "but totally unphotogenic."

The keener-eyed Carol Philips got Carmen up to *Vogue* in a hurry, and it was star-is-born time. In her first issue, she had seven full pages. She had covers. "I saw the first cover on my way to dance class. There was a stack of *Vogue*s at the newsstand. I thought, Ugh! What a terrible picture. So I lifted up the top *Vogue,* hoping the one underneath would be better . . . and I lifted the second and the third . . . ugh! . . . I just dropped them and ran."

A minority opinion. To the rest of the country—who evidently failed to notice that she "had ears like sedan doors and feet like coffins, and my chest was so flat it was concave, and the boy I had a crush on never looked at me"—Carmen Dell'Orefice was bigger than China. And everybody looked at her. Ali Khan looked. William Astor. Joseph Kennedy, Senior, looked—a little closer than the others. "Little did I know when he took me up to a lovely apartment on Park Avenue, in the Fifties, and asked me, Wouldn't I like my mother to have a better life? . . . I mean, I was fifteen, a scrawny kid in brown Oxfords. And I was truly naive, which is the ultimate protection. You

know what I said to him? I said, 'Oh, *yes!* My mother has worked so hard. I really do want her to have a better life.' 'Well, you know,' he said, 'she could live here.' And I said, 'She could? She'd *love* it!' He nearly fell through the floor; he didn't expect me to be *that* naive, and he took me right home."

As a matter of fact, both of Carmen's parents had had a hard life. Her father—"my wonderful, artistic, tall, green-eyed Italian father"—was a symphony violinist whose work was just about washed out by the Depression. Her mother, a former ballet dancer, is Hungarian, a tough-spirited woman who went to work at a radio factory and two weeks later was promoted to foreman, in charge of wiring shortwave radios. She was a mother-knows-best mother; when Carmen, not too long before her break into model-

---

"I'm the kind of person who—if I had a black eye—would put matching shadow on the other eye."

---

ing, came down with rheumatic fever and had been in bed a year, Mrs. Dell'-Orefice said, Enough. Ignoring doctors' orders, she slipped her daughter into art classes (Carmen got a scholarship), into swimming classes (Carmen worked up to Olympic-swimming trainee), back to ballet classes (before her illness, Carmen had been a scholarship student at the Ballet Russe). A few years later, Carmen was a *Vogue* model, earning $100 a day, which is taxi fare for a top model today, but it was big money then—more than enough to send her mother to college (where she made Phi Beta Kappa and graduated in three years). And a few years after that, when she was eighteen, she became—and remained for ten years—the Vanity Fair girl, thereby elevating lingerie advertising to the ranks of high fashion. The "scrawny kid in Oxfords" was, as Walter Winchell said, "the hottest . . . model in town."

Like any woman who has ever gone the distance in this business, Carmen is totally honest with herself. Everything proceeds from self-knowledge: "I know my body very well. . . . I know my face. I know, when a makeup man is doing my face, that if he's putting a black line under the eye, he's closing it in, which is going to elongate my already elongated face. And if he makes a mouth that is long from side to side, it's going to accentuate my jawline. . . . I'm not complaining. I'm just speaking technically—architecturally. I do it all the time; I have to. And I'd like to encourage all women to do the same, to look at themselves this way; they're not going to be penalized for it. 'Women: Look in the mirror, a front mirror and a back mirror. See yourself the way other people see you. It's so shocking. It's so funny. Don't worry. The important thing is to be open, re-examine, redo. The process is fun.' "

For Carmen, the process is ongoing: "It's a pleasure to keep myself happy, which means keeping in shape. It's all part of the same package. I sleep with a feeling of joy. I get up with a feeling of joy. I look forward to the morning. I do exercises before I get out of bed. If I didn't I'd fall on the floor in a faint, because I have very low blood pressure. So I do some stretches and sit-ups in bed, and when I can focus on the pictures on the opposite wall—nowadays I need glasses (nature has been kind to me; after forty I started having diminishing eyesight, and if I look in the mirror without my glasses I keep looking the same)—when I see everything clearly, I get out of bed.

"Then I go and brush my teeth and, holding on to the sink, I do twenty or thirty deep knee bends. Then I do stomach exercises on the floor and general stretches. Once a week, I work out with Kounovsky. Basically, he's retired, but there's a private group of ladies that he has known forever, and he keeps on helping us. I would exercise on my own all the time, but I need a professional to correct what I may be doing incorrectly. I don't agree with people who think, I'll get this exercise book and do it myself; it's too easy to

reinforce a negative. Even if it's only once a month, you should go to a pro; you need someone to look at what you're doing.

"It's getting better, but America has been pretty sedentary. At least running has gotten people to move; it's something. For a woman, the more she moves, the better: the better the circulation, the better the complexion, everything. I would heartily recommend to any mother of a daughter, whether your daughter is going to be a dancer or not, very early on in life put her at a ballet barre. She will benefit all her life from this discipline."

Carmen has delicate, beautiful skin, and she cares for it almost exactly as she learned to do when she was just starting out as a model. "Mineral oil is what I use at night. I could afford it even when I couldn't afford anything, and I buy it now, when I can afford a great deal more. . . . Water is the great-

est free healing thing we have. I think any doctor will agree. If your skin is 'oochy' and you want to soothe it, dilute whole milk in water—half and half. If my skin feels especially dry, I use more whole milk and a little less water. It makes a very refined emollient —like a moisturizer—for under makeup. . . . If I have dryness around the mouth, where those little lines come in, I open a vitamin E capsule and smooth it in, plus some mineral oil. . . . I'm the kind of person who, if I had

"I know my body very well. . . . I know my face."

a black eye—a real purply, greeny, garish shiner—would put matching shadow on the other eye. Otherwise, I don't wear much makeup. My skin doesn't like it. I don't like it."

Carmen has been married three

times (by her first marriage, she has a daughter, Laura Miles, now twenty-eight) and divorced three times. "I wanted the first divorce; I was grateful for the second; and the last was my turn to feel devastated. For nine years it was a marriage made in heaven. Then we ran into the sixties, which was a very strange time, a kind of diseased time . . . the drugs . . . everything that went on in the sixties was such an external pressure that I had to make a choice. I had to redirect my life." Carmen is friendly—"not intimate, but caring"—with all her former husbands. She knows their wives; their children have gone on holidays with her. "Marriage and people's fantasy about marriage need to be redefined. Where I come from, we were told marriage is a fifty-fifty proposition. I think you're doomed with fifty-fifty. If each person gives a hundred percent, then, I feel, you have a fifty-fifty chance."

"Being a well-brought-up Catholic girl, I hadn't heard that I didn't have to marry every man I fell in love with."

For the last seven years, "I have been single—quote, unquote. But I have never been busier or felt more love from friends or felt a closer connection with my daughter. So my life feels full, even though I don't have a live-in anybody—not even a cook or a maid." Recently, Carmen decided to come back to modeling. And it's beginning to happen for her . . . in French *Vogue*, in *Harper's Bazaar*, in *Town & Country*. She did Michael Volbrecht's kickoff fashion show for the Coty Awards presentation dinner and walked away with it; at the finale, in a drop-dead pailleted sheath, she had the whole house— which included most of the hottest young models in town—on its feet cheering, blowing kisses, welcoming her home.

"You know, Dorian Leigh said in her book, 'I don't want to be the oldest model in captivity.' I'm so relieved, because you know what? I do! I want to go out doing it when I'm seventy, eighty, ninety—however much time I have left on this earth, that's what I want to do." Will she do it? Is the Pope Catholic?

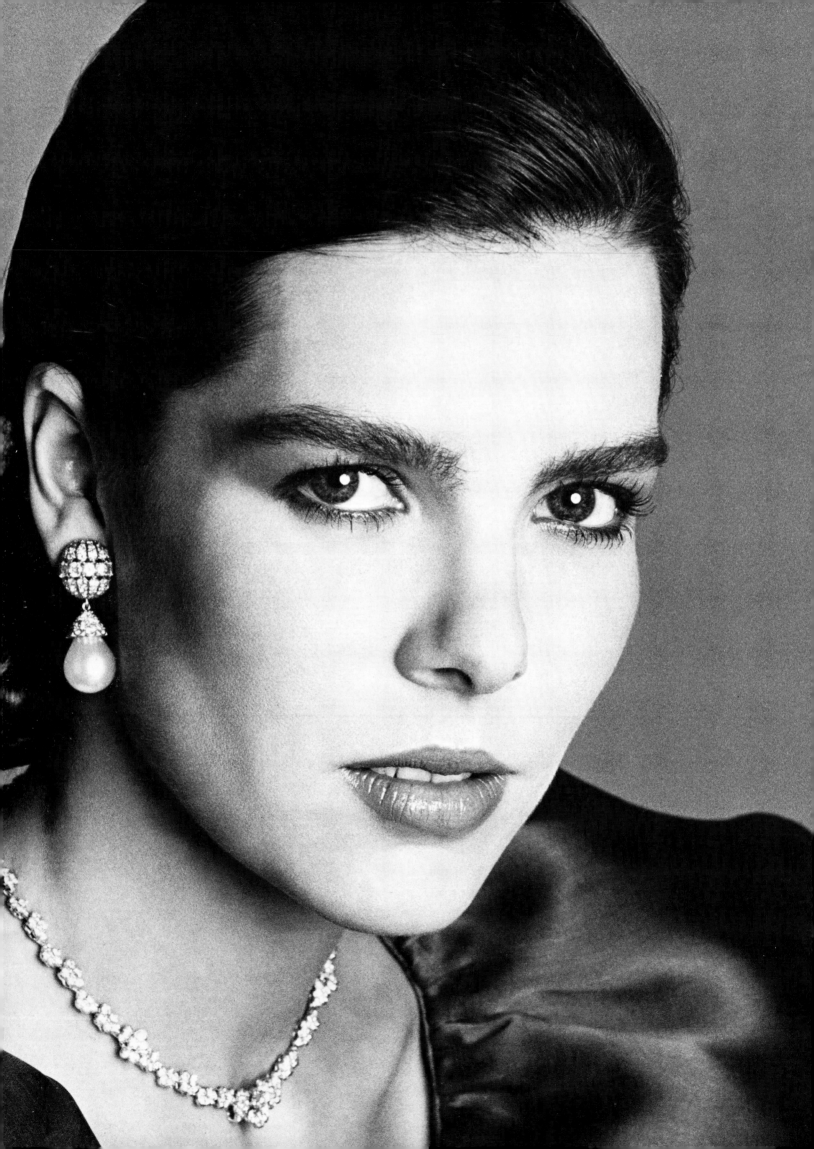

Princess Caroline of Monaco

We are none of us strangers to the fantasies of children. Having been there ourselves, we know all about little-boy cowboys on broomstick horses and little-girl princesses trailing through make-believe palaces. More glamorous than this it isn't possible to be—keeping in mind, of course, that one child's fantasy is another child's reality, and that there's nothing especially magical about, say, princesses and palaces if that's what you are and where you live. In which case, your fantasies might incline more along the lines of a Princess Caroline of Monaco: "My brother and I used to pretend to be poor orphan children. . . ."

Princess Caroline, as practically the whole world knows, is the daughter of the former Grace Kelly—of whom she is a taller brunette version—and Prince Ranier. At twenty-three, her daydreams are less melodramatic than they used to be, but just as wistful. "For the last five or six years, I've desired only to be anonymous. . . . I just thought it rather boring, you know, having 'important' parents—very strict parents—and not being allowed to do this or that thing. And I used to lie about who I was and who my parents were. Even in school—they'd say, 'Oh, but you speak English,' and I'd say, 'Yes, I'm American.' And of course, my name was Grimaldi, which can be

an Italian name. And they'd say, 'Are you Italian?' And I'd say, 'On my father's side—we have family,' or whatever. I'd just sort of improvise.

"There are ways of keeping a low profile, of leading your own life. Yet, in these stories, I just *love* to go out and party, which is absolutely untrue. What I like more than anything is to stay at home and have a very quiet life. And I do lead a quiet life, except for occasional things that I have to go to. Then, of course, they take nine thousand pictures and use them all the time, at weekly intervals. . . . I'm living in Monaco now, and no one bothers me there. It depends on where you go, what circles you move in. And sometimes you get trapped in a circle . . . and it's just very difficult."

"What I like more than anything is to stay at home and have a very quiet life."

Conversely, relatively little is heard about her work for UNICEF during the Year of the Child, in which she was instrumental in getting children involved in the actual work; or about the foundation that she helped to start, which will finance special projects developed by underprivileged youngsters in the south of France. Still too new to have a name, the foundation has already sponsored a cinema club organized by students at a *collège technique* and a Monegasque teenagers' mountain-climbing expedition in South America.

Caroline learned early on that the

public is less interested in her good works than in her marital problems (solved) and prospects (of which all that is known for the moment is that Prince Charles is no longer among the candidates; not that he ever was: "Honestly! Do you know, in the Houses of Parliament, they still refer to Catholics as Papists?").

While she has never observed a formal dress code, "I was brought up to realize that certain things are . . . well . . . anything too plunging, anything too transparent, anything too . . . you know. And nothing too wild. It doesn't look right on me; I'm sort of a big girl, and it all magnifies—amplifies—on me. I don't like ruffles and frills. I like very simple, very classical clothes, and solid colors. I

like Dior a lot" . . . and she wears, just like your average princess-next-door, "jeans most of the time." And very little makeup. "I generally just do my eyes. I put some brown on my lids, and a bit of mascara, and kohl inside the bottom lashes on the edge of the eyelid. That's all I do. It takes me five minutes—and I have to put a little pink on my cheeks because I'm so pale. Except, I usually don't. . . . Usually, I just pinch my cheeks to look rosy. Sometimes, for a whole week, I think, 'Ah, I should really do something. . . .'" No, she shouldn't; she's just right as she is.

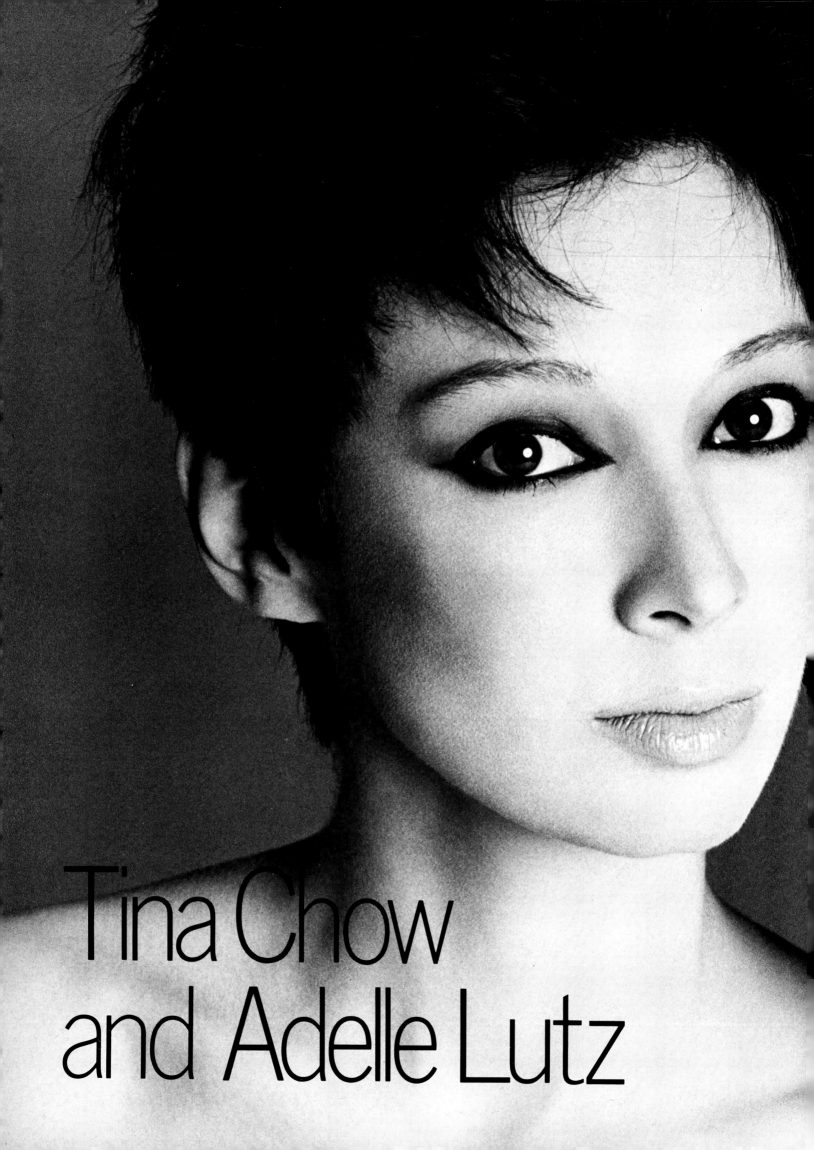
Tina Chow
and Adelle Lutz

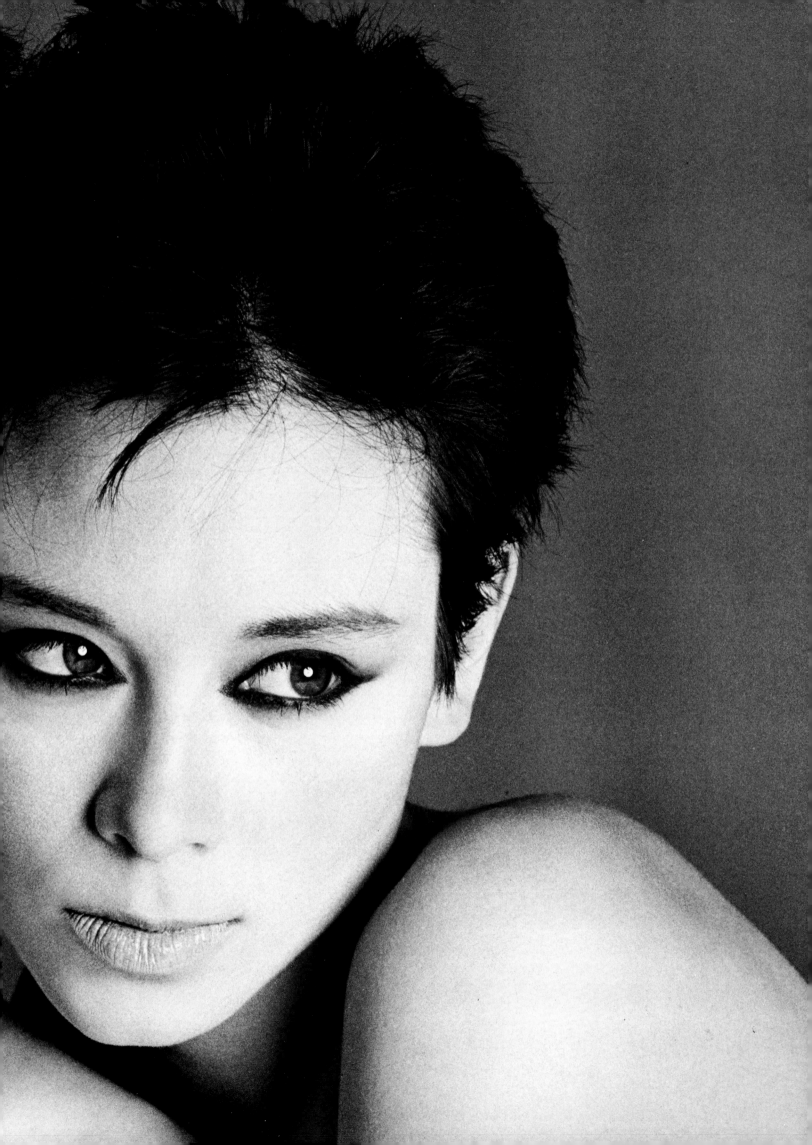

Tina Chow

"The English seem to feel that they've already gone through their greatness, so they sit back and relax. . . . In America, we feel we have to accomplish something whether or not it has a purpose or a value."

Y ou don't hear people talk about elegance anymore; at least, not in the sense of a physical attribute. Women today have a dash, a look, a vitality, an excitement, an allure. But elegance is something else. It has to do with line and gesture and carriage. And with a certain sophistication of taste, which in turn suggests self-knowledge, self-discipline . . . maturity.

To me, Tina Chow, barely out of her twenties, has elegance, by anyone's definition—even her own: "Having your own chic . . . it isn't the only elegance, of course." But it's key. And one way you learn is by "finding out that the things that are the most fashionable and most distinctive—certain looks that a designer has for one season —are the things to avoid. Because everyone will remember exactly the date, and if it's just a passing phase it may look awkward or ugly later. Learn how to do your own version, but don't buy those major fashion 'statements.' Buy subtler clothes, instead, or the more classic ones that no one takes much notice of.

"You just have to look for clothes that transcend a particular season. It's difficult in New York; here they think that if you're dressing in a classic manner it's too boring, that you have to keep up with fashion. I don't do a lot of shopping in New York. I don't do a lot of shopping. And I never shop with the idea of getting a whole new wardrobe. It's just finding something that's going to fit in, or look right, or amusing. The best thing is to find the perfect sample and get it copied in Hong Kong."

Elegance, for Tina, has also to do with "a beauty that doesn't just hit you straight in the eye. . . . I don't think women are trying to make themselves beautiful right now. When China Machado was modeling, for instance, there was a whole different attitude toward fashion, more studied, not so spontaneous or carefree. That image has changed. And the grooming has changed—letting everything hang out is not very attractive. Maybe it was too studied before, but I suppose I miss it."

She has two indelible images of a beautiful woman. One is "the crown princess of Japan . . . very thin, with graying hair, and so elegant . . . always in kimono of either gray or celadon, very quiet green colors." The other is Silvana Mangano, who came to dine at Mr. Chow, in London: "She was almost ghostlike, so pale, so thin. I was seeing her as though she were in a Visconti film. The air seemed to change around her. She was wonderful. The

skin, porcelain. Just so white. And so elegant and thin."

Tina—five feet seven and a half inches tall, 118 pounds—would like to be thinner. I can't see it. She says it's because of her jaw. "I have a terribly strong jaw, very square, and I tend to clench it. Sometimes it's too hard and unforgiving. But I guess it's my best feature . . . it makes me look thinner than I am." She wants to lose ten pounds, which "is all concentrated below the waist. So what I've been doing is starting to fast again. By fast,

"Letting everything hang out is not very attractive."

I mean stop eating. Seriously stop eating for three to five days. Three days is very easy; it's those extra two. But there are some schools that say you have to fast for five days before it really does your system any good. . . . What I want to do is first lose the weight and then start exercising. Because if you have too much fat and you start exercising, it can turn to muscle. So I want to trim it away first and *then* let it turn to muscle. That's my own philosophy. I don't know whether it's true or not, but it's how I feel."

She has her own makeup philosophy: "Black eye disease around the eyes. Which consists of a kohl pencil all around. And over it, very dark charcoal-gray matte eye shadow. I bring it out to the sides, rather than up—my eyes go up enough already—and sort of phase it out to the hairline. . . . No blusher. I went through the period of too much blusher, really lots of color. And the blusher under chin to define the jaw; remember that one? . . . I use a very light base, halfway between a cream and a liquid. It's sort of a flat

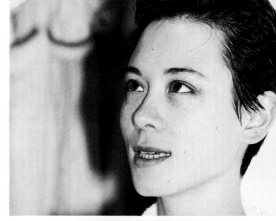

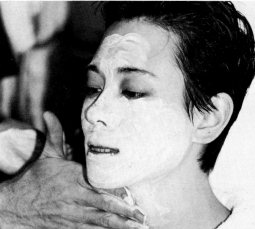

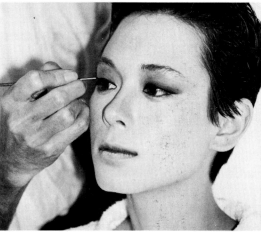

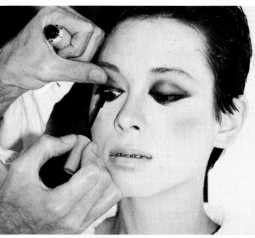

1. No makeup
2. Very light base for dramatic effect
3. Black eyeliner to elongate round eye
4. Mascara side to side for lush effect
5. Pale lips to emphasize eyes

beige, with a bit of yellow in it—my skin tone being oriental and not too pink."

She doesn't go to skin-care salons, but she's a believer. "I do it myself—a lot of facials, a lot of masks. Just to cleanse and tighten your pores, there's nothing like a nice herbal mask and steam. Whether it works or not, it feels great." Whatever beauty tricks she may have learned as a model, she claims to have forgotten—except one: "Knowing what things work best on you and staying with them, instead of rushing out to buy the latest mask or the latest color of eye shadow or the latest whatever. I guess you have to go through a phase of experimenting, not only with makeup but with clothes. It can be expensive. . . . I went through a phase of shopping after moving to London and having nothing to do—in the sense of nothing to do all day; there was the restaurant at night—so I would go shopping. In one month, I bought three dozen sweaters—that's thirty-six sweaters. I think I kept five; the rest I discarded. A costly lesson."

don original, plus Los Angeles and New York) and retired from modeling. "I was fed up. It was getting to me. Also, being a half-breed, knowing that I'd never fit in completely as half Japanese and half American. If you're half anything, they really look upon you as something else. Even if you're traveling in a sort of international circle, which means you get away from that, there's still never a feeling of total acceptance. So Adelle and I got out."

No one place has a monopoly on half acceptance: "It applies very much in Japan. It also exists in Hong Kong, in China." And she grew up with it in Ohio. "The hair didn't curl, I wasn't blond-haired, blue-eyed. It bothered me. I think there's much more acceptance in Los Angeles or New York. But Cleveland—well, it's a nice midwestern town, and very provincial. That's why I enjoyed living in London for so many years, and why I avoided living back in the States, not knowing how it would be. . . . London is a whole different mentality, a whole different way of life. The English seem to feel that they've

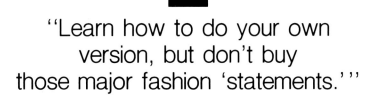

"Learn how to do your own version, but don't buy those major fashion 'statements.'"

already gone through their greatness, so they sit back and relax. Even if the country is falling apart. In America, we feel we have to accomplish something whether or not it has a purpose or a value. Things can get a bit frenzied, especially in New York.

"I had forgotten that living in New York was so unlike growing up in Cleveland, and it took me a few months to get used to the fact that I wasn't sort of singled out. In New York, once you hit the street, no one singles anyone out. It's strange. And it's wonderful. I'm very happy here."

In London, Tina married Michael Chow (there are now two small Chows: China, six, and Maximillian, three, and three Mr. Chow restaurants, the Lon-

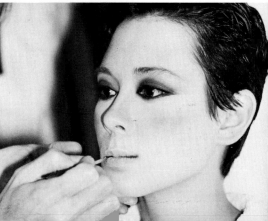

Adelle Lutz

Adelle Lutz and Tina Chow, born in Cleveland, Ohio, are the daughters of a Japanese mother and an American father of German descent. Geneticists ought to make a note of the combination. They are *exquisite*— flower faces—with sheer white skin, black hair, and huge hazel eyes that turn up at the corners. I don't expect that Bay Village had ever seen anything so exotic; in Japan, of course, where they lived for several years in their teens, it was their Western-ness that stood out. And Japan being a country that's trading out in a big way, it figures: Both girls took off as models. Both had contracts with Shiseido, the Japanese cosmetics company that sells around the world, though "Tina was always more high fashion; I was the commercial one. . . . I did Japan Airlines for years, and I did a *lot* of Coca-Cola. I was the all-American Japanese girl."

Adelle is on the left, the one with the cheekbones (Tina says she doesn't have cheekbones, just a face). Adelle is also the one with all the hair, in the single picture. "I went through a period when I thought I would like to have Dorothy Lamour hair. It's funny, I wanted short hair; Tina has had it short for a long time, but she has a tiny head and a baby face and a long body. I'm shorter and bonier, and also my jaw is quite prominent—big-looking, really. With short hair, I thought I would have this face just sticking out."

Which was precisely the reason to go short—to show that face and bring out those bones. And when she was in the makeup room, with Way Bandy and Harry King, we talked her into letting Harry cut it. What a difference! For me, all that hair was completely lacking in style. If you're going to wear black hair long, then wear it straight. Otherwise, off with it. Just look how much more important her face is now

. . . how much more extraordinary! Even more to the point, Adelle adored it right away: "It gave me more energy immediately. And it's so much easier; you stick your head under the faucet, and you don't have to walk around for hours with wet hair."

For photography, it's always the same thing: hair, eyes, mouth. . . . As he usually does, Way first plucked and shaped the eyebrows, then penciled them in a little bit. The eyes are shaded in red, with the black outline extended at each corner to emphasize the long slanting shape. And paled, glossy lips.

"I was the All-American Japanese girl."

The rest is simply light, moist foundation and pink cheeks.

Adelle does her own makeup very well, and now that she's living in New York she wears it most of the time. "I have to, simply because of the air: the cars, the buses, and all the dust flying around. Makeup gives you a layer of protection—against the elements and the sun, as well as pollution." She uses a liquid foundation, paler than her own skin, and over it puts a dusting of loose powder. The color, an ultra-pale lavender and white, is "Tina Chow's Special Blend . . . we found in London a company called Makeup à la Carte; they will blend your powder for you and keep the formula on file so you can get it there any time."

She does a taupe eye, very subtly. "I put the shadow right under my eyebrows, and shade it into the bridge of my nose. I feel that my face is very flat there, and this adds a bit of depth. Or, from time to time, I'll put it right on the brow, just brushing straight up. It accents the slant . . . pulls the eye up a little. Way has *the* great taupe shadow. It's a stage makeup, made by some man in Massachusetts. And it's not iridescent. That's the thing I think is wrong with all the cosmetics out now—everything is pearly and iridescent, and you can't get a clean, flat color."

Adelle finds what she likes anywhere on the map and stocks up. For lip color, "there's a Japanese thing that I love—a little red cake that the Kabuki actors use around their eyes. It's put on like watercolor. You dip your brush in water, and you paint it on your mouth.

has "temperamental skin and a lot of allergies. If I go to my ballet class, my perspiration will make me break out. If I dust my house, I get hives—or if I'm blowing my diet, or if I'm around the wrong chemicals, or if I put on the wrong makeup. . . . I can only use things on my face that aren't perfumed or don't have lots of lanolin. I like Clinique cleanser and tonic, and then I throw on Clarins moisturizer—it's French, I think. . . . If I feel that I need a mask, I get out my sponge and scrub with soap. And once in a while, I go to Georgette Klinger—just to get my face clean. Plus, it's a treat."

thinking about service, about tables, the presentation, is the food correctly prepared, the people waiting at the bar. Plus, the chefs are so busy; can you see me going down there and saying, 'Hey, you guys! I'm hungry. You'd better make me some prawns right away.' I pick on the bartender instead. I take out my Naturaid soya protein powder, and say, 'Who's ready for a protein shake?' And then, it's easy: just a tablespoon of the protein powder, a little bit of orange juice and milk, some ice, and just whiz it up."

As you might have guessed, Adelle's ultimate goal is not to be a restaurateur. Nor is she planning to model. What she wants is to act. In Los Angeles, where she was helping to run Mr. Chow when that branch was new, she studied with Jack Garfein and Martin Landau and did a bit part in a TV play. (She played a nurse in an intensive care ward, all covered up except for her eyes. "People who came to the restaurant said, 'Wasn't that you on that show?' They recognized my eyes.") Now, in New York, she takes five classes a week with Stella Adler.

"In Ohio, you grow up on Fritos and Twinkies and pizza. In Japan, you go naturally to fish and very beautiful vegetables . . . you appreciate food more in Japan."

And it doesn't move—you can go through your day, you can go through your hamburger or your whole dinner, it doesn't move off your mouth. If you want it moister, you can put lip gloss on top. . . . I've got lots of these little cakes all stacked up.

"If I don't use the Kabuki cake—if I don't want that bright a red, for instance—I must use a lipstick pencil to outline my upper lip. I outline in a darker shade, then I fill in the whole mouth with a lipstick just one shade lower, like a plum or a pink. I find that most lipstick tends to slide. This way it stays. . . . Someone told me a fantastic makeup trick that I promised I wouldn't tell. She said, 'You'll knock the men out this way.' Hmm, I can't wait. But. What she taught me to do, whether I just wore lip gloss, or a flesh-colored lipstick, or pink, or whatever: Line the lining of the mouth in red. Brush on—or use a lip pencil, because it's much drier—a deep true red or scarlet, so that when your mouth is closed or open, there is just that little sensuous kind of blush. It makes such a difference, it really does—it gives you a glow. And it's a surprise."

It often seems to me that when God gives women beautiful skin, He always throws in a kicker so they won't get too vain or complacent. Naturally, Adelle

Going from Cleveland to Tokyo made the first big change in Adelle's eating habits. "In Ohio, you grow up on Fritos and Twinkies and pizza. In Japan, you go naturally to fish and very beautiful vegetables . . . you appreciate food more in Japan." The second change was triggered by the discovery that she had a low blood-sugar level. And this meant turning around her whole way of eating. In the past, her pattern was one big meal a day, eaten whenever she happened to be hungry. Now it's six mini-meals spaced through the day to keep her blood-sugar level running evenly. "And it's hard. It isn't easy eating a boiled egg or a handful of nuts or carrot sticks or a piece of Jarlsberg cheese. I want to sit down and *eat*. But it's worth it; it changed the way I was feeling right away—the way I thought, my energy, everything. The trouble is, I love starches. I love rice. I love pasta. I like sandwiches."

Especially it's trouble if your brother-in-law is Mr. Chow, proprietor of the famous Chinese restaurants in London and Los Angeles, whose latest New York branch you are helping to run. I know I'd have a hell of a time trying to stick to a diet at Mr. Chow. Adelle evidently doesn't. "When you run a restaurant, you don't have time to think about feeding yourself. You're

Also, four or five times a week, she does ballet. "I danced when I was little, then I didn't for years, then off and on in college. But when we lived in Japan, and when Tina and I started modeling, we didn't know anything about it and we weren't with an agency. We had to teach each other what to do, so we went to all the fashion shows we could, and we watched all the models. We would see who was good and who was bad, and what they did to make them good. Then we'd go home and practice and practice. And I just decided that if I knew how to dance, I would be able to move without thinking about it. And it's true for photography, too. . . . A lot of the modeling classes try to teach these young girls how to walk, but I really think they should throw them all into dance classes and make them aware of their bodies. And of their posture. I think the most important thing in beauty is posture. . . . Often, you'll see the most beautiful person walking by with slumped shoulders, and it's a real tragedy. . . . And, plus, you need so much stamina for modeling—all that jumping around, doing this and that, and running on the beach. Dancing builds stamina . . . it just gives you a freedom. And a grace—most people don't have it naturally. You learn it." Frankly, I think Adelle had it all along.

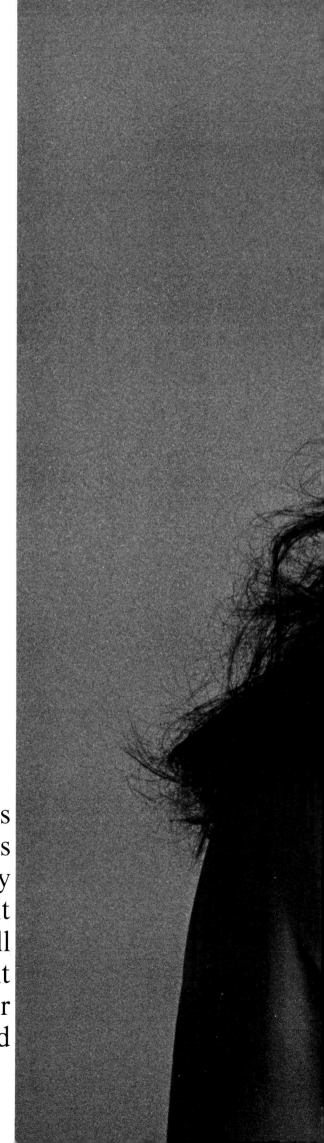

Minimal makeup for a newly
self-confident beauty

Judy
Collins

"My whole approach to life has changed. What I put in my body has changed, what I do with my body has changed. And I can see the result in an emotional and mental as well as in a physical way. I've never felt better, and I know that I've never looked better—my skin is better, and my hair, and my figure."

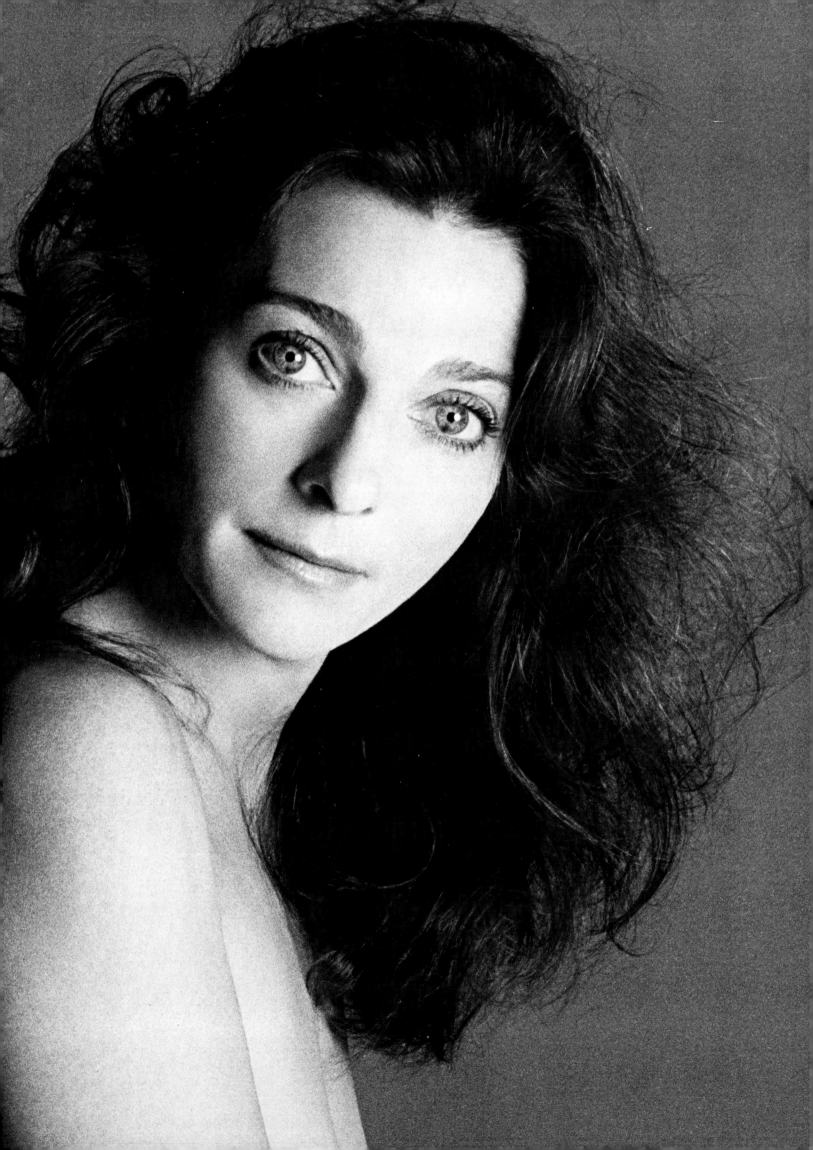

Judy Collins

The first time I photographed Judy Collins was for the cover of a record album called *Judith.* Earlier pictures I had seen of her had been done in what I think of as typical folksinger dream style: soft-focus meadows with lots of mist and grass and Judy in the distance, wearing something folksy and a big floppy hat. You couldn't see the girl for the atmosphere. . . . I said to her, "Let's see *you,* for God's sake!" Especially, let's see those eyes. Judy has the most incredible eyes—six different colors at least, grays and blues and greens, and the light just seems to pass through. When I look in her eyes, I feel I'm looking through to the other side of the universe.

Judy was ready for a change. Like most people who come to me, she didn't just want to be recorded as she was or as she had been; she wanted a new image of herself. So we gave her the full glamour treatment—hair, makeup, clothes, the works. She adored the finished picture—eventually. When she first saw it, she was shocked. Why wouldn't she be? She had never seen herself looking that way, or imagined that she could.

The idea for doing our second album cover as a nude was Judy's: "You won't believe this," she said, "but I want to be photographed nude, and I want very little makeup." And I think this had to do partly with the fact that the success of our first sitting had given her a new confidence. But basically, her assurance was the result of dramatic changes that she had made for herself, all by herself; they turned her life around.

The first thing was: "Two and a half years ago, I stopped drinking. And at that point, my body—although I had been exercising for ten years and was physically in good shape—my body underwent a drastic change for the better, which also had to do with a total change of diet. This was because when I first quit drinking, I craved enormous amounts of sugar—if you have a lot of alcohol in your diet, you're getting a lot of sugar. So I went to a nutritionist who is also a holistic doctor. He looked at my whole dietary pattern, and he said, You don't need sugar, and you don't need dairy products, and you don't need cheese. Except that he wanted me to have liver once a week, he said that red meat should come out of my diet (out of anybody's diet!), and salt; you take kelp to get the iodine you need.

> ### "Caffeine is not good. . . . Among other things, it dries out the skin."

he put me on a very mild thyroid medication, which cleared up various internal problems that I had—hair falling out, irregular periods. . . . I used to get colds all the time. I haven't had a real cold in a year; the most was a little sniffle maybe four or five months ago. I used to be anemic; I haven't been for two years.

"He also feels that caffeine is not good—a couple of cups of coffee a day

> ### "I stopped drinking. And my body—although I had been exercising for ten years and was physically in good shape—underwent a drastic change for the better."

He ran all the tests: the blood tests, the hair tests (hair registers very quickly what's going on in your system). He found that my thyroid was functioning at practically zero level, so

should be anybody's maximum. Among other things, it dries out the skin, and I tend to have very dry skin. Still, coffee would be major for me to give up. So I make a compromise: For every cup of coffee I drink, I drink three glasses of water. In other words, I try to wash it all out of my system, and I'm working on cutting it way down or out."

If you go to Judy's for dinner, most likely she'll "take a bunch of bean sprouts, onions, mushrooms, some green vegetables, and sauté it up, with sunflower seeds sprinkled in, put it in a wok, and serve it with broiled chicken or fish, and a nice fruit salad for dessert (mainly I use melons, grapefruit, strawberries, papayas—that is, negative-calorie foods, which only means that what's in the food when it goes into your system takes more energy to digest than the calories, with the result that you can eat as much of these things as you want)." . . . Once in a while, you might even get "something chocolate . . . I'm not really such a spartan."

"I see a totally different person from the one I see when I look at photographs of myself a few years back."

In addition to her dietary regime, Judy does a meditation program and twenty minutes of aerobic exercise—swimming, jumping rope, running ("I don't sleep well otherwise; rather than suffer insomnia, I will put on my jogging shoes, which don't make much noise, and run in my apartment"). She has massage regularly: Shiatsu, or a technique called bioenergetic therapy, which is related to Rolfing but gentler. "It's dealing with the body in a way that releases a lot of tension. I started doing it at a time when I was very locked up—so off the wall, so anxious, and so hysterical that I was everywhere but 'here' at any given moment. It was marvelous for me."

There is no question that she has turned a corner: "My whole approach to life has changed. What I put in my body has changed, what I do with my body has changed. And I can see the result in an emotional and mental as well as in a physical way. I've never felt better, and I know that I've never looked better—my skin is better, and my hair, and my figure (I'm twenty pounds lighter now than when I stopped drinking). I'm learning a little bit about balance in my life."

For me, of course, the clearest evidence of the change in Judy is what I see in the pictures I take of her. As she says, "I see a totally different person from the one I see when I look at photographs of myself from a few years back. That person was frightened-looking . . . driven, sort of panicked . . . you know, tomorrow maybe the stove. . . ." Today, she is light-years away from that person. And secure enough so that we don't have to do the big glamour number anymore. When I work with Judy now, I just go with her. We keep her look very natural—minimal makeup. The key word is: eliminate. And I keep the talk very soft, very easy; I don't want to trigger the old habit she used to have of setting her mouth in a thin, nervous line. (This is a trick even an amateur photographer can learn: Don't tell your subject that her mouth, or whatever, looks tense; mentioning it only adds to the problem. "Talk" it away—soft words turneth away tension!)

At forty-one, Judy is getting the whole picture into perspective. She talks with joy and pleasure of her twenty-two-year-old son, Clark Taylor, the child of an early marriage that ended in divorce. She has a man she's in love with ("Louis Nelson is my wonderful boyfriend/lover/companion/friend"). And she is high on her career: "I think my work is getting stronger and stronger. My technical ability is now to the point where I can do just about anything I want in terms of material. And I'm more comfortable on the stage than I have ever been. I have put the guitar down . . . actually put it away and come out from behind the crutch. With a guitar, you don't really have to show yourself . . . don't really have to stand in front of the audience. I didn't. I had this big *thing* over me all the time. I took it off just two years ago . . . that has been a fantastic experience!"

"I'm learning a little bit about balance in my life."

Rita Coolidge

Believe it or not, both of these pictures of Rita Coolidge were taken on the same day. All afternoon we had been shooting the cover for her first rock album, and we had gone for glamour all the way. Way Bandy had done her makeup, with lots of smolder to the eyes; Harry King had curled and teased her newly shoulder-length hair; and we put her into gold lamé. Everything about her look in this photograph stands for a break with the past—as she wanted.

Then, just as she was leaving the studio, she turned to wave goodbye. She had taken down the makeup to almost nothing and had brushed out the curls, and she had on a soft, black woolen cape. I can't tell you how glorious she looked!—proud, beautiful, and very much in the spirit of her Indian heritage ("My father's mother was Indian, and there's Cherokee on my mother's side, so I have Indian blood on both sides of my family"). Everybody had left—Way, Harry, the whole crew—but I pulled her back into the studio and shot one roll of film. They are my favorite pictures of Rita.

They are also Rita's favorite pictures of herself. To me, the way Rita is in this photograph is the way she was when she and Kris Kristopherson were married and working together. Then, her music was country and her look was Indian: lots of turquoise, lots of silver, and four feet of straight black hair pouring down her back. One by one, each of these signatures has been dropped. "I cut my hair after I saw a back shot of Kris and me on the *Phil Donahue Show*. I looked like that guy on *The Munsters* and I said, Nobody needs that much hair! . . . When I got pregnant [Casey, her daughter by Kristopherson, is now six years old], my hands and feet started swelling, and I had to take off the turquoise. And one day a girl walked up to me and said, 'You look like Rita Coolidge, but you couldn't be; you don't have any turquoise.' So I stopped wearin' it for good. I think you've got to discard certain images that become so attached to your personality they start to mean more than what you're doing as an artist. And I like to keep changing. Change is real important."

"I cut my hair after I saw a back shot of Kris and me on the *Phil Donahue Show*. I looked like that guy on *The Munsters*. . . . Nobody needs that much hair!"

The biggest change, of course, has been the switch to rock and the forming of her own group. But it's less of a turnaround than you might think; she's been there before. "I'm really back to what I started out doing—the style of music and being in charge of the whole organization; I helped pay my way through Miami State University by singing, and for a while I had a band: RC and the Moon Cars. It's from an old southern saying—RC being Royal Crown Cola, and the moon car was one of those chocolate-coated cookies with marshmallow filling. It used to be my very best favorite snack, so that was what I named the band.

"When Kris and I were together, it was more his show; I was like a guest artist. Also, our music is very different. My music is more properly hard rock or rhythm and blues; he's definitely country. I never really considered myself to be a country singer. I never listened to country music when I was a kid in Nashville. I listened to R and B, and I grew up with a love for that music and for artists like Sam Cooke and Ray Charles—much more than for Hank Williams."

Rita was born in Nashville, Tennessee, the daughter of a former schoolteacher ("she taught me to be an achiever") and a Baptist minister. The youngest of four children—one boy and two girls preceded her—she made an unusually precocious debut in her father's church, singing with her sisters. "We had a trio; Priscilla was five, Linda was four, and I was two. . . . My mother says I sang before I talked, words and all." She remembers herself as "a real scrawny kid. And when I was thirteen, I was in a bad automobile accident. I had sixty stitches in my face—across my nose and one whole eyebrow. As I've grown older, it's faded, and I can cover what's left with makeup. It took me a long time, but I learned to overcome it. I think now that it was one of those mountains, as I call them, that God has blessed me with. Yes, blessed; I would not be as rich a person if I didn't have those things to go through." There have been other "mountains": "I lost a baby about three years ago. I was five months pregnant, and the baby died. That was a hard one. And my marriage didn't work. There have been a lot of things; it's never smooth. But I wouldn't have it any other way; it's what makes me strong."

This interview with Rita was done in New York, near the end of a month-long tour that had begun in San Francisco and would wind up somewhere in South Carolina.

One thing you can count on: Hell or high water, the lady is going to be out there, singing her heart out for no less than an hour and fifteen minutes, maybe more. And once in a while, she's going to be tired; once in a while the

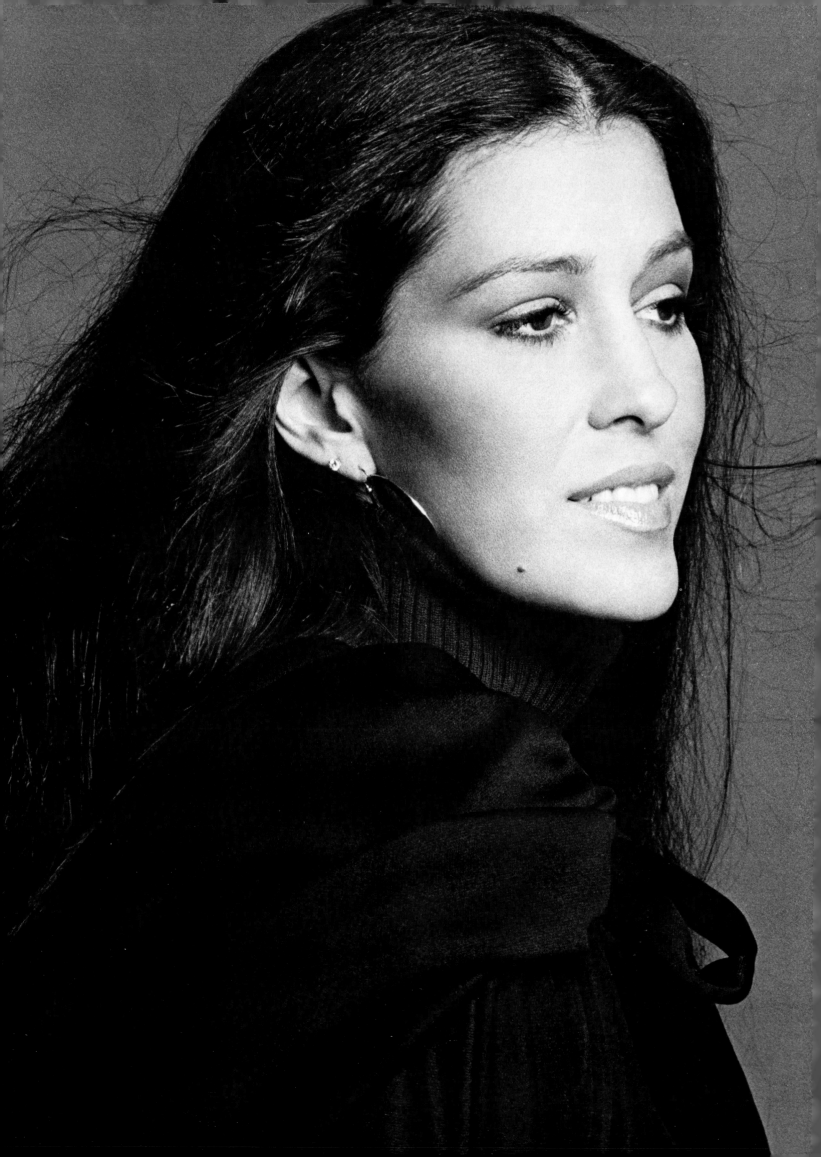

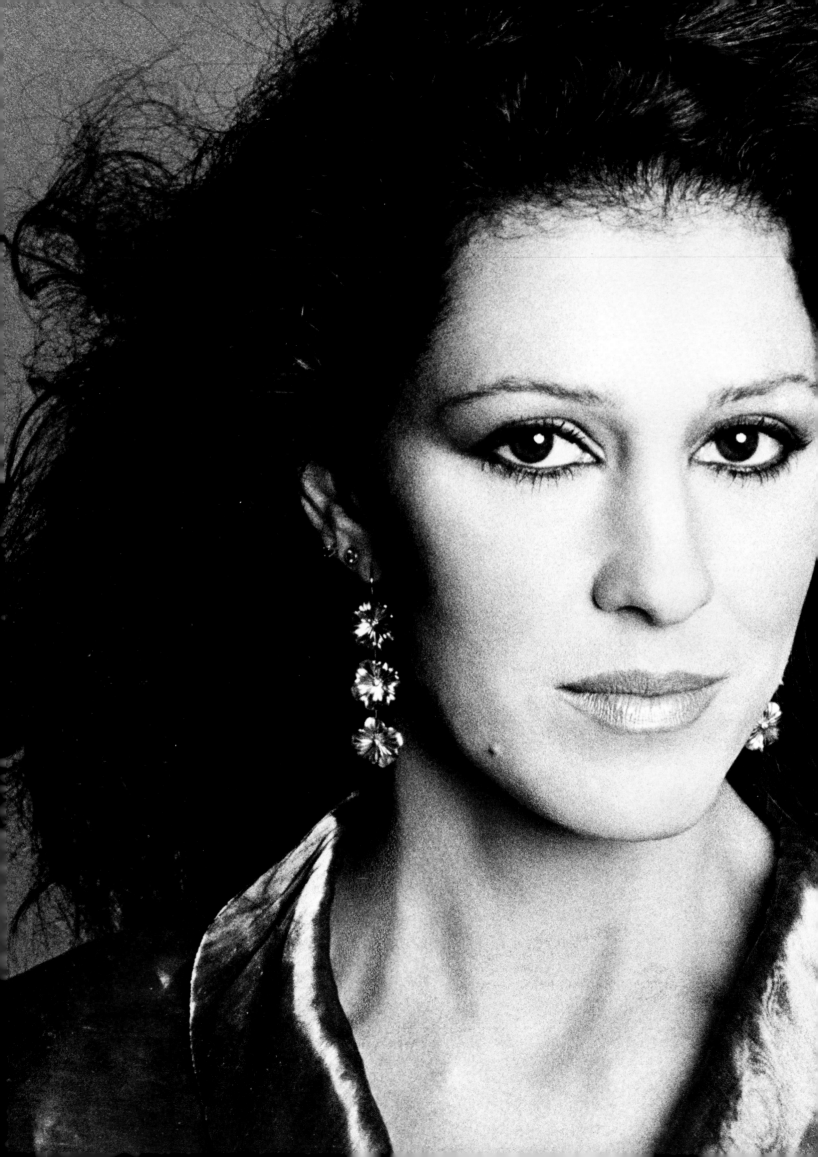

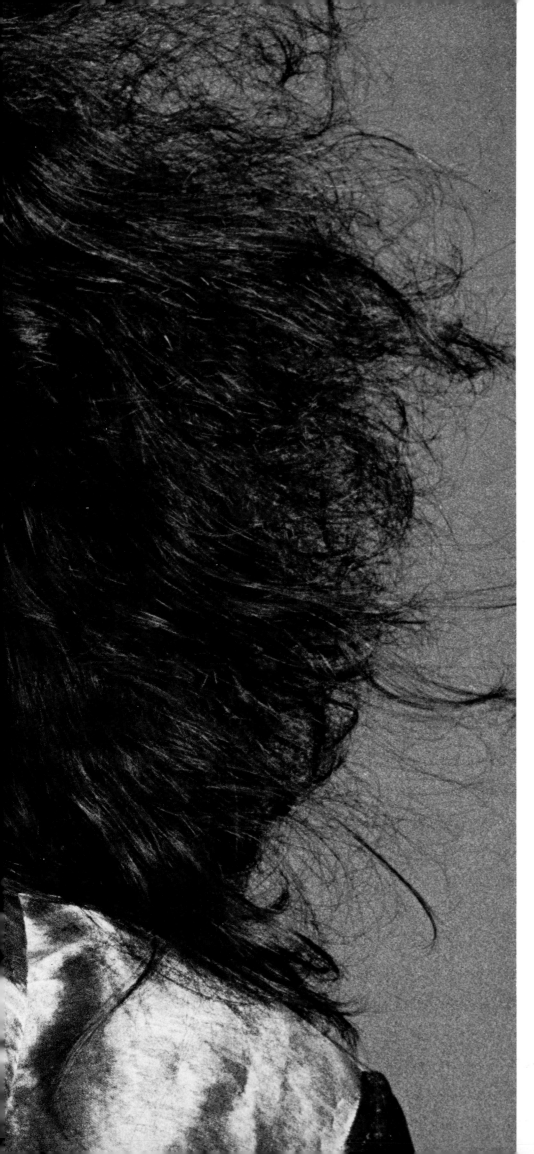

Rita Coolidge

whole crew is going to be tired. "Maybe we didn't get enough sleep the night before, or we had too much wine. And we come out to do the show, and we all just start trying to kick each other in the butt—you know, challenge each other. Somehow, those shows are the best."

Don't ask how she unwinds: "You couldn't print it! We meet in somebody's room or in a bar and talk about the show, and about how we can make it better. Sometimes, we teach each other dance steps. A lot of the time, we sing till we're worn out, and then we go to bed. . . . Touring is difficult; you wouldn't believe how many vitamins I take. And I get six hours' sleep a night. But I feel the drain.

"I have about four shirts in different colors, and I use one or another. And jeans. I've always liked working in jeans. I can be as trendy as anyone; I went through the Indian period, and I went through ties and vests. But I don't think clothes matter so much anymore. I look in the mirror and I can feel when I look right for a show. It may not be what's happening this very minute, but it might be happening tomorrow because I did it yesterday. . . . I have a kind of vision of myself in the future as an old lady—a wonderful old lady, in wonderful hats with feathers. I would just like to get more outrageous as I grow older, because I started out as a real shy, skinny kid. And look at me now! I feel a lot more free about myself than I ever did, about who I am and what I do. I'm a young thirty-five, and I'm engaged, and I'm havin' a wonderful time!"

Rita once described for me a visit from her Grandma Coolidge, her Indian grandmother: "She came up from Texas to Tennessee when I was about six years old. And she had such great flair; she always wore very colorful clothes, and I remember she had on this red taffeta skirt, a bright-colored blouse, and lots of petticoats with ruffles. And, oh!—she was *beautiful.*" It could be Rita talking about Rita. To me, it's the image of her that is truest and best. Of course she felt it had to change before she could turn her career around; that's only natural. But now that she's home free, I'd love to see a little of that Indian fire and finery again. It is *her* look. And it's a smash-eroo!

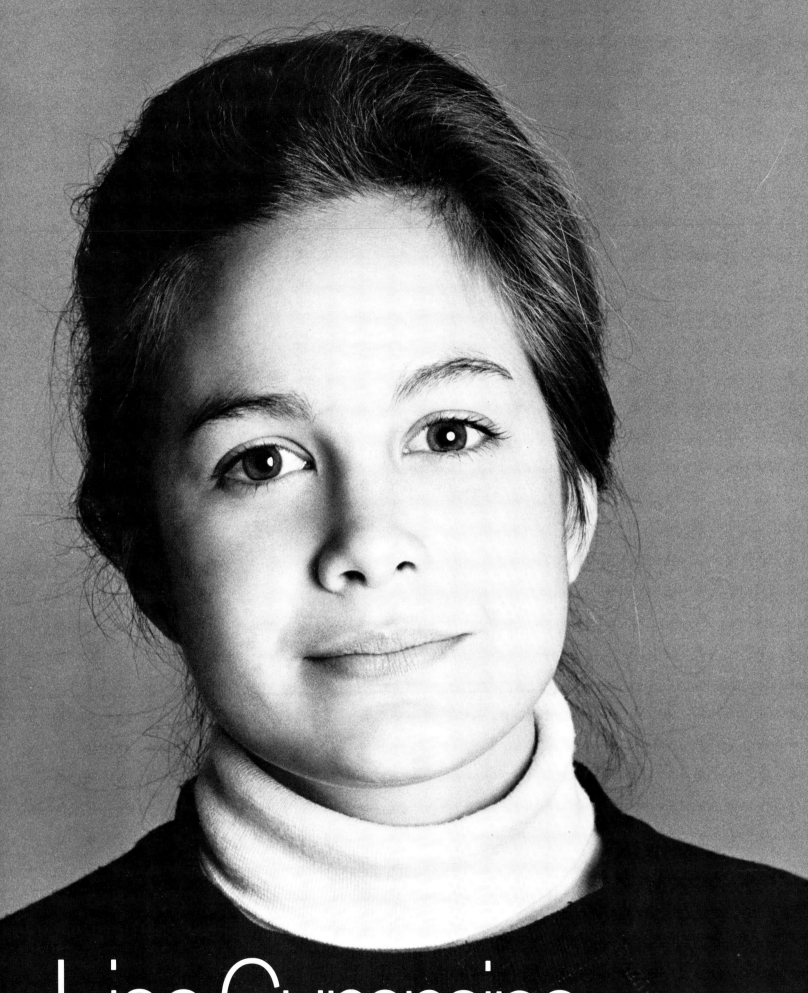

Lisa Cummins

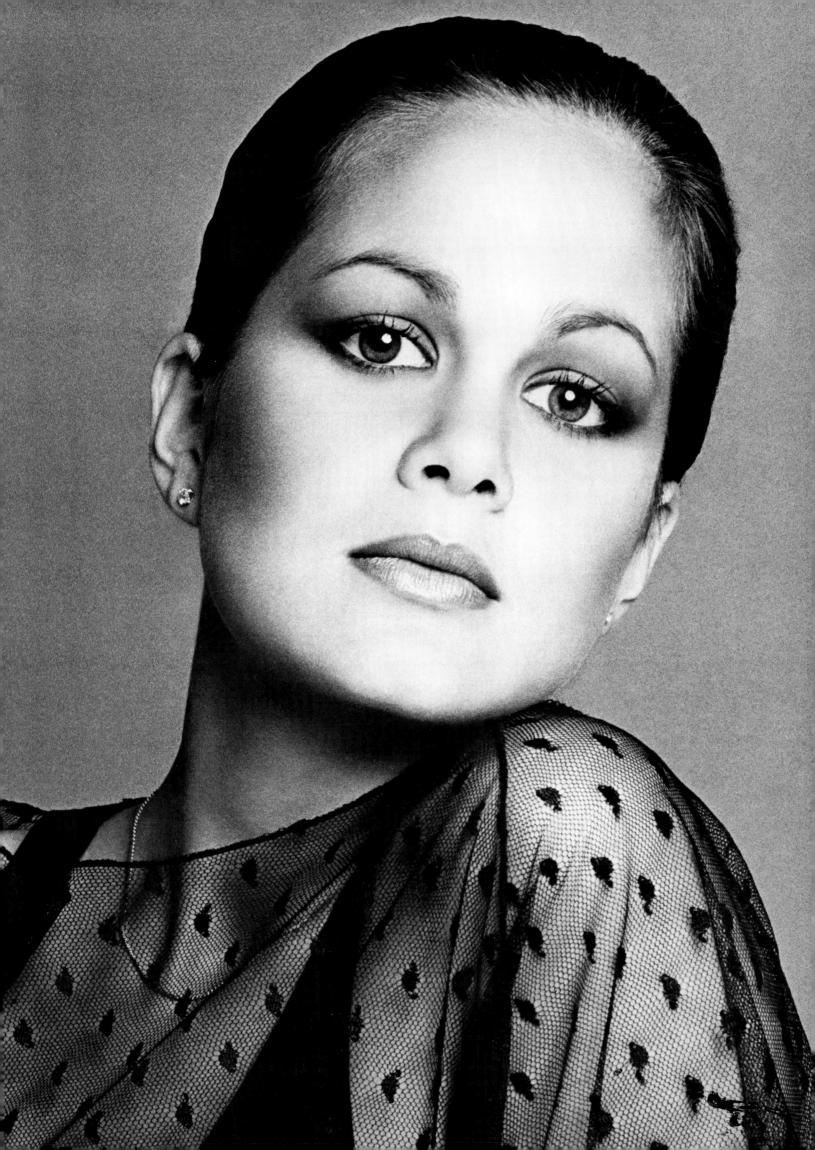

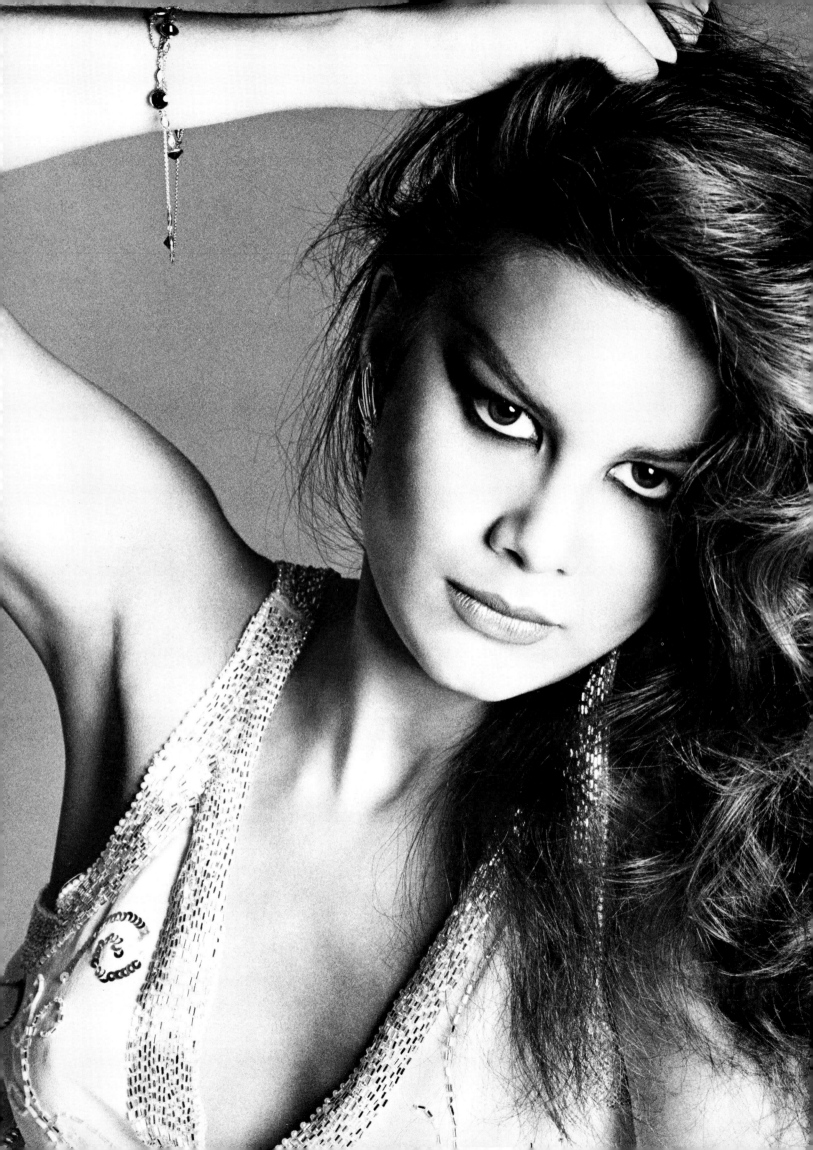

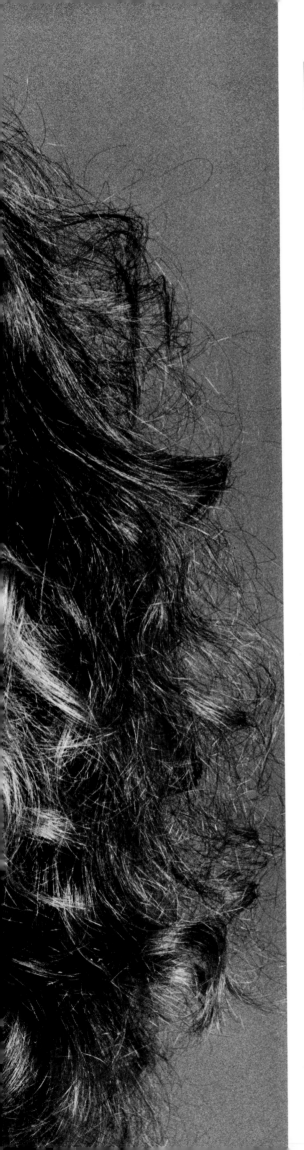

Lisa Cummins

Lisa Cummins is the perfect example of the pretty little girl who puts on makeup and, without a single other transition, steps instantly into womanhood. In the first pictures I did of her (with pulled-back hair), she was fifteen—without makeup, fifteen going on twelve. With makeup—with her eyebrows defined and slightly extended, her eyes enlarged and shaded out at the corners, and the baby cheeks slimmed down with contour rouge—she is a beautiful, sexy young woman. This sitting—when we combed out her hair and put on different clothes—resulted in Lisa's first *Cosmopolitan* cover. Her most recent is the third photograph here: three years older, three years thinner—a knockout!

hate wearing it. Every time I do, I can just feel the pimples creeping in. It's like my skin is crying out to breathe."

Lisa is blond, blue-eyed, and, as models go, tiny—just a shade under five-seven. Both parents are a strong influence in Lisa's life. "My dad was the one who encouraged me to model. And he always kept me thin; he was the first to tell me, 'You're getting fat.' Mom was always fashion-conscious, and she would buy me the clothes. But both have always stressed that I be smart. They want me to do well academically, because they always have. . . . My mom was very strict, and she doesn't like my dating too much—she didn't really let me date until last year. When I was younger, I used to come down with colds a lot, so she kept me in for health reasons. And later on, I was always studying. Then, when the boys started getting interested, that's when she had to take control and say, 'No, you can't go out.'

"At the time, I was mad. It's hard; you're so young, and you don't understand why you can't go out, why someone is bad for you. . . . My mom has always the idea of a reputation—she

"Sex for just sex is . . . you might as well run out and take a jog."

Lisa is not one of those girls who falls out of bed in the morning, pulls on a pair of scruffy jeans, and goes into her day with nothing on her face but a smile. There is a lovely, old-fashioned word for Lisa's look; it's well-groomed. Makeup is part of it. Except when she has a tan, she wouldn't dream of going without. She started wearing it at thirteen, "as soon as I got my contact lenses and got rid of my glasses and could see my face. I'm very critical. I look at my face in the morning like a blank canvas that needs to be painted. I try my best and hope that it comes out all right. . . . I like to look nice for other people. I feel better when I think I look nice."

It doesn't take much to make Lisa look very, very nice—maybe the lightest touch of color; otherwise, she says, "I feel bland. I have monotone coloring—my lips are the same color as my face—so I have to have the blush and the lipstick. And I've worn mascara since I was fourteen. . . . Base is like uck! I

says a tarnished reputation will always follow you, so watch it. She says—and it's so true—women have to take all the risks; a man doesn't have to be as careful. . . . So if a guy dates me, I don't say it point-blank, but he gets the idea that I'm not that type. If he wants that, he can gladly find another girl. There are enough girls who do fool around. I just happen to not. And I respect myself more because I don't. I put more value into it. A lot of my friends don't. I mean, sex for just sex is . . . you might as well run out and take a jog."

The way Lisa figures it, she won't be getting seriously involved for at least a few minutes. This year, with the idea of becoming a plastic surgeon, she transferred from Swarthmore to Cornell. If her plan holds, she will move from premed to medical school to two-year residency. "I want to get married, but I intend to have my career. That's my first priority." That is, of course, "unless there was a diamond like *this*. . . ."

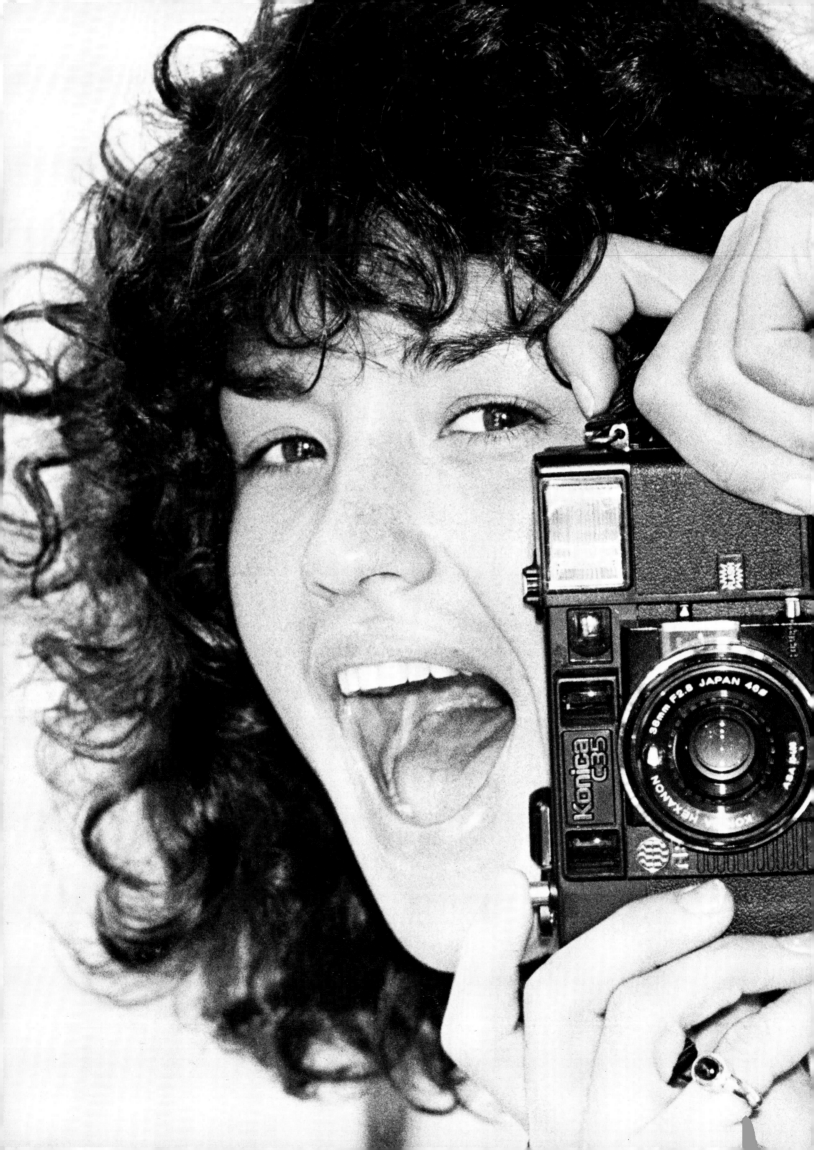

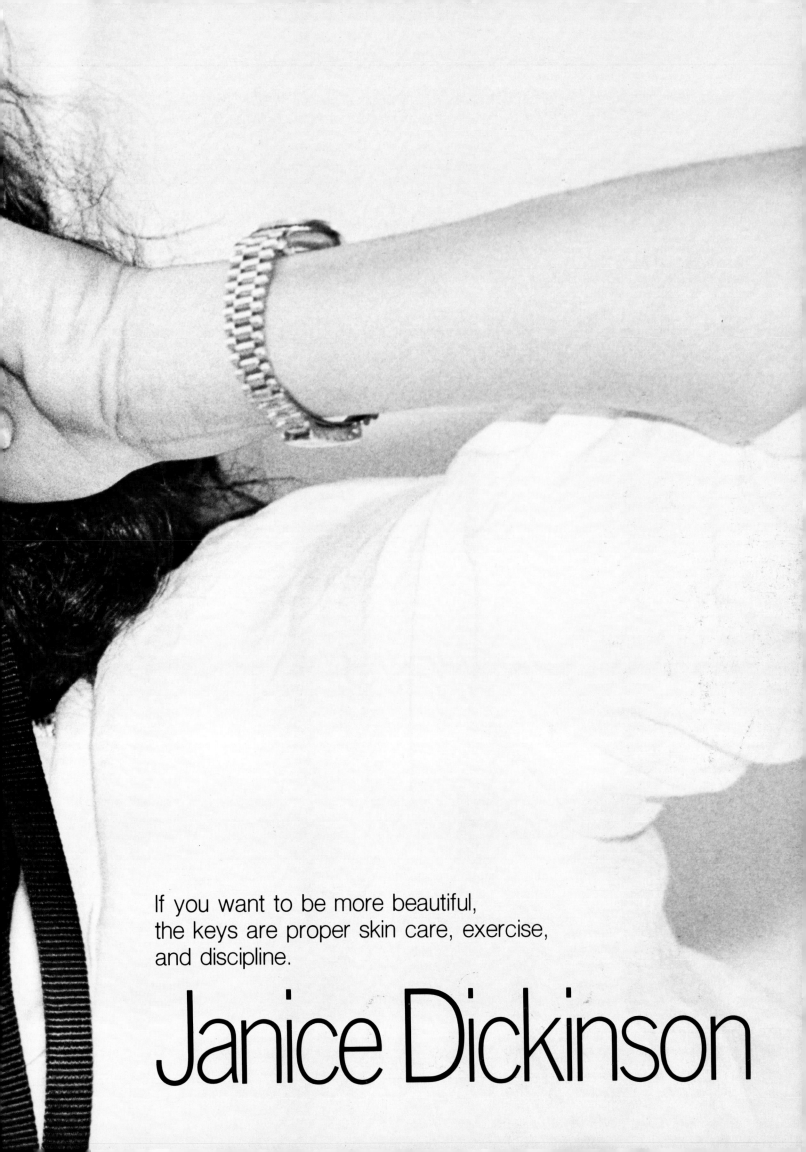

If you want to be more beautiful,
the keys are proper skin care, exercise,
and discipline.

Janice Dickinson

"I usually fall back on the natural, simple things. I use Albolene cream. . . . Then I use tepid water and an oatmeal soap with no detergent in it. I never rub, I never squeeze. If one of those things is growing on my face, I let it come out. I go to a sauna or I put a warm washcloth on the little abrasions. . . . After that, I'll make a bit of freshener with apple cider vinegar and warm water. Then I use a nuclear protein cream. . . . Whatever I'm doing, it seems to be working."

No matter what you may have heard, not every great model is a great beauty. Janice Dickinson is a perfect example. She is not classically beautiful in the sense of, say, a Rene Russo. Neither is she in the sexy/wholesome/cheerleader tradition of a Cheryl Tiegs or a Kelly Emberg. Her lips are too full, her expression too exotic, too sultry, too languorous, too . . . you name it; it doesn't easily conform to conventional standards of American beauty.

Yet there is no question that Janice is a great model. For more than eight years (an eternity in fashion), she has been in every magazine (though not yet on the cover of American *Vogue*), here and abroad, editorially and in ads. I love working with Janice, but I handle her with kid gloves. I use soft, direct lighting—Paramount lighting—on her, and I always ask the makeup artist to tone her down. I don't want her to look like a black crow, or hard, or obvious, or tough. And Janice can look all of these things; her face is a rubber band and she can pull it into any look she wants—she's got a whole gallery of monster faces. Those I tell her to save for the other photographers: "I want you very soft and alluring, very beautiful; think that way today."

And she does. Every time. And that's what it's all about, of course. Janice is simply a stupendous performer, and she has the controlled energy to sustain a performance; no matter if she's been up all night or coming down with a major flu, she always comes through with that shine. And when a model can give you that . . . it's like Barrie's definition of charm in *What Every Woman Knows:* "If you have it, you don't need to have anything else; and if you don't have it, it doesn't much matter what else you have."

An interesting thing about the modeling business. The girls who make it to the top usually do it right away. They don't languish around. After all, we have our eye on the "in" look. Photographers, editors, agents—we're all on the lookout for a new face. Nobody was looking for Janice. She remembers: "I knocked on every door for eleven months . . . it was solid rejection all over town." What she had to show were "three bad pictures and twenty-

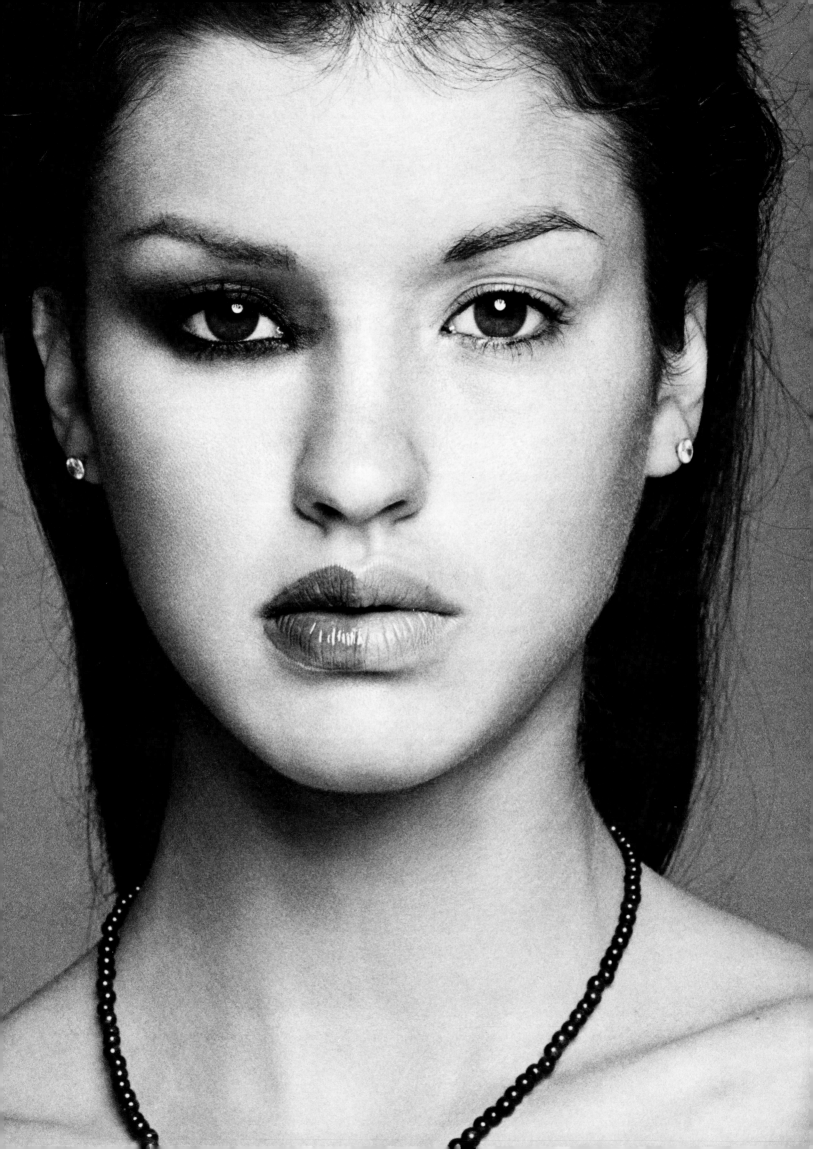

Janice Dickinson

five pounds more than now. . . . I was a big, pudgy girl. . . . Someone at *Vogue* said my eyes were not the right shape to sell magazines in America."

So here is this girl with wrong-shaped eyes selling Max Factor eye makeup as though it were going for free. . . . Ironically, it is those eyes and those full, pouty lips that have helped zoom her to the top: "Every ethnic now has a face to identify with . . . you can't believe the letters I get, the mail I receive from black women, Puerto Rican women, Cuban women . . . 'We like to see your face, keep going,' signed Carmelita Dadadida from the South Bronx. . . . Someone I know was doing a story on a tight-security prison in San Antonio. He sent me a Polaroid, with about twelve men lined up, pointing to a picture on the wall—the *only* picture. And it wasn't Farrah Fawcett; it was a *Glamour* shot of me in a bathing suit. So he said, 'Why do you have that girl's picture on the wall?' And one of these guys—these are rapists and murderers—said, 'Because I think she's some dynamite chick!' I guess they identify with me; I'm their dark muchacha."

Some dynamite chick grew up in Hollywood, Florida, one of two children (Debbie, her younger sister, is also a successful model) of Polish Catholic parents. What stands out in her memory is that her schoolmates made fun of her lips and that via Debbie she got into sports. Debbie was on the Junior Olympics gymnastic team and Janice was the one who chauffered her to the gym, where she didn't just hang out: "I did the basic exercises for gymnasts, which is not your average basic exercise . . . and I did karate . . . and swimming."

The habit stuck (which is probably why, when you ask her to name her best feature, she says instantly, "My body"). . . . "I work out like a fiend, one reason being that I'm very tense. So in order for me not to bring home any kind of tension—as well as just to feel good and that I've accomplished something—I've got to do some cardiovascular exercise every day. . . . When it's warm, I sometimes go up at five thirty

in the morning to an Olympic-size pool in the Bronx. . . . Or I go up to Columbia University. They have a great pool and an indoor track. I work out with the real jocks up there. . . . Even though I had a bad accident and quit for a year, I still do professional biking . . . really hard, not a nice normal jaunt through Central Park."

"I can't live and work with someone; it's just not possible."

Janice doesn't worry about her looks, but she cares . . . she cares about her skin: "My closet looks like Boyd Chemists; it has *everything*. But I usually fall back on the natural, simple things. I use Albolene cream now. I mean, my mother used to use that, and I'd say ugh—you know, it's not expensive enough. But it gets the gunk that I put on my face . . . sometimes there's five or six layers of base. So I start with Albolene, and if I don't happen to have any, a little baby oil is fine . . . you don't have to spend seven dollars a bottle for anything when you can get baby oil for thirty-nine cents. Then I use water, water, water, water, water, water: tepid water and an oatmeal soap with no detergent in it. I never rub, never squeeze. If one of those things is growing on my face, I let it come out. I go to a sauna, or I put a warm washcloth on the little abrasions if they happen to squirt. After that, I'll make a bit of freshener with apple cider vinegar and warm water. Then I use a nuclear protein cream that I get down at Health Nuts . . . they have a mixture of collagen in almond oil that's good, too.

"Whatever I'm doing, it seems to be working. Also, I'm very happy. You know, you can be the richest woman in the world and go to the best facial salon, but if you're not happy, forget it . . . my facial is working up a sweat every day. And going to a sauna. And getting laid once a night."

Happiness has a lot to do with a model/actor/sailor/triple black belt in karate, jujitsu, and ikito named Charles Haugk, who "makes me feel like a queen. He gives me breakfast in the morning. I mean, I can't believe it! I thank him all the time. He said to me, 'My God, what kind of men were you living with?' "

Janice was married at eighteen to the "man who played piano for B. B. King . . . the white piano player in an all-black group . . . we used to tour the chitlin' circuit, up and down the deep South. Modeling was a cup of tea after that." One night, Janice walked in and found her husband in bed with another woman. She didn't shoot the piano player . . . but she left in a hurry.

For five years, she lived with Mike Reinhardt, the photographer: "A wonderful, wonderful person. But our egos clashed. Insecurities were coming out of me like crazy: The models would come in with their portfolios, and if he wasn't paying attention they'd maybe pick the skirt up a little and stick the leg out. I love these girls, but I was furious. . . . I can't live and work with someone; it's just not possible—he'd be taking my picture from nine to five, so how could I be alluring? Then I'd take my makeup off, and maybe my nose would be bright red. . . . I know that real beauty comes from within, but I mean! . . . And then I'd have to go and cook dinner."

In her next incarnation, Janice would like to direct films; before that, she would like to be on the cover of *Vogue*. Meanwhile, she is happy with life as it is, and it follows: "If you're happy, you don't have to stay out at discos all night, you don't have to snort cocaine every second. I'd much rather be in the sack with Charlie, drinking red wine and eating a big salad, with French bread and country butter, and watching TV, than go out somewhere and stay up late. . . . But then, there are times, you know, when there's a nice little party. . . ."

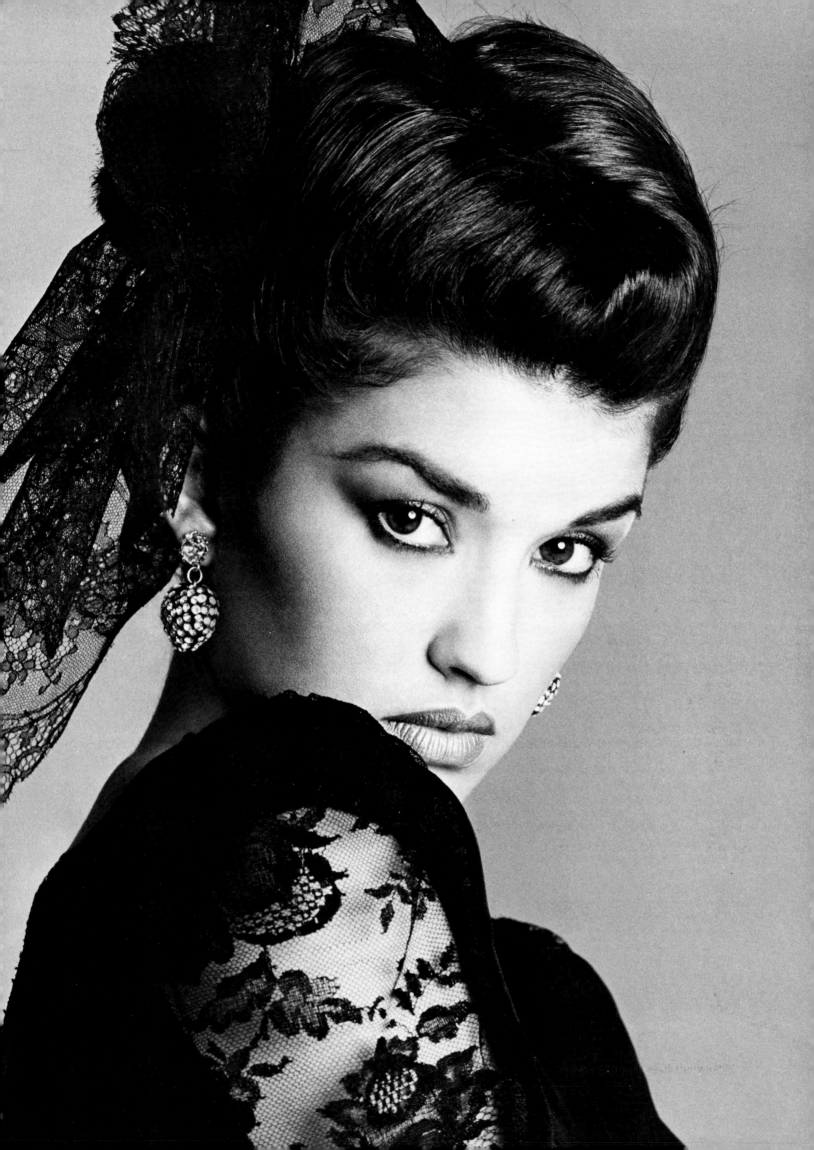

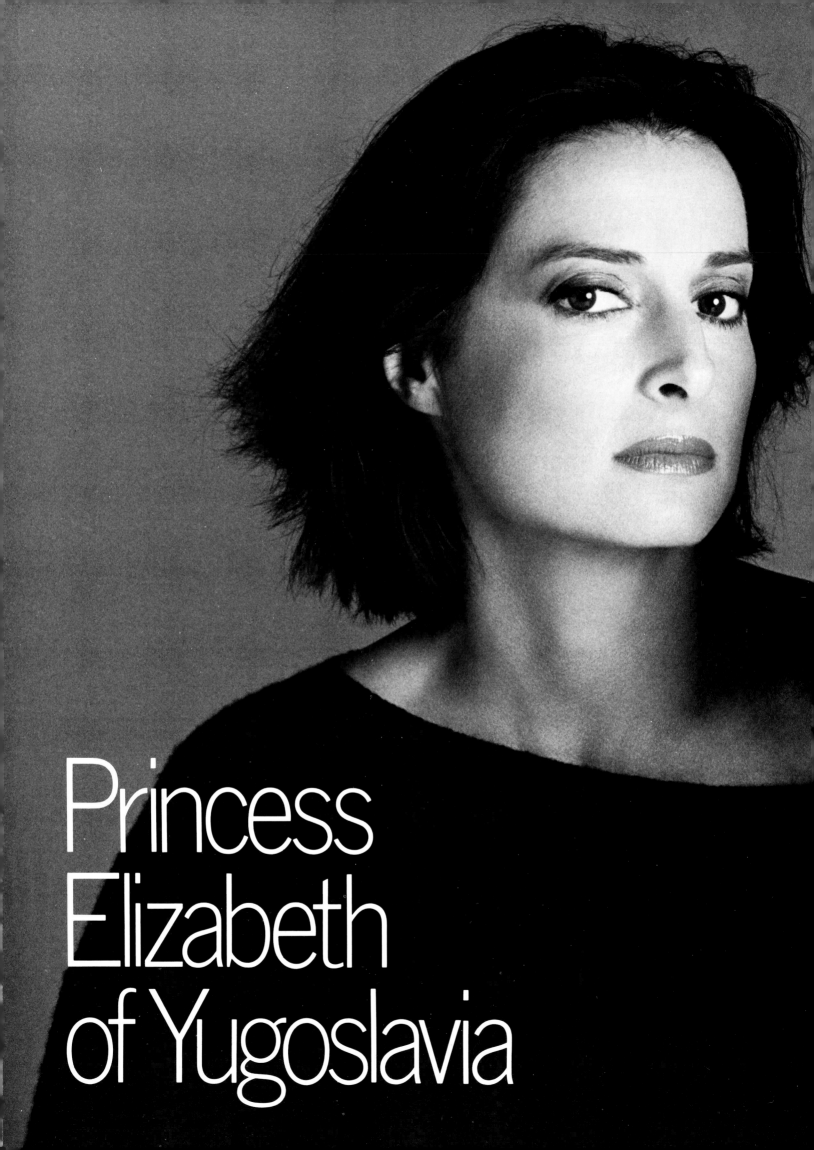

Princess
Elizabeth
of Yugoslavia

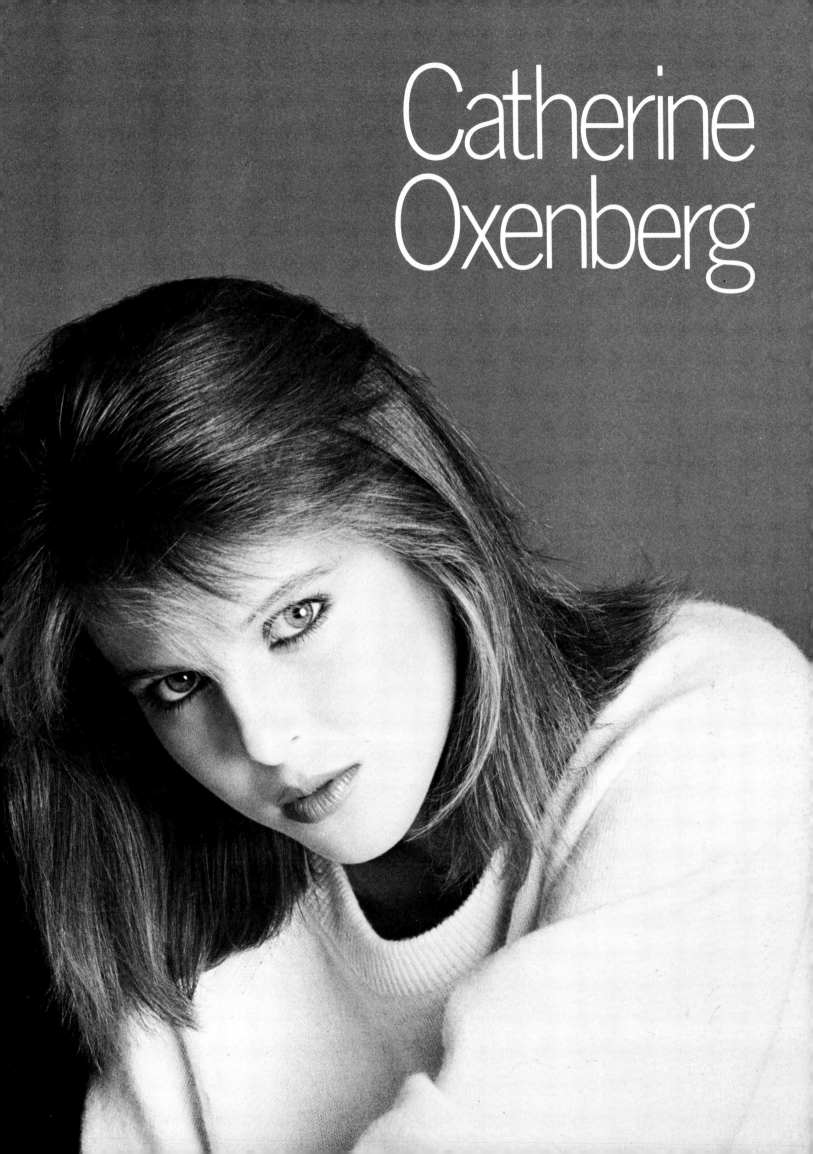

Catherine
Oxenberg

Princess Elizabeth of Yugoslavia

Princess Elizabeth of Yugoslavia is descended on her father's side from a Serbian hero called Karageorge, who led an uprising against the Turks in 1806 and founded "one of the few ruling families in Europe that came from the people." Through her mother, a Greek princess and a sister of Princess Marina of Kent, she is closely related to the British royal family; Prince Charles is her second cousin, Princess Alexandra her first.

In 1941, during the German invasion of Yugoslavia, her family moved to Africa, where Elizabeth grew up. Since then, she has lived all over Europe and in the United States, rooted in no particular place, at home everywhere: "I can fit in anywhere with anybody of any nationality. I'm totally adaptable." Everywhere, her reputation is unvarying: She is, without question, one of the great beauties of our time.

By her first husband, Howard Oxenberg, an American, she has two daughters, Catherine, nineteen (see photograph and text), fashion model and college student, with her own apartment in New York, and Christina, seventeen, who goes to school in Colorado. Following the breakup of her marriage, Elizabeth moved to London and married—and later divorced—Neil Balfour. Their son, Nicholas, ten, is at boarding school in England.

> "I can fit in anywhere with anybody of any nationality. I'm totally adaptable."

Two years ago, in the middle of a successful career, wholesaling American fashion accessories in England and Europe, Elizabeth took a giant step: "I decided to change my life. Totally. Bang, bang. Give up England and come to America. America is so interesting and exciting. It's the country of right now, whereas Europeans live in the past. Europeans have a general lack of enthusiasm and desire to change their life pattern, and the people tend to live in a comfortable, albeit boring, rut. In New York, if you don't find something interesting to do, you should be locked up! . . . There are millions of courses to take—I'm going to take a photography course, for instance. And modern-jazz dancing. Also, I've gone back to acting school. . . . In a way, it's like having a second childhood; and with all the children away from home, I can do exactly what I want."

One already completed project: She has changed her look "top to toe, from haircut and makeup to type of dress and type of shoes. To begin with, I found an excellent hair stylist called Neil, at Gerard Bollei. He has done something so clever with my hair that I can wash it twice a day and never set it and never go under a dryer. I can go swimming and come out of the water looking as though I'm going to a dinner party. . . . And then, after making me up for this sitting, Way Bandy gave me some hints about how to do a more modern makeup than I had been doing. Mostly, it was a question of brown tones on my eyelids. I used to do purple; I'd just stick my finger in the pot and put a patch of purple on each lid. Now I shade, the way he taught me, using browns and a gray-black pencil liner. He also gave me a lighter, more orange-y lipstick that's much softer than the dark pinky-purples I used before.

> "You should have a hot and cold shower every morning. It's very stimulating for the body. And it helps you to digest your breakfast."

Last summer, for the first time in my life, I wore strapless tube tops and very short shorts. And I wore flat sandals, which I always thought I was too short to wear. Of course, it's not true; five-feet-five isn't that short. It's just that my attitude about clothes was stuffier; my summer uniform was high heels, a T-shirt, and skirt. I've also started wearing blue jeans. I bought my first pair this year—Jordache—I love them."

Princess Elizabeth is very fond of active sports; the day before we did this interview, she had played six hours of tennis. "At Bendel's, I go to Pilates gym, where Kathy Grant keeps an eagle and expert eye on my every move."

Since coming back to New York, she has gotten into swimming in a big way. "What it does is incredible; my legs have improved a hundred percent. England isn't exercise-oriented like America. And if you go to France, forget it! —the French don't even *think* of sport. And they look it. They're always green in the face from overeating and lack of exercise."

wonder what color they'd turn at the thought of Elizabeth's diet: "No meat. No sugar (which is a simple carbohydrate). I am a great believer in complex carbohydrates as a source of energy and nutrition—and I eat a lot of bread, mostly whole wheat, and a lot of brown rice. I like spaghetti and baked potatoes and don't find them to be fattening. I rarely eat cheese anymore, as I find it is very fattening and very indigestible. Except for apples and grapefruit, I don't eat much fruit. But I love all the green vegetables, especially leafy ones like spinach and salads." Most of her nutritional habits were shaped by a naturopath. What he said "made a lot of sense to me, and when I changed to a vegetarian low-sugar diet, it changed everything. I used to have bad circulation, for instance; I was always cold in winter— cold hands, cold feet—but all this improved and suddenly I wasn't cold any-

more. Not even in England."

On her own, she figured out that "milk is a *disaster!* All baby animals, once they're weaned from milk, never go back to it, because milk is a food for the growing process. I think human beings should follow the same pattern. I took my children off milk as soon as they caught a cold, and I reduced their milk intake in general—to the consternation of various in-laws who would think, 'Poor things, they can't have milk.' Nonsense! Milk is awful for you, especially if you have a *cold;* it helps the germs multiply. In fact, many Mediterraneans are allergic to it. I used to drink coffee with milk when I was a teenager, and I felt sick every morning. It took me years to puzzle out why." Elizabeth rarely gets sick; when she does it's over in a flash: "The last time I got the flu, I threw it off in exactly twenty-four hours" (eating only raw foods with lots of onions—as she was taught by the naturopath); she doesn't take masses of vitamins, though she does take some when she remembers.

for oily spots, followed by a superfatted soap and fifteen splashings of water. "I happen to be a committed washer—I am *always* scrubbing!

"Another thing. The same naturopath taught me that you should have a hot and cold shower every morning. It's very stimulating for the body. And it helps you to digest your breakfast; if you just crawl out of bed and eat, your system is half asleep. I used to force both my daughters to have a hot and cold shower as soon as they got up. They hated it, but I was very fussy about all of these things. Their hair always had to be perfectly clean, and I taught them how to take care of it. Thanks to Philip Kingsley, I showed them how to do their nails. Fuss, fuss, fuss, nag, nag, nag. But it worked."

It seems to have done so without an iota of damage to their relationship. "I suppose it's normal for mothers and daughters to be in opposition at times, but on the whole there is excellent communication. If I'm annoyed with Catherine about something, I call her up

"I am a great believer in complex carbohydrates as a source of energy and nutrition."

She doesn't use moisturizers on her skin; she thinks there is more to be said for having a humidifier in her apartment. Besides, moisturizers are contraindicated by Janet Sartin, the New York skin specialist by whom Elizabeth swears. She has Sartin facials twice a year, uses Sartin preparations every day. Most of all, she loves the cleansing routine, which, for dry skin like Elizabeth's, consists of an oil to remove surface dirt, plus an astringent

and scream at her, and she screams back. Most of the time, she listens to me. . . . I'm glad she's found a career that's put her on her feet so young; the world is tough, and you might as well get used to looking after yourself as early as possible. I don't think modeling will go to her head, as Catherine is a very level-headed girl." . . . Like her remarkable energy and marvelous looks, it's clearly a characteristic inherited from her mother.

Catherine Oxenberg

Catherine Oxenberg is her mother in pastels: the same wide, pointed cheekbones, plus blond hair, fair skin ("in winter, it goes *newt* white"), and eyes that are "sometimes a sharp blue, sometimes steel gray, and other times bright green." Her favorite thing about her appearance is that "I think I look a little bit like a cat—the shape of the eyes, and the cheekbones —which is nice, as I *adore* cats. The rest is pretty ordinary. I tend to see my face as a canvas as opposed to a finished product; it's very blank—a nose to be worked with, a mouth that has to be painted in, and sort of white areas around the perimeter. . . . I'm really immune to physical beauty in terms of model-type looks, because I'm surrounded by them. Every day you work, there are other models there. You go on 'cattle calls,' and there are hundreds of little blond turned-up noses and blue eyes, and smiley five-foot-eleven giants." Catherine is five-feet-six—the mighty midget of modeling.

With a Harvard acceptance in her pocket, she lucked into ten full color pages in *Vogue.* Whereupon, she deferred from Harvard, found an apartment in New York, enrolled at Columbia, and established herself as a working model. She is in it, frankly, for the money. "I want to pay my own way through college, and that is the only reason I'm doing it. I think it's embarrassing, in fact, that one can make so much money off the way one looks. You need no prior training, no special talent, no credentials whatever, except what you look like, which makes modeling a very easy way to start off in the career world."

Easy? Her first sitting was with a photographer who "shoots like a machine gun." The second photographer she worked for "takes like two pictures a day, and you're on the floor for four hours for each of those pictures. I was *devastated!* It was agonizing—just the strain of concentration and the emotional interplay between all the people involved: the photographer, the editor, the makeup artist, the hairdresser. It's an odd business. But I like actually working in front of the camera. That's because I love acting. I'm a moody person—I don't mean bad-moody or good-moody, but moody in the sense that I react strongly to the environmental mood. And if the photographer is right, and the situation, and the place, then I come across well. Other times— for a catalogue, say, where you're doing fifty shots a minute, and you really can't put your whole heart and body into it—it doesn't come off. These sittings always make me feel so frustrated and terribly guilty when I hand in my voucher, because I'm a perfectionist; I want to give as much of myself as there is to give."

tea, and everyone else is Pygmalion. And a girl with a strong sense of herself just isn't going to accept the script easily. "It's degrading; they have always got to change you so that you are their creation, as opposed to being yourself. They forget that you're a human being, and they try to make a statement on you . . . try to do something that obviously doesn't suit your look. With me, for instance, for the all-American commercial look, people always want to curl my hair. And I look idiotic with my hair curled. Sometimes they really friz it up, and then I look like an absolute asshole! . . . I had this problem in Paris. I went over to do the collections, but I didn't end up doing them, because they wanted to cut all my hair off.

"People are always suggesting things: Why don't you wear this instead of that? Why don't you change the shape of your eyebrows? Why don't you tan your body the same color as your face? . . . You're always too dark, too light, too green, too purple, too hairy. Or you've got baby fat. There's

---

"I cannot even think of eating red meat without thinking of eating rotting flesh. . . . I love chicken and fish. I love good bread. I love cheese. I love salads."

A curious aspect of this business, which quickly becomes apparent to young models—as it did to Catherine—is that it's basically a two-character play; the models are all Gala-

always something wrong with one. A Swedish photographer said to me, 'You've got legs like a cow'; well, thank you very much. And then, the other day, another photographer said, 'You have lovely legs,' and I almost fainted, because it's so rare. But I have no hard feelings; I know it's just a job."

She takes "just a job" more seriously than you might expect. "I'm very competitive—hate to be number two. Whatever I do—schoolwork, modeling —I apply myself to the utmost. And I've got a lot of ambition, which in something like modeling could cause me to go completely nuts. Because, of course, I am also very paranoid; if I ever have a day without a booking, I flip: 'Ah, this is the end, I can't stand it!' " There have been very few of those days. Mostly, she works. And she learns. "I've learned how to contour. I put a horrible dark-brown, pasty line all the way around under my jaw, which sort of brings out the bones and creates a hollowed illusion. It gives me that eighteen-year-old look as opposed to the thirteen-year-old look. Then I brush some dark powder blush under the cheekbones, in an up-and-out direction, and I slap some pink right on the smiley bones. It looks ghastly in real life, but on camera it looks quite normal."

In real life, she wears almost no makeup. Occasionally a base (like her mother, she uses Janet Sartin; the base is a colored astringent, very, very light), but usually just lip gloss and mascara. "I get tips from all the makeup artists about the best mascaras, which happen to be the cheapest. The *very* best, they say, is the Maybelline one that comes in a Locust Valley pink-and-green container; it's called Long Lash something or other, and it never comes off, not even if I cry."

Being her mother's daughter, she is "manic about being clean, feeling clean

---

**"I'm a perfectionist;
I want to give
as much of myself as
there is to give."**

—clean hair, clean hands, clean nails. I was *drummed* to wash—to be very hygienic—by my mother. Thank God, because one finds that a great many females aren't that clean, especially in Europe." Also like Princess Elizabeth, "I never eat red meat, not ever; my mother brainwashed me. When I used to eat it, she would say things like 'How can you eat a dead cadaver!' or 'How can you put rotting flesh in your mouth!' I have a rather vivid imagination, and that stopped me. I cannot even think of eating red meat now without thinking of rotting flesh. I just cannot eat it—ecch! . . . I love chicken and fish. I love good bread. I love cheese. I love salads. Once in a while, I'll go on a potato binge or a whipped-cream binge or a chocolate binge. . . . I hate processed foods, canned things, Twinkies—all that sort of junk food, I hate it, hate it, hate it."

Mummy puts her foot down. But for the rest of the time, she says, 'I have great faith in you. I trust you and I trust your judgment, and I know that ultimately you'll survive. Therefore, do what you think is best.' " Her relationship with her father, Howard Oxenberg, a retired textile executive, is not quite as idyllic. As Catherine sees it, it is the classic situation of possessive father versus suddenly grown-up daughter. Plus, "He's very old-fashioned in certain ways. I think he really thinks that a woman is only an extension of her man—when he heard that my boyfriend was coming to New York, he said, 'Why can't you live off him?' I almost *died!* I said, 'You must be joking!' " ("Of course he was," says Elizabeth; "he is *totally* proud of her.")

Catherine doesn't see herself as an extension of anyone. "I hate even the symbolism of a woman giving up her

---

**"I have to create a self strong enough
to assume credibility."**

The problems that often beset daughters of celebrated beauties seem not to have touched Catherine. For one thing, she and her mother are exceptionally close, and "being so close, I never thought of her as beautiful. She was just Mummy. She's a very strong, domineering person, which can be daunting. But, although I don't have much self-confidence, I do have quite a strong character—I'm strong within me—and I was never crushed by her. My sister was. Christina is about fifteen months younger, and maybe because she's dark and looks more obviously like Mummy, she always felt that she wasn't as pretty. I think she somewhat resented my mother, and that took the form of being jealous of her on a physical level, as well. They're just incompatible; whatever Mummy wants her to do, Tina does the opposite."

It's easier for Catherine. "Sometimes

name in marriage. It's giving up part of your identity. I won't have it. I have to be myself—or, rather, I have to create a self strong enough to assume credibility. . . . I want to be known, if known at all, for some wonderful merit, for some wonderful talent that I have, for some wonderful thing that I've done, as opposed to having a passive celebrity, which I consider a model's to be, and which isn't what I want at all."

For the moment, however, "I'm satisfied if I work every day and make the rates that I'm getting now." But tomorrow: "I might have something to do with dealing in Chinese art. Or I might become head of Mongolian oil. . . . That's the joy, the luxury, of adolescence: You can be a character dilettante and play around with all sorts of different identities." I hope she sticks with the present one for a while—it's a winner!

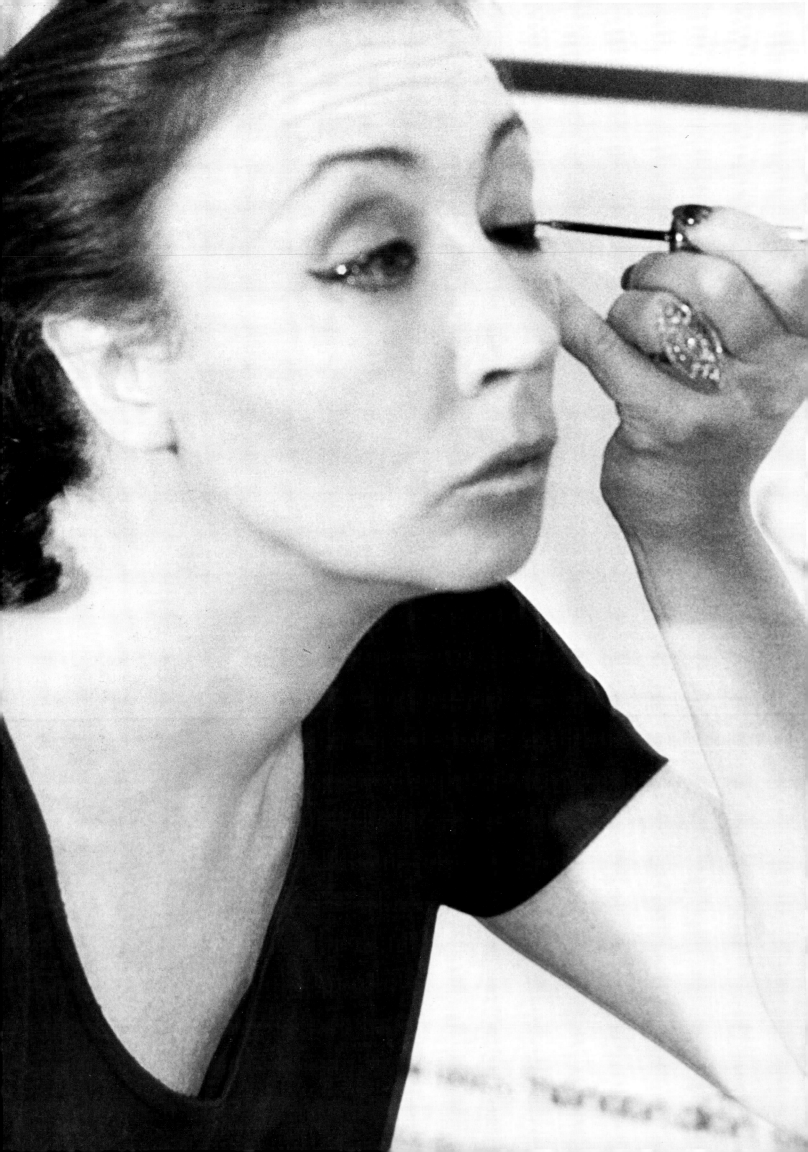

Oriana Fallaci

This photograph of Oriana Fallaci, the Italian writer, whose first fame in the United States is as a political interviewer and journalist, was done for *Vogue* at the time of the American publication of her novel, *A Man.* Stubborn, intense, fiercely principled, this small, pretty woman, who covered the Vietnam war at the front lines, who was shot down in the 1968 student uprising in Mexico, who threatened to walk off the set of a TV talk show if the host persisted in questioning her about her celebrated interview with Henry Kissinger instead of discussing the present novel—and walked ("when I am furious, I am *very* furious")—this remarkable woman couldn't understand why I would want to put her in a book that had to do with beauty and glamour: "A woman who is always in a hurry and always in trouble as I am, a woman who has been involved with a man the way I was involved with Alekos [Alexander Panagoulis, the hero of *A Man,* with whom she lived for three years until his death in 1976]—to call me glamorous! If tragedy is glamorous, then I am glamorous. I don't live glamorous. . . . I don't dress glamorous.

"I have never been obsessed with what they call beauty. I don't agree with its rules. A person who is stupid, for instance, is to me automatically ugly, as is a person who is a coward. Of course, I could never find attractive a stupid man, a cowardly man, and this goes also for women. I hardly find attractive a woman who has not intelligence and courage—which is not something that usually, especially in the past, has been required of a woman. In the world I came into, in the kind of culture which was imposed on me as a child, a woman had first of all to be beautiful. Then she had to be sweet. Then she had to be decent. Then she had to be a wife and to make children. Well, I don't think this means to be a woman. It means to accept the moral and aesthetic rules that this society established for its own interests. And I am not the kind of person who accepts rules because they are rules.

"Of course I do not like to look ugly, to look sloppy. Of course I like beauty and grace and elegance, in any field, thus in the person. Who doesn't? Beauty makes life more acceptable; it's a caress on the eyes. Besides, you

"Beauty makes life more acceptable."

would be surprised to discover how much I love jewels—I even wear them with blue jeans—and how much I love perfumes. I collect perfumes. But I simply refuse to associate the beauty with the fashion and the eyeliner and the nail polish. Even more, I refuse to associate that stuff with being a woman. I don't give a damn for the fashion. I never did, I never had the cult of it. I always dressed myself with care yet ignoring the dictatorship of the dressmakers, and I'll tell you more: When something is in fashion, I don't wear it as a principle. I mainly wear slacks and jacket. I always did; I started in my early twenties when a woman wearing slacks and jacket was not admitted in a restaurant. I hate the dresses, the knee-length dresses, I think they cut the figure and I don't have one of them. Finally, I don't give a damn for the makeup. It takes time, it takes patience, it glues the skin, it disturbs, and I am so unaccustomed to it that even when I am on TV I refuse any makeup. I proudly face the studio's lights with all my little wrinkles unhidden.

"Of course, nobody likes to have wrinkles. Not men, not women, nobody. When you begin to get wrinkles it means that a good part of the splendid adventure called life has been spent, and walking along the road which drives to the end it's hateful. Yet I would be lying if I said that I am obsessed by wrinkles as some women are. There is something chic in the wrinkles, a kind of severe chic. I mean, a cute wrinkle may be as elegant as an elegant dress or an elegant combination of colors. Besides, wrinkles aren't necessarily a mark of decadence. Sometimes they are a mark of sorrows, difficulties, intense life. All things I had abundantly, and now more than ever. I also have bags under my eyes. I sleep so little, and I live under such pressure. But I do nothing to hide those too. My friend Anna Magnani didn't either. She said, 'They are my medals!' Well, mine too. When someone advises me to do something against my bags and my cute wrinkles, I laugh and shout, 'They are my medals!' "

Throughout the makeup session with John Richardson, Fallaci resisted anything that might seem to falsify her image—eye shadow, mascara, foundation ("I cannot move my face when I have that stuff on"), rouge. ("No! I hate it on every woman—the red on the cheeks, like a doll. Why? Do they think it looks healthy? Healthy! Who says that looking healthy means to look beautiful? Hasn't literature taught us about those fantastically seducing women who were consumed by tuberculosis? Think of Greta Garbo when she dies, as pale as a white lily, in *La Dame aux Camelias.* Being ill is so *interesting.*")

Despite her misgivings, she let John continue: "I don't want you to cry for that," she said, "so do it a little, just a little, then you will see, I am right." As it turned out, she was. Makeup would have turned her into a cartoon of herself; without it, she is fabulous. And this is how I photographed her: almost no makeup at all, just her own liquid eyeliner—two black, bold, unsmudged lines, self-applied ("I do like that—*tac, tac, tac,* very quick")—which exaggerates the surprisingly Oriental shape of those gray-green eyes. The liner has become a signature: "I always go around with it. For a reason. Because although with aging it has changed a little, I have

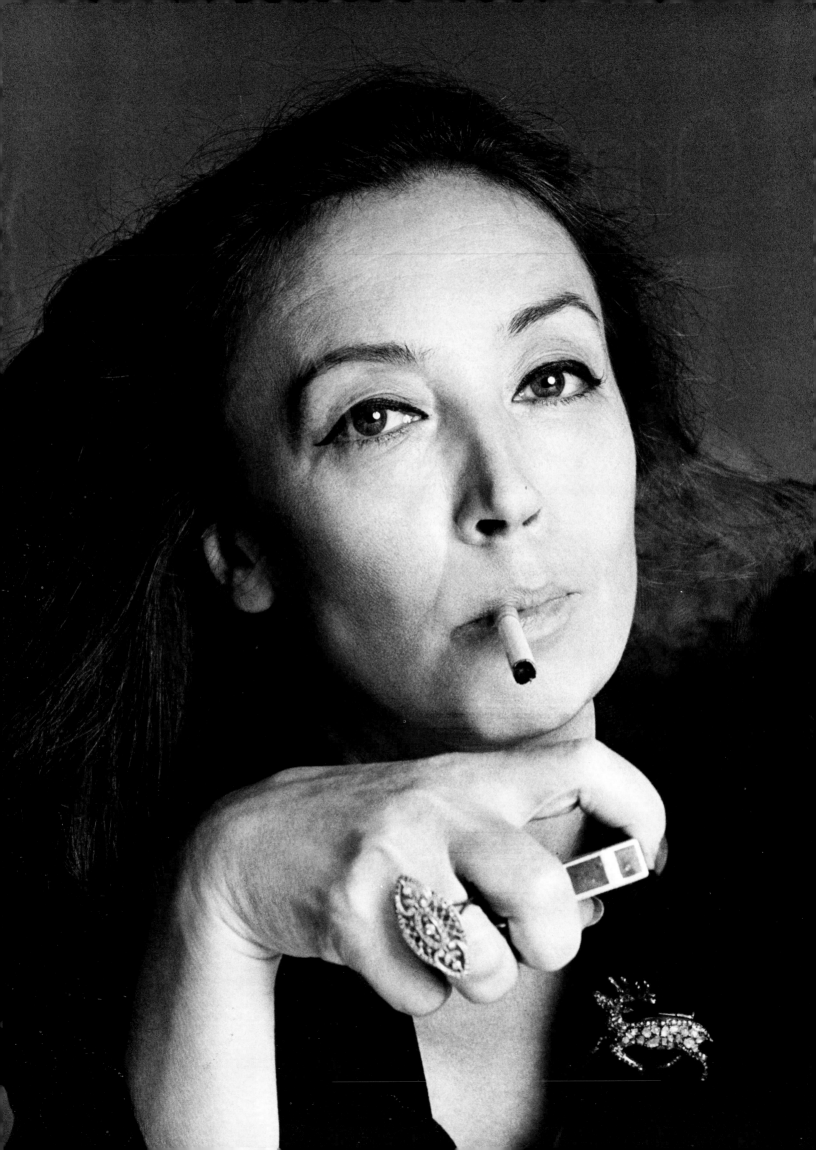

Oriana Fallaci

■

"I am not the kind of person who accepts rules because they are rules."

■

always had a kind of Asiatic features and Asiatic eyes—I should say Florentine features and very Florentine eyes. I am the most Florentine thing you can ever imagine. If you see, for instance, the frescoes in the churches of Florence, you see many Orianas . . . if you see the terra-cotta busts of Andrea della Robbia, they are my portraits. This means I have a typical Florentine face. And typical Florentine eyes are like Asiatic eyes, with lashes that are straight. So I cannot put mascara on the lashes; this liner is more than enough. Besides, doing it amuses me so much. One has to have a very firm hand to do it, like shooting. Look how firmly I do it, and quickly. One, two, three, and *voilà!*"

Just out of camera range in this photograph of her is another Fallaci signature: the very large sunglasses that she wears even when it's dark or when it's raining. "That's because I have gray-green eyes, very clear, and people with very clear eyes cannot stand excessive light; it hurts. Moreover, I feel protected by sunglasses. Kind of hidden. When you wear the sunglasses, people don't recognize you too easily so you can remain alone with yourself. I am asocial. If you want to make me unhappy, real unhappy, you have only to invite me to a cocktail party and listen to those questions. How do you do, where do you live, what is your next book about, did you really take off the *chador* in front of Khomeini—I get sick. I can even faint out of boredom at a party. Once I fainted. It was so boring, so unbearably boring, that I fainted. When I am alone, on the other hand, I never get bored. I like to be alone."

Then, the cigarette. I could no more photograph her without it than I could photograph her face without its features. It's part of her: "a tic . . . a vice." She smokes an average of two packs of Larks a day, unless she is writing. "When I wrote this last book, I reached seventy or eighty cigarettes a day. Smoking helps me to think, but I must admit I like the taste also. The Lark taste, I mean. Listen. Life is too short to give up something that gives one pleasure and that is innocuous to others [sic!]." Predictably, the antismoking campaign has had a reverse/perverse effect on her: "The moment they start breaking my bones—don't smoke here, don't smoke there—I say, OK, then I smoke double!" It isn't always possible; in Italy, where smoking is now prohibited in most taxis and in all movie theaters, she waits a long time for a ride and, she says, never goes to the movies anymore. Last year, she stormed out of an Air France ticket office when she was asked not to smoke —"To hell with you and with all Air France," she said—and booked with a more permissive airline.

The most desperate she has ever been for a smoke was in June 1970, during the invasion of Cambodia: "It was bad that day, bad, bad, shooting, bombing, shooting! And I had no cigarettes . . . I had no Larks. I was going around asking the soldiers, asking the officers. And they offered me *marijuana!* Finally, I got to a major. He was so nice, so sad. Good person. I said, 'Major, *please* get me some cigarettes.' He said, 'Yes, ma'am, at once.' Then he came back with a big parcel of marijuana cigarettes and gave them to me with a triumphant smile: 'Here they are.' I looked at him in despair. 'Major . . . don't you have a Lark, major?' But he hadn't and, besides, I couldn't offend him with a refusal. Could I?" So she accepted the gift and put it in her knapsack, where it remained for days, untouched, all the days she spent at the front lines searching for news and Larks.

"Finally I return to Phnom Penh. I get to my hotel, the Royal Hotel, and these marijuana cigarettes seem to me heavier than a five-hundred-pound bomb. I don't know what to do with them. I mean, on one side I felt guilty at the idea of throwing them away because there were people who would kill to have them, and on the other side I didn't want to keep them because I never understood people who dope themselves. But just as I am walking down the hall with my problem, I bump into an old friend of mine, the Italian ambassador in Saigon, Vincenzo Tornetta. And he looks at me with bewilderment, and he asks, 'Where do you come from?' From the Fish-hook area, I say; from the field. 'Oh, that's why you look so tense, so nervous,' he says. 'No,' I say, 'I am tense because an American officer has given me a parcel of marijuana cigarettes and I don't know what to do with them. What do I do with them, dammit?' He bursts out laughing. 'Let's taste them!' Well, we did. We went to my room, we shut ourselves in there like kids who taste tobacco for the first time and are afraid to be caught by their parents, and we lighted a cigarette, and . . . was it bad! Did it smell! It smelled like incense. I felt as if I were in a church, and I don't get along very well with the churches, you know. Any church. So I took the parcel and went in the bathroom and threw it into the water closet. All of it. Then I flushed."

She smiles happily. "The rest of the story you wouldn't believe it. Because the Lark people wanted me to publicize it. But I did not, of course." No need to explain that her negative answer wasn't dictated by health reasons. "You know, four people in my family have died of cancer. Yet they did not smoke. With all my smoking, instead, I'm still alive. Well, I cough a lot. Very lot. But I am one of those people who are all the time ill and who will die at ninety. We have a proverb in Tuscany. When people are all the time ill we say, Yeah, that one will bury all of us. I always say that if they don't shoot me, if they don't kill me, assassinate me, I have many probabilities to last . . . just because I smoke all this good tobacco." Who in his right mind would argue the point with Oriana Fallaci?

Spectacular looks improve
with a more natural approach

Farrah Fawcett

"I'm a person who be-
lieves that 'less is more,'
the total made-up look
just didn't work for me.
The more natural look is
better. Don't change my
bone structure or eyes,
because this is the way I
am. Sure, my look has
changed, but if I had
known then what I know
now my look would have
been what it is now."

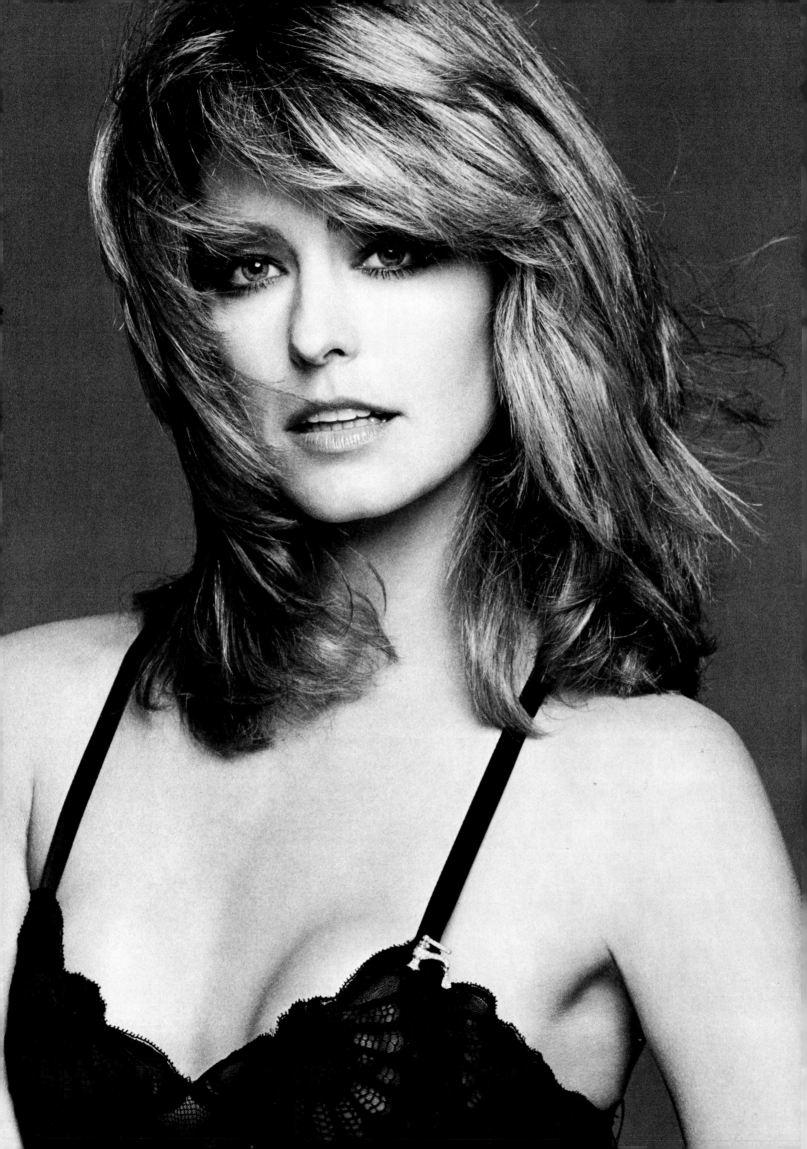

Farrah
Fawcett

1978

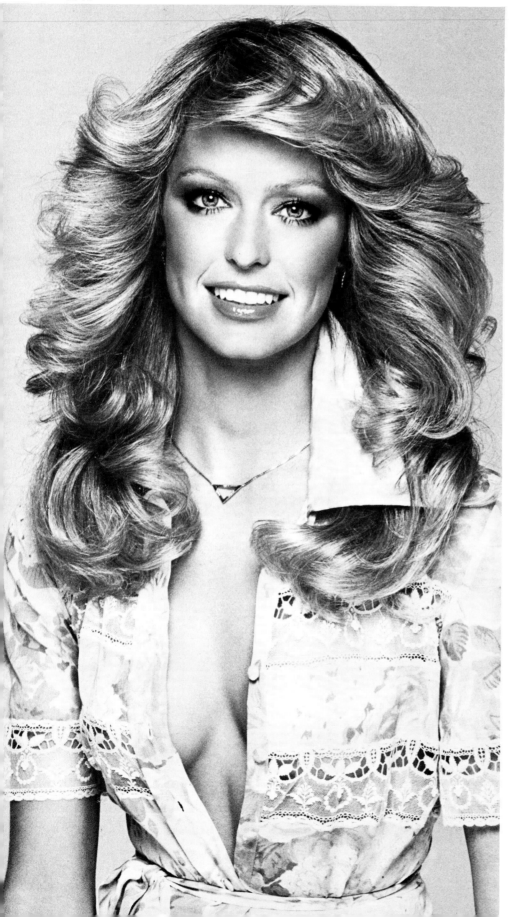

Farrah Fawcett is America's sex-and-sunshine girl—clean as the ocean, sparkling as October, wholesome as corn flakes. I think of Farrah on a tennis court, looking great after a million sets—looking great when she sweats. Looking fit and healthy and sexy. She makes good on all those promises that parents bait their children with: If you brush your hair a hundred strokes, it will grow thick and shiny. If you get lots of fresh air, you will have rosy cheeks and a beautiful complexion. If you brush your teeth twice a day, you will have a gorgeous white smile and be very, very popular.

She is. Her appeal catches everyone, even women. That famous Farrah poster, which has probably outsold Picasso by now, isn't bought just by men: "A lot of women ask me to sign my poster for their husbands, and they say, 'I'm glad he likes you. I like you too.'" In fact, she got her first big break because the thirty or so secretaries who sat in on the final selection for the Wella hair commercial liked her best: "When the agency people told me that I was the girl, they said, 'You know, you didn't offend the women.'"

Farrah and I go back to her commercial days. She came to do a Wella ad, and when I saw her it hit me: Here was my next *Cosmopolitan* cover. So I got Helen Gurley Brown on the phone and told her, 'I want to shoot the cover right now, and I'm going to do it with this unknown girl.' That cover sold more copies of *Cosmo* than any previous issue. Shortly after, she went into the TV series *Charlie's Angels.* And by the time she made her first movie, *Somebody Killed Her Husband,* she was the third highest-paid actress in films—"only Barbra Streisand and Faye Dunaway got more.

"It all just happened for me. I kind of slipped in the back door—I didn't train, I didn't study. But I had a manager who made all kinds of demands. And I think it went to his head. I think it went to the heads of a lot of people around me. But not to mine. I was too busy working. I got up at four thirty in the morning, I went to work, I worked all day. On my lunch hour, sometimes, I shot a cover. I flew to New York on weekends: I did six pages for *Vogue.*

"You don't appreciate it at the time it's happening. You don't realize that you are the hottest poster girl in the country, that you are in the top TV series, that you are on the cover of *Vogue,* on the cover of *Time.* I was just too busy working, too busy learning my craft, trying somehow to find enough hours to get in my run before going to the studio in the morning, to keep up my energy, to take the right vitamins. . . . My parents, too—it was a total whirlwind for a while. The phone ringing all night long. I couldn't walk down the street; I got mobbed. We all went through a terrible time. I became too available: too much publicity, too many covers.

"I don't mind at all getting older, but I would like to age gracefully."

Then, finally, I had to say, 'OK, that's it; now I want to be selective. I want to do a talk show only when I have something to say, when I can talk about a new film that I'm proud of—I mean *proud* of.' So I've become a little more exclusive." And a lot more independent. "I now dress for myself. I don't allow the wardrobe people to dress me. And I don't allow the hairdressers to say more about my hair than I want to say about it. The same is true about my makeup. It was a different story when I did that first *Cosmopolitan* cover; I was very disappointed with my makeup. It changed the shape of my eyes, and because I'm a person who believes that 'less is more'; the total made-up look just didn't work for me. The more natural look is better. Don't change my bone structure or eyes, because this is the way I am. Sure, my look has changed, but if I had known then what I know now my look would have been what it is now. Actually, I did know then; I just didn't feel I could say anything about it."

For this second *Cosmopolitan* sitting, Farrah had her say (she also had Way Bandy to do her makeup and Harry King to cut her hair, which didn't hurt at all). "And not the Farrah Fawcett hairdo. I try not to slip back into that. Now it's all more one length. And I've stopped streaking it; I don't like to have it so blond anymore. I want to go into a more natural look. Just for a change. Since the interview, I've had it cut again [for her *Bazaar* shooting with me] on the top—it's slightly 'new wave'; I'm constantly changing.

"It isn't that I decided, 'OK, now I'm gonna change my look.' But I think I'm changing as a person, as a woman. I think I've made the transition from ingenue to woman, and with that you have to change. I see changes in my face. My face has gotten thinner and—well, wiser-looking. I'm sure that comes with just getting older; your face gets older. I don't know that I see distinct wrinkles and lines, but I see the beginnings of them; I just hope that tomorrow I don't see giant bags and everything. I don't mind at all getting older, but I would like to age gracefully. I think this is why I exercise and try to eat properly—though one day I'm a health-food nut and the next day I eat totally junk food."

Before coming over to do the sitting, Farrah ran from her hotel, at Fifth Avenue and 60th Street, all the way up to 90th and back again . . . then she walked to the studio. Fast. She is almost as famous for fitness as she is for her hair and her smile. "It's a big part of my life. I get up and run every morning. I don't really set a goal for myself, the way most dedicated runners do. Sometimes I do five miles, other times I'll only run a mile. If I get up and play three games of racquetball, then I won't run. If it's really bad weather—bad enough to keep me in—I'll do sit-ups, plus fifteen minutes of other exercise. Just as long as I get my exercise.

"Everything that I like to do, you get sun. No matter how much you try to keep it off you—which I do try to do for the sake of my skin—it's always there. I play a lot of tennis, and I wear a visor to keep the sun off my face. And then I like to swim, and I like to play racquetball, and I like to run. I wear sunscreen, but it still hits you. I just do the normal things for my skin. I mois-turize. Also, when I go into the sauna I have special cream masks that I put on. The one I have now is a eucalyptus mask that draws out the impurities. I do that—the mask in the sauna—once a week, and I keep trying different ones. While I'm in the sauna, I also put Farrah Fawcett conditioner on my hair and let the heat from the sauna help make the conditioning effect even better." After the sauna, I always moisturize my face and body. Like makeup, I'll try one kind of moisturizer and then I'll try another. Basically, I think they're all rather similar."

Farrah's beauty also comes from a profound commitment to health. She is the national chairperson of Women Against Cancer and she travels across the country doing commercials, fundraising, and speaking for the organization to educate women about cancer prevention. "When you have your health, you have it all," says Farrah. "I firmly believe that beauty comes from within and that it's just as crucial to take care of yourself internally as externally."

Farrah's love of beauty extends to art and sculpture as well. Farrah majored in art and sculpture in college and still paints and sculpts. "Art's an inseparable part of my life, not just in dress or surroundings but everywhere. Even on a set or visiting friends at the beach, I always have my sketchpad with me. I keep hoping that one day I'll find a role that will incorporate my love of art with my acting, a role that would allow me to express my love of both."

Farrah's acting career shows no sign of a slowdown either. On the contrary, last year she received critical acclaim for her performance in the four-hour television drama of the documentary novel *Blood and Money.* In this, Farrah plays (with her hair pulled back) Joan Robinson Hill, a high-spirited Texas heiress, who—according to her father—was murdered by her husband, who in turn was murdered, allegedly by the father's paid assassin.

Farrah also comes from Texas. She was the first freshman ever from the University of Texas to make the list of the ten most beautiful girls on campus. "So they put my picture in the paper and a Hollywood publicist saw it and called me saying, 'Come to Hollywood . . . you have a great smile . . . you'd be sensational in commercials.' I really wasn't ready at the time, but the following summer I hadn't made any plans and didn't really know what to do. So my parents encouraged me to give it a try, what could I lose? They sure never expected I wouldn't come back at the end of the summer. It's funny how destiny is, you know?" I know.

Breaking the rules to develop a personal, comfortable style

Ruth Ford

"I don't believe in rules and generalizations. I don't believe in fashion, I don't follow fashion. I think that's boring. . . . I don't go in for heavy makeup. . . . You have simply got to try to develop a sense of yourself."

Ruth
Ford

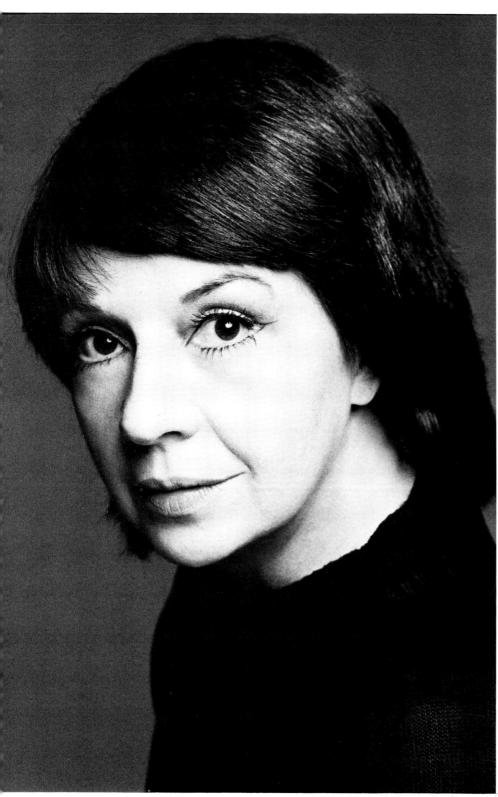

1970

Thirty years of photographing women has made me extremely skeptical of any hard-and-fast rules about who should wear what or at what age one should stop doing this and start doing that. For the most part, I think it's all garbage. I know tiny women who are sensational in big, bulky "tall women" clothes, redheads who are terrific in red, grandmothers who look like a million bucks in leather jeans and a trench coat. It isn't that they are exceptions to the rule; it's that every woman is an exception, an individual. And the woman who understands this is going to look damn good all her life.

Actress Ruth Ford is the perfect example. If Ruth has ever heard that a woman over forty shouldn't wear black, shouldn't wear her hair long, shouldn't dye it blond, she just isn't having any: "I don't believe in rules and generalizations. I don't believe in fashion, I don't follow fashion. I think that's boring. I canceled my subscriptions to *Vogue* and *Harper's Bazaar* and *Women's Wear Daily* a long time ago. I don't go in for heavy makeup because I don't think it's becoming to me now, not because a magazine says that makeup should be lighter as one gets older. Neither do I need a magazine to tell me that if I'm short-waisted and rather big-waisted, which I am, I would be stupid to wear anything with a waistline . . . you have simply got to try to develop a sense of yourself. I don't care what colors are in or out; black and red are my favorites and I wear them all the time (I had five red evening dresses in college); I don't like yellow or Kelly green and I never wear them. . . . I used to enjoy decorating myself—I bought all my clothes in thrift shops—but I don't feel in a very eccentric mood at the moment; right now, I like to be comfortable. Though I might go back to all that, who knows? . . . Since 1949, when I had to go blond for *No Exit,* I've gone back and forth —blond to brunette, long hair, short hair. I would find it boring always to look the same . . . after all, life is change."

An interesting thing about these photographs of Ruth. People usually guess the dark, short-haired picture to be the more recent. The truth is, I did that one about ten years ago; the blond, long-haired Ruth is the Ruth of today: a happy woman, enthusiastic about everything, bursting with health and vitality, and looking—incredibly—even younger than she did a decade earlier.

I don't know Ruth's exact age—*Theater World* gives her birth date as 1915; a book about the production of *Requiem for a Nun,* the play that William Faulkner wrote for her, gives it as 1912 and suggests that it is probably earlier—and wild horses couldn't drag it out of Ruth. "I'll tell anything except my age," she says. "No woman should—until she's ninety. Then she should knock off twenty years. If she has taken care of herself, she'll get away with it. What I hate is this obsession with youth that so many American women have. I think we should all stay as young and beautiful as we can, but when it becomes obsessive it's a bore."

In her unboring, unobsessive, unorthodox way, Ruth Ford takes care of herself. "I don't sleep well, but I don't worry about it, and I don't take pills. I don't take any medicines. I take masses of vitamins—E, A, D, C, B-complex—plus desiccated liver, pantothenic acid, dolomite. . . . I never take a drink when I'm alone, but I enjoy a glass of wine when I'm with people, or a vodka on the rocks. I smoke to this extent: I'm a serious social smoker; it goes with a drink, at parties. If I really *smoked,* I'd stop. I wouldn't do anything that I thought was bad for me. . . . Frankly, I've always been kind of smart. And I've been blessed with good health. I like to eat. I love everything on earth, provided it's cooked well. Except lung. And German food. I'm not a health-food nut, but I'm very nutrition-conscious (in high school, in Vicksburg, Mississippi, I took a course in nutrition; I was the only one in the class). I eat fresh fruits, vegetables, nuts, seeds, yogurt, wheat germ. I drink low-fat milk, rose-hip tea, and only one cup of coffee a day. No nitrates, no nitrites, no white bread, no fried foods. . . . I'm a good cook. I haven't really 'entertained' since my husband died, in 1965 [Ruth was married to Zachary Scott, the actor], but if people want to come and sit in the kitchen with me, I'll give them a lovely cold borscht in the summer and lentil soup in winter.

"I would like to weigh ten pounds less. I have never gone on a diet. I have never exercised. I don't swim, ride, jog, or play tennis. I love to dance; I have my whole life. . . . I do what gives me joy and pleasure. Living in New York does; I think it's the most wonderful city in the whole world. I once lived—briefly—in Hollywood; I wouldn't do it

again for all the bucks in the bank.

"Fifteen years ago, I got out of the sun; that's one good thing I did for my looks. And the best thing I do for my skin—apart from putting on Lubriderm before I put on makeup—is: I don't pay attention to it. I don't have facials. I think they're destructive. All the women I know who have regular facials have old-looking skin, sagging flesh, wrinkles."

sponge (to soak up the excess powder; applied with a puff, powder tends to stay on the surface and leave nasty little deposits that can make a superficial line photograph like the San Andreas fault), and water finger-patted all over so that everything stays dewy and light.

There is also this about Ruth: In front of the camera she is totally unselfconscious and outgoing; it's all positive energy bouncing off that face and body.

"I'll tell anything except my age. . . . No woman should— until she's ninety. Then she should knock off twenty years. If she has taken care of herself, she'll get away with it."

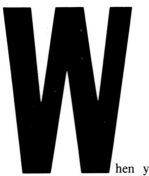

hen you look at pictures of a woman taken ten years apart, and the ageing process seems not just halted but reversed, you look for a reason. And in Ruth's case, there are several: some physical—light hair, for instance, brings light to the face; soft hair softens it—some psychological—the first sitting took place only a few years after the death of her husband, and I think the sadness she still felt is reflected in her face. All traces of grief are absent from the second photograph; she is upbeat and relaxed, and her face shows it. . . . It happens to be a very, very good face—good eyes, good contours. I'm not one of those photographers who go crazy over bone structure, but I don't knock it. Good bones hold the face up, hold it together. Ruth has good bones. As John Richardson, who did her makeup for the second sitting, says, "It's a face that is kind of *there.*" It doesn't want a major makeup production. Mainly, it was a question of simply following the natural contours, bringing out the cheekbones and accenting the line of chin and jaw by shadowing lightly underneath. At the end, a touch of baby powder patted on with a flat cosmetic

She likes being photographed ("It's part of being an actress; I want to show off") and has been all her life, both as an actress and as a beauty. At the University of Mississippi, where she did a Master's degree in philosophy, Ruth was an official campus beauty. Later, through her brother, the poet and filmmaker Charles-Henri Ford, she met and posed for such illustrious photographers as Man Ray, Steichen, Hoyningen-Huené, and Cecil Beaton, and became celebrated herself as "one of the ten most beautiful women in the world."

To be known as a "beauty" early on is a dicey business. I have seen so many of these women who are frozen in the attitudes of their first bloom: the same look of hair, of makeup, the same style of dressing, the same way of thinking. They are like clocks that have stopped. Ruth Ford is ticking all the time. When she isn't reading scripts, she is cataloguing her art collection; Ruth and her brother own, jointly, the largest Tchelitchew collection in the world. . . . In the theater, she has played Shaw, Sartre, Faulkner, Lorca, Giraudoux, Albee, Mark Crowley, Tennessee Williams. She has done Shakespeare's Ophelia, Desdemona, Lady Macbeth; she did Portia on TV. . . . Not everything she touches turns to gold. Recently, on Broadway, Ruth starred in a production of *Harold and Maude:* "It cost half a million dollars and folded in four nights. . . . Tragedies have to make you stronger if you're going to survive. I am a survivor. And I guess I'm an optimist." . . . She is in the best tradition of southern belles: true grit and no syrup.

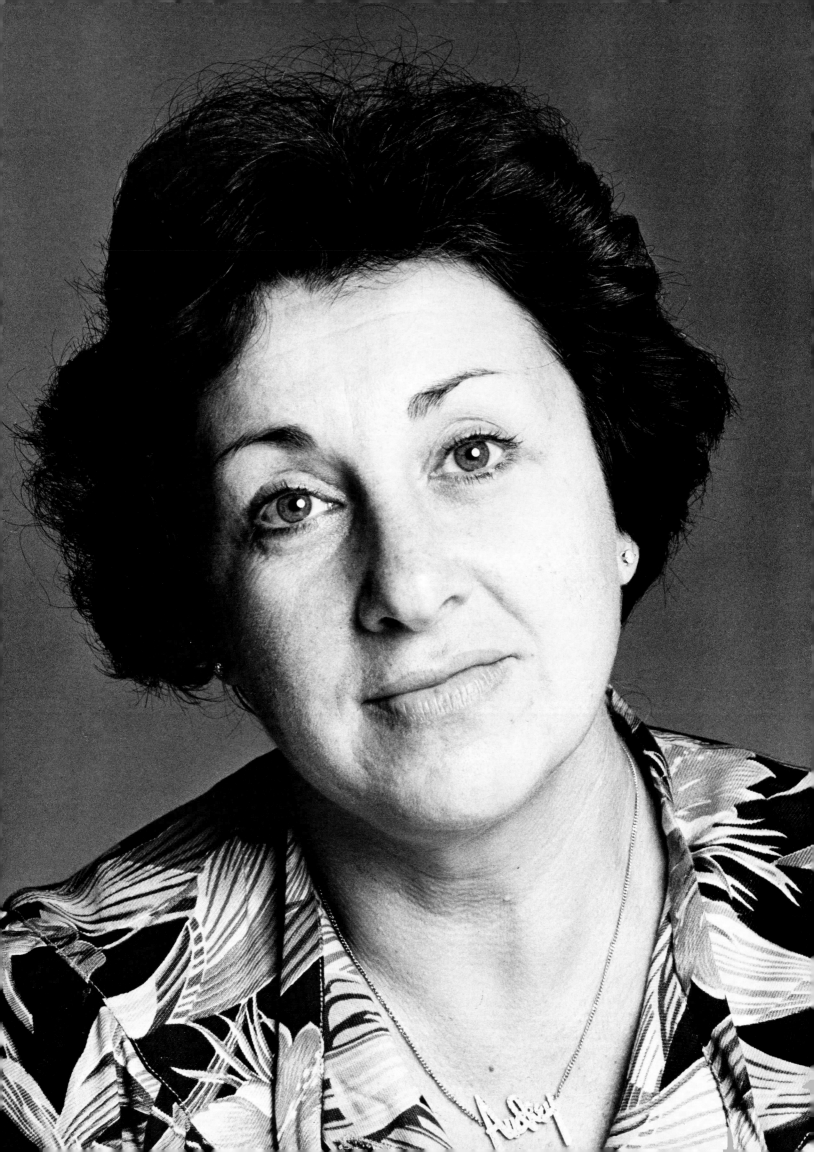

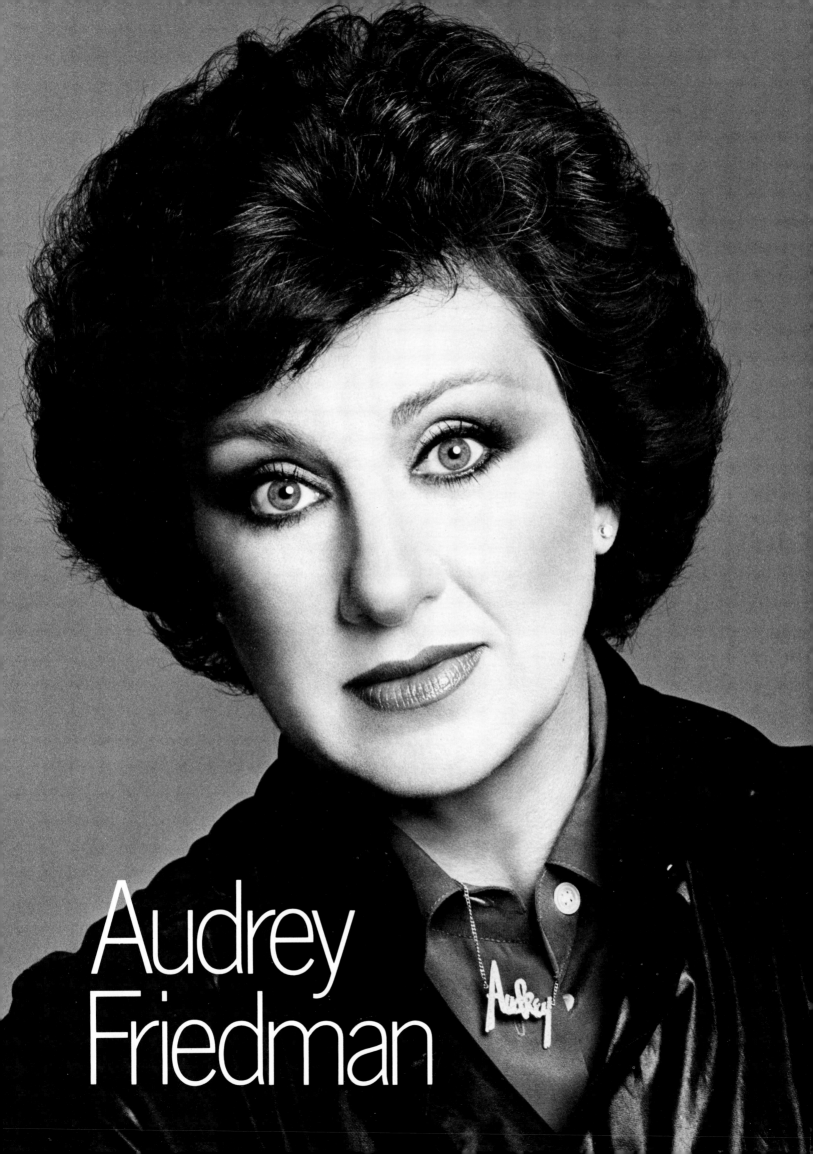

Audrey
Friedman

Audrey
Friedman

"I have a woman who comes to the house to give me facials, manicures, and pedicures. . . . I'm very particular about my toenails and my feet. . . . I think it's awful to get into bed with a man and put your callused feet on his back. I mean, that has just got to be disgusting, right?"

W

hen Audrey Friedman saw her finished portrait, she said, "I'm going to take this picture to a plastic surgeon and ask him to make me look just like it." Which is a nice compliment, but it's based on a false premise. The truth, of course, is that the portrait does look like Audrey. It couldn't look like anyone else.

After all, it's the same woman—except: Instead of the dowdy, nondescript print that adds years and pounds, she's wearing shiny black, which shoots up light to her face and clarifies it . . . instead of the shapeless, boring, old-looking haircut she came in with, she now has a cut by Harry King that is young and nifty and doesn't drag her features down . . . instead of invisible eyes and wispy eyebrows that she had plucked almost to the point of extinction (no woman should do this job herself; to do it at all, you have to work

---

"My children ate Beef Wellington when they were two years old; they grew up on stuffed artichokes."

---

close up, but to do it properly you need to stand away—i.e., you need a professional), Way Bandy has blended lots of sooty, smudge-y grays and browns to bring up the size and sparkle of her eyes and used a soft brown pencil to feather in eyebrows along the natural curve of her brow.

Contouring under the chin and on the cheeks makes her face appear slimmer than it actually is. But if Audrey were to lose weight, these are the contours you'd see; they are there. Makeup can bring out, enhance, accentuate, or diminish; it can make more of what's good, less of what's not good.

And I use it for all it's worth, not to

get a picture of something that doesn't really exist, but to show what is already there—potentially. The heaviness, the unflattering haircut and print dress aren't important; they're easy to get rid of. I go with the positive. With Audrey, it was her eyes and mouth and a vitality that she has, a sort of glow.

"I'm going to take this picture to a plastic surgeon and ask him to make me look just like it."

Now this, more than anything, is what you want to get in a photograph: this glow. It's not difficult with models; they're used to projecting all kinds of moods and emotions. Most women, though, find it harder. . . . But as I found out, Audrey Friedman is not most women.

For one thing, she is a woman who, in 1973, without a day of working experience, started a business from zero and built it into the largest of its kind in the world. For another thing, since 1977 she has been happily married to a man who is thirteen years her junior.

Until these events changed it all, her life was as conventionally domestic as a breakfast food commercial. For twenty-two years she had been a housewife and mother (she has four children, now twenty-five to fifteen) and, according to local reputation, "the best cook in Dallas, Texas. All my creative energy went into cooking . . . my children ate Beef Wellington when they were two years old; they grew up on stuffed artichokes."

Like most people who love to feed other people, Audrey also set a pretty table. The way some women collect gold rings and cashmere sweaters, she collected placemats—when she could find them. Attractive placemats were practically as rare as white truffles, until Audrey took over. That happened when her favorites wore out, and,

unable to replace them with anything nearly as nice, she ran up her own. Her family were charmed. Her friends were charmed. And it occurred to Audrey that a lot of other people might be. So she took her samples over to Neiman Marcus and Sanger-Harris—and came home with enough orders to warrant contracting a fabric cutter and a team of home sewers. Within a year, "Audrey" was a big name in table linens . . . within five, the biggest.

Inevitably, when a woman who has been solely a wife and mother for more than half her life suddenly veers off in a whole new direction, there are going to be complications—school meetings that conflict with business conferences, family occasions that get pre-empted by clients' deadlines. Audrey remembers "the children suffered a little at first, but they came out of it beautifully." Her marriage didn't. In 1974, Audrey and her husband were divorced. And three years later, she remarried. The bride was forty-three, the groom thirty—a statistic that seemed of far greater concern to outsiders than to the principals: "I got all these articles from well-meaning friends, something they had read in this or that magazine about older women and younger men. . . . *People* magazine interviewed me, ostensibly because I was a woman who had never worked and had built this phenomenally successful business almost single-handedly. But when they learned that my husband was so much younger, they wanted to do the whole story on that." Among the severest critics of the marriage was Audrey's first husband, which was curious in view of his own second marriage—to a woman thirteen

years his junior, the same age, in fact, as Audrey's new husband ("And wouldn't you just know, people said to me, 'At least he didn't marry a young girl!' ").

Audrey's life since her second marriage has been smooth as honey. Her daughter is an advertising executive in New York, her eldest son works with her in her business, another son is in college, and the youngest lives with Audrey and her husband in Dallas (there is also a California beach house in Malibu and, for business trips, an apartment in New York).

There is a kind of unobsessive vanity about Audrey that I find refreshing: She likes looking nice for her man. Before her marriage, for instance, she had cosmetic eye surgery: "I had it done before I needed it, but I felt it was coming, and I was in a period when I was more vain . . . I had just gotten divorced and was getting into a new relationship with a younger man."

And she treats herself to small, pampering luxuries: "I have a woman who comes to the house to give me facials, manicures, and pedicures. . . . I'm very particular about my toenails and my feet. . . . I think it's awful to get into bed with a man and put your calloused feet on his back. I mean, that has just got to be disgusting, right?"

There are women who go to bed with makeup on; Audrey would rather die first. In her whole life, she has done it exactly once. And that was the day I did her portrait. What we put on her face—eyes, contouring, the works—stayed on all the way back to Dallas and to bed that night ("It didn't look terrific next morning—but, oh, how I adored it!").

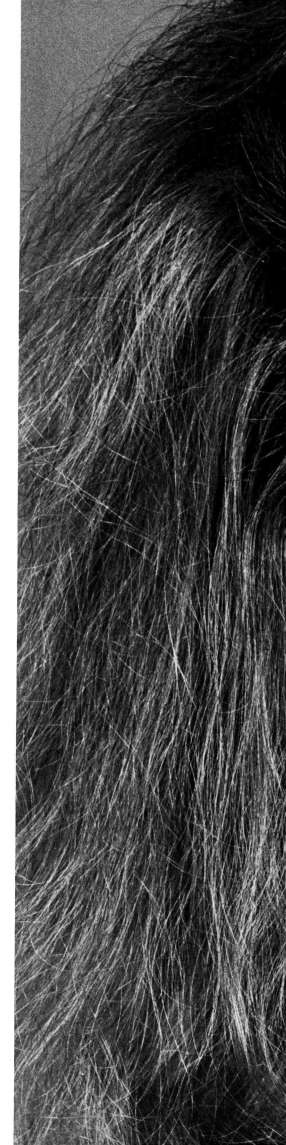

If your eyes are your best feature, emphasize them with makeup and keep the rest understated

Anne Hearst

I was photographing for *Harper's Bazaar,* and Anne, who had been working at the various Hearst magazines, turned up as a kind of bonus. She reminded me of Margaret Sullavan, who was one of my favorites: the hair, the face, the slightly husky catch-in-the-throat voice. She was fabulous to photograph. And easy. Harry King didn't change the look of her hair. Way Bandy didn't do a lot of fussing with her face, just filled in her eyebrows, did a good eye makeup, and a pale, pale mouth—Anne's lips are somewhat thin, and if you make a thin mouth dark you exaggerate it, which would make her look hard. So he kept the mouth pale and concentrated on the eyes, which are her best feature.

Anne has dry skin: "I use lots of creams and lotions and an oil instead of soap when I shower. I used to go out in the sun and bake and burn and didn't care. But I'm twenty-five now; my skin is already dry and just too pale to risk it. If I were to keep on baking my skin as I used to, it would be ruined by thirty."

What I suggest for dry skin is Evian water, not only before putting on makeup but all through the day. Lots of women carry a spray bottle in their purse. Plus a purse-size moisturizer. Of course, you can't keep putting moisturizer over makeup. But I don't think any woman should wear makeup in the daytime, except on the eyes. It's rarely an improvement. And dry skin, like Anne's, is usually the prettiest kind— smooth-textured, evenly colored. It needs moisture, not makeup.

Anne's is really a *face.* . . . I like her style, her Anglo-Saxon cool—with a little steel in it. I like her loyalty to Patty (in a close-knit family of five sisters, Patty and Anne are third and fourth respectively, and only a year apart) and her forthright way of dealing with the inevitable questions: What was it like being Patty Hearst's sister? What really happened?

When Anne talks about the events that pulled her whole family into a nightmare of public scrutiny and easy judgments, it is with honesty, a leaven of humor, and angry disbelief at the malice that seemed turned against them all relentlessly, like machine-gun fire. "After a while, people began coming out for Patty; William Buckley was one of the first. But before that, there was no one. It's very depressing not to have anyone at all behind you. When we were in the real heat of publicity, it seemed that things couldn't get worse, and they always did. It wasn't the sort of publicity that surrounds glamorous people. It was unfriendly . . . like being hounded. The media were especially hard; they made me ashamed to be part of the press. Of course, there were times when the press were decent and professional. There were a lot of tender moments, too. And a lot of dramatic moments. There were also a lot of amusing things. When life gets that bizarre, you are bound to run into them, all sorts of crazy things happen that seem very funny: psychics, who can be very weird indeed . . . people running in and out of the house all the time . . . bodyguards . . . the FBI. The FBI lived in the house, in a den downstairs that we began calling the FBI room. Long after they left, we were still calling it the FBI room.

"It's so nice that it's over. I know Patty has nightmares; it's the one real scar. But mostly, I think, everybody has come out of it well. Patty is married, happy, living a normal life. In a funny way, I think it helped having to sit in court and retell the story in front of a million people, telling it again and again and again until finally she learned to come to terms with it. She couldn't even try to block it out— she didn't have the chance."

Lena Horne

Lena Horne says that her mother was "the most beautiful woman in the world." She undoubtedly was beautiful. Just as, without doubt, Lena Horne is one of the great beauties of our time. Yet she rarely talks about her looks, and when she does it's usually to say, "I'm pretty good for an old broad," or to credit the makeup and hair stylists. The truth is that Lena Horne is *fabulous,* one of the rare women who has it all to begin with. She's alive, vibrantly so. When she walks into a room—those marvelous eyes flashing, sparkling with vitality— she radiates an energy you can't help responding to. Her face is definitive: high cheekbones that defy time and gravity, eyes that are eternally young and glowing, dazzling teeth, a smile that simply bowls you over, and a laugh that can be so earthy it's almost sinful!

Her remarkable career as a performer has spanned nearly half a century, yet as a performer she's constantly growing and regenerating. The critics practically ran out of superlatives for her recent tour de force on Broadway, *Lena Horne: The Lady and Her Music*—not to mention that she wowed standing-room-only audiences night after night and was awarded a special Tony for her show-stopping performance. Lena Horne is a star, and she has been one for years. Yet her voice sounds better than ever and her understanding of lyrics is more profound now than in the past. Today, in her mid-sixties, Lena Horne has a clear sense of herself as a woman and as a performer. "It's only been in these last few years that I've wanted to be a success for me."

Her evolution from colored chorine to star, from mannered, icy singer (her reputation at nightclubs here and in Europe in the 1950s) to this earthy, funny, wise, warm, let-it-all-hang-out knockout performer, took some doing, some elemental rearranging of psyche and soul. Lena Horne fought to become her own woman, and getting there was one incredible journey.

Lena started in show business at sixteen, as a dancer at the Cotton Club, a then-famous nightclub in Harlem. Characteristically modest, Lena says she made it on her youth and looks. "In the old days at the club, their attitude was if you weren't tan and great-looking you couldn't get it. You should have seen the girls there. Now *they* were beautiful. I was nothing more than average."

"It's only been in these last few years that I've wanted to be a success for me."

Perhaps her reluctance to define herself as beautiful partially stems from that period when she first saw the ways beauty could be misused. Of course she was beautiful then as now, but she also had an abundance of talent, brains, and guts—which came in handy on her steady, often painful climb to fame. Along the way she set precedents and broke more than her share of barriers: She integrated big-band music, touring in 1940 with Charlie Barnet's until then all-white band; went to Hollywood and became the first black woman to be celebrated there for her beauty and the first to receive public recognition from white audiences. She was also the first black actress to break the stereotypes of Hollywood casting— no maid or mammy parts, thank you. She was the pin-up black GIs carried with them during World War II, and she refused to entertain white troops unless blacks were also admitted (later demanding the same of the nightclubs she performed in). Yet by refusing to allow herself to be a stereotype, she found herself thwarted in her dream of developing as an actress.

As you might imagine, Lena's memories of her Hollywood years are sometimes tinged with a bittersweet note, such as the story about the time a studio commissioned Max Factor to create a makeup just for her. Factor called it Light Egyptian. As Lena tells it, "then they went and put that makeup all over Ava Gardner (a friend) and gave her the role I wanted as Julie in *Showboat.*" Still, her impact on screen is evident in the two highly praised all-black films she starred in, *Cabin in the Sky* and *Stormy Weather,* both of which make regular appearances in revivals as well as on television. Watching her in them it's clear that, had she been given the right vehicles, Lena Horne would have been as big a star in that medium as she is on stage.

She has been married twice, first to Louis Jones, a preacher's son, educated and very conventional, while she was still in her teens, and then to musical arranger Lennie Hayton in the 1940s. Her first marriage produced her two children, Gail and Teddy . . . and some penetrating insights about the unique role of black women in marriage: "A Negro man needs more, expects more from his wife than other men do. A Negro woman . . . has to be terribly strong. She cannot relax, cannot simply be a loving wife . . . she has to be a spiritual sponge, absorbing the racially inflicted hurts of her man. Yet at the same time she has to give him courage, make him know that it's worth it. . . . It isn't easy being a sponge and an inspiration."

After her marriage to Jones disintegrated, Lena went to Hollywood, making a string of movies which usually found her leaning against a pillar as she sang. Her cameos were all carefully set up so that she could be easily edited from the films before they were sent

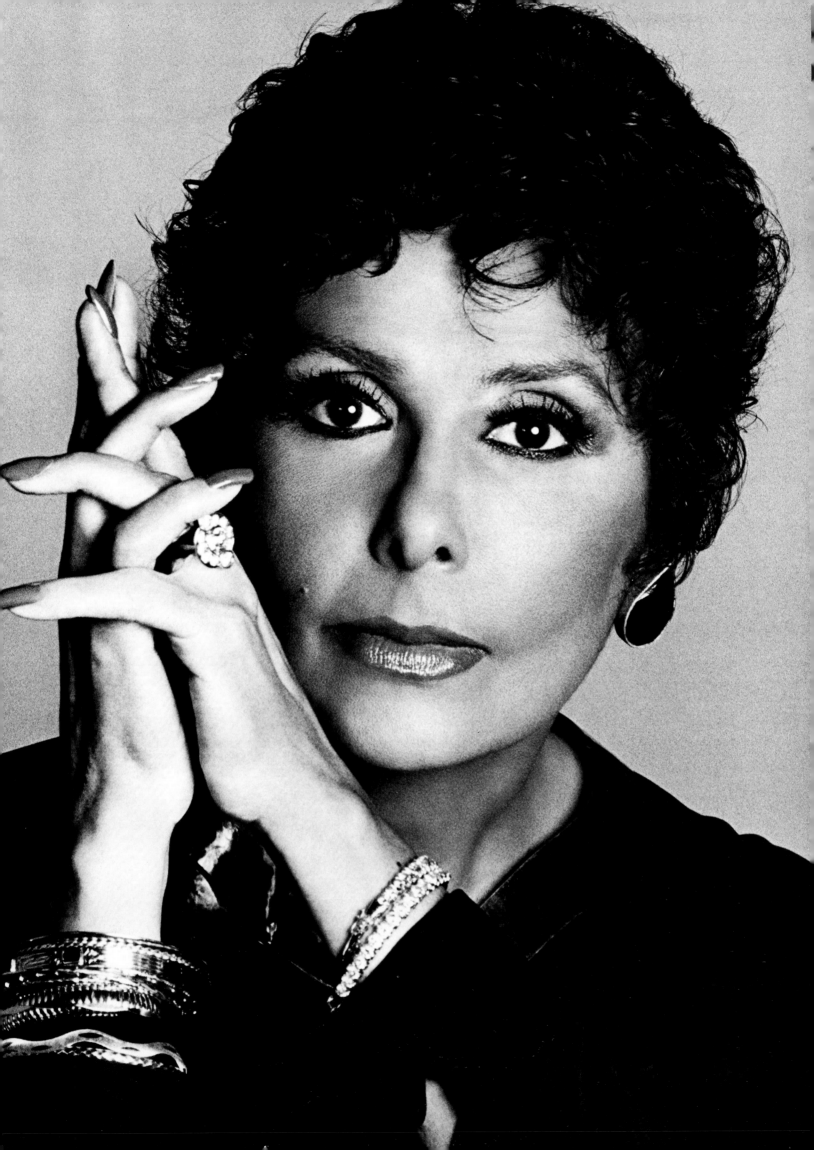

Lena Horne

South or anywhere else where a black woman's appearance on celluloid might be criticized. So when her secret marriage to Lennie Hayton was revealed in 1950—at a time when interracial marriages were a felony in most states and anathema to both races—a firestorm of controversy broke. Marrying white did not fit the image of a woman who had become a symbol of her race. For a time in the early 1950s, Lena Horne was persona non grata in the United States: Her marriage to

of a heart attack). "The pain of that opened me." That she wasn't shattered is very much a statement of her dynamic will and the fierce determination that saw her through so many times in her career.

Talking to Lena Horne about her life, the battles fought and won, the applause and adulation, the many accomplishments, the deeply loving woman shines through. Nothing gives her greater joy than her relationship with her daughter, Gail Lumet, a talented writer ("I'm somewhat in awe of her"), and being grandmother to Gail's and her late son Teddy's teenage children. When she speaks of them her face glows and her voice softens, almost purrs with pleasure. Her dreams for them and her pride in her family are obvious.

voice, as Way Bandy discovered when he did the makeup for this photograph. Way went to her dressing room at the Nederlander to make her up before a performance and, though it was a hot summer night, the air conditioning in the theater had been turned off to help protect and warm her voice; to help open her vocal cords, a steamer with eucalyptus oil was kept going in her dressing room.

Lena is a pro at doing her own makeup, and Way changed relatively little. The false eyelashes she uses for stage were replaced with fresher, more flexible sets. More shade was added around her eyes to bring them out even more, then a red for her lips (which she prefers); the tops of her cheeks were lightly highlighted, and her cheeks were warmed with rouge. With her dark, flashing eyes, striking bone structure, and flawless skin she needs only the slightest touches in hair and makeup. Even from a distance, the beauty and strength of her features are all the presence she needs. Like many truly beautiful women, Lena Horne knows that less is sometimes very much greater than more.

> "In the old days at the club, their attitude was if you weren't tan and great-looking you couldn't get it. You should have seen the girls there. Now *they* were beautiful. I was nothing more than average."

Hayton and her well-known friendship with Paul Robeson left her vulnerable during the McCarthy era, and as a result she was listed in *Red Channels* (a directory of entertainers accused of being Communist); so the Haytons went to Europe, where they remained for years. Returning to the United States in the 1960s, Lena encountered a profound change: the civil rights movement, the murder of Medgar Evers, the marches, and, above all, the rise of black consciousness—mirroring so much of her own personal struggle —opened her up, personally and professionally. Instead of the glamorous "chocolate chanteuse" in a sexy gown, she started to appear on stage casually but elegantly dressed in slacks and blouse, singing songs like "It's Not Easy Being Green," Kermit's song from *Sesame Street,* and making it a moving emotional testament for everyone who ever felt different, outside of, and apart. She made it her song.

In the early 1970s, Lena's strength was tested again. Within a thirteen-month period, "the three most important men in my life died"—her son (at thirty-one, of a kidney ailment), her father, and her husband (unexpectedly,

No doubt her family, like her millions of fans, continue to be awed by Lena. Seeing her perform these days—when she sings "Stormy Weather" you wonder how anyone else will ever dare sing it again—her talent and her beauty are more striking than ever. Her face commands your attention; she lures you with her eyes and smile; when she moves across the stage it's obvious that this woman with the stunning, lithe figure is at home with her body and herself. She doesn't smoke, drinks sparingly if at all, and dances for exercise as well as enjoyment. Her beauty regimen is simple and moderate. Although she loves the sun, she rarely goes out without a hat and sunscreen—"I freckle easily." And, not surprisingly, she pampers her

When you think of the impact this legendary woman has had and continues to have on her audiences, and on women in particular, it seems odd at first that only recently did she come to genuinely love performing; for years she did it "more to please others." Today, Lena Horne has a very sincere desire to show 'em what she can do and more . . . a new feeling of "closeness" to her audience. Which is very much what the lucky people who have seen her perform come away with—a sense of closeness, of being part of something memorable. From time to time Lena, a New Yorker by birth who still admits to "being intoxicated" by the city, speaks of retiring and spending most of her time puttering around her home in Santa Barbara or with her family. Marriage is not in the picture—"it's too demanding"—yet somehow it seems impossible to imagine this vital spirit not performing, not giving and getting that incredible exchange of love that takes place between the lady, her music, and her audience every night of her show.

Lena Horne's greatest beauty secret? The radiance that comes from being unself-conscious about her looks and the confidence of having become the best singer a woman could possibly be. She's kept growing as a person and a performer. And the spectacular result is that what's externally beautiful is more than matched by what's within. I'll say!

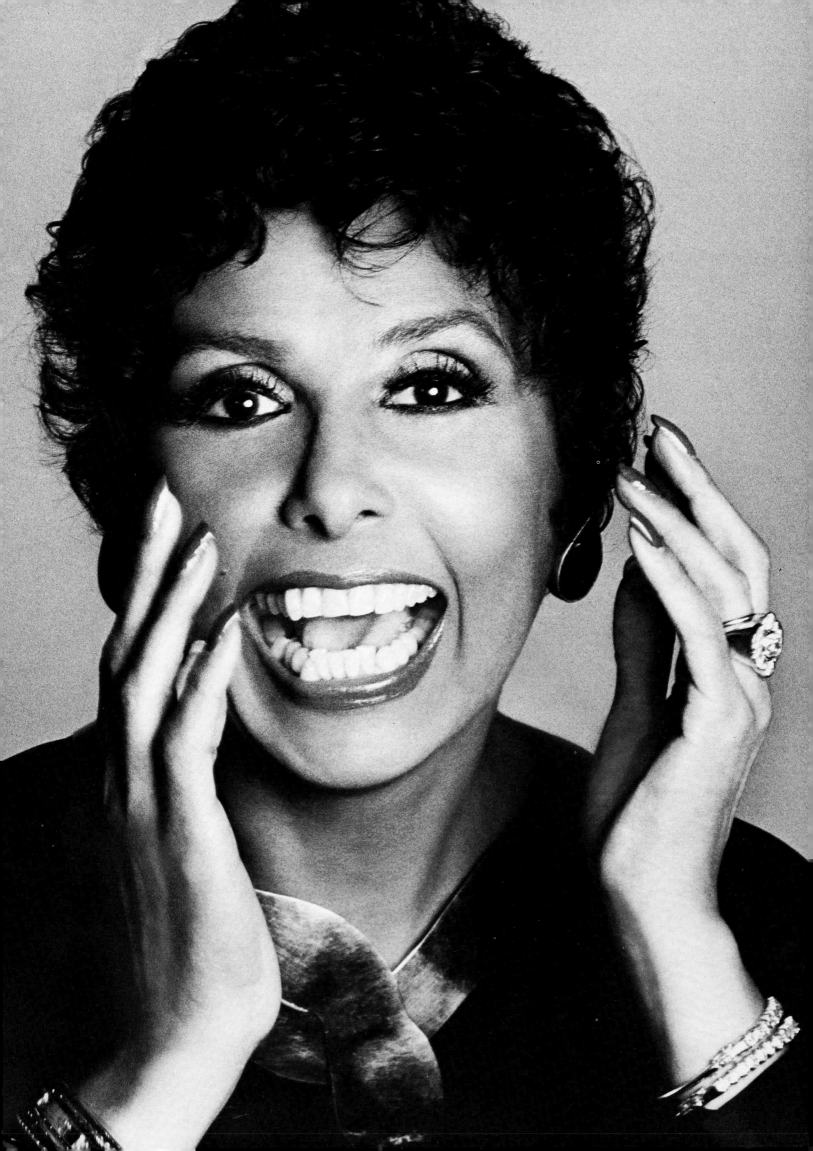

If you have a busy working life, keep your makeup and clothes quick and easy.

Norma Kamali

"I'm never into the same thing from one minute to the next. I do something, create something, and I get very excited about it. And then I want to do the next thing.... That's learning; I learn every day from what I did the day before.... I'm the type of person who always wants to break the rules and do something different."

People who only know her clothes —the exaggerated shoulders, the drapery, the parachute jumpsuits—usually assume that Norma Kamali must be some extravagantly tall, exotic space queen of a woman who, when she isn't cooking up far-out things for other far-out women to wear, is dancing off her six-inch heels in ten different discos a night. It couldn't be further from the truth. The real Norma Kamali is a little bit of a thing, five feet four inches tall, with big, beautiful brown eyes, a strong jaw, and a wistful manner.

Not only does she not make the disco scene ("I stopped about ten years ago; it wasn't fun any longer—my work became more fun"), she hardly goes out at all. ("I don't get invited anymore, because I don't go to anything. But I haven't the patience even to think of going to a party when I could be having a good time working. I'm getting more pleasure out of it than out of most movies or anything else that's supposed to be entertaining. My work is my entertainment.") What's more, if she were to go out, it wouldn't be in six-inch heels. She doesn't wear them; in fact, often she just wears sneakers. Plus, she wears her hair long. She does lots of things that short girls are told they shouldn't do (looking at Norma, you think that maybe they should), which doesn't mean she won't do something else tomorrow: "I'm never into the same thing from one minute to the next. I do something, create something, and I get very excited about it. And then I want to do the next thing. It's not that I jump from thing to thing. It's that one evolves out of the other. That's learning; I learn every day from what I did the day before. . . . I don't have rules that I feel I have to stand by, because I'm the type of person who always wants to break the rules and do something different."

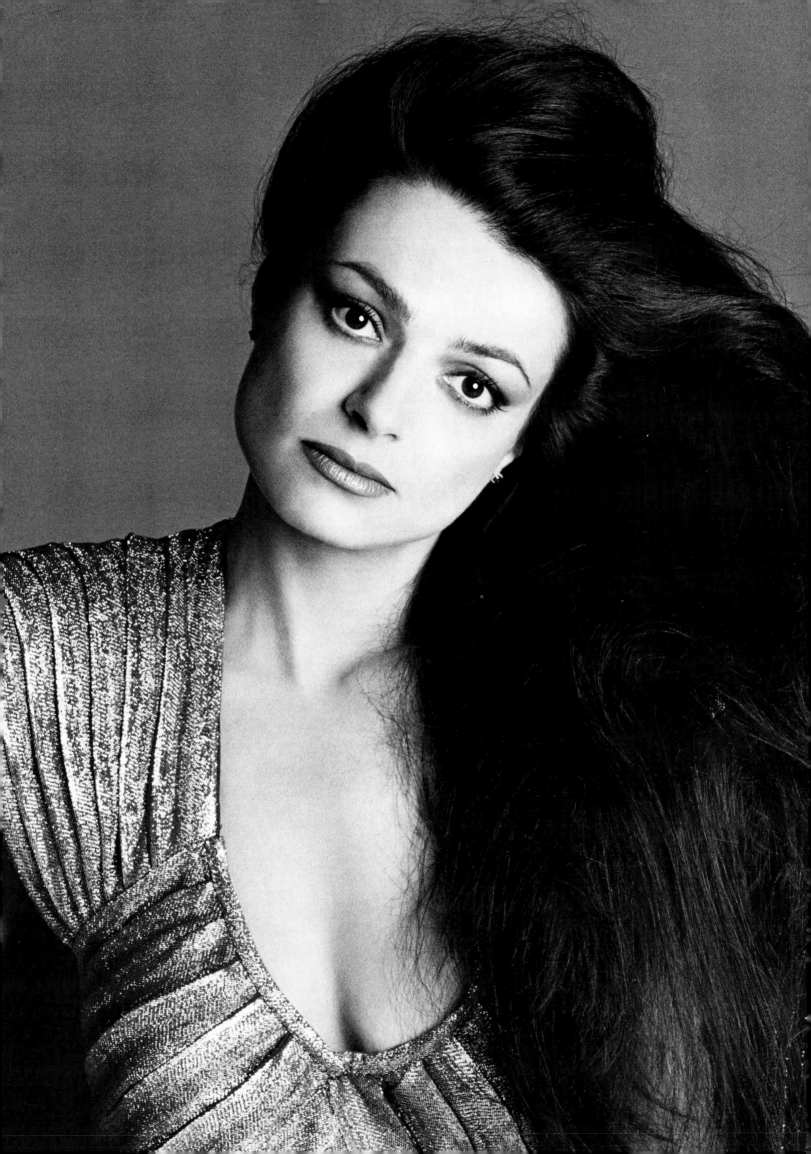

Norma
Kamali

1980

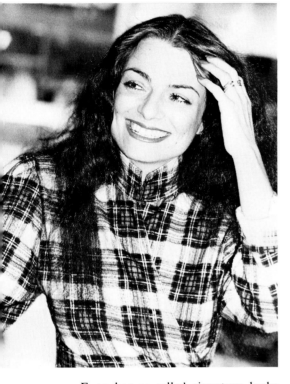

any age—"sixteen, seventeen, forty-five—and the older I get, the older they'll get. I'm thirty-five now, and there's a whole group of women my age or thereabouts who are going to go right along with me. . . . The range of prices is also wider than people tend to think. Sure, there are some very expensive things, but I don't do them in great quantities, maybe four or five, and if somebody needs something to perform in or for a special occasion, it's available to her. But a jumpsuit can be around one hundred dollars. I think very much about what a person can afford."

Doctors wear Norma Kamali. And bankers. And lawyers: "If you work in a law office, and if you prove that

may not want to draw attention to it. But if you're confident about the book, you're going to feel very good about somebody opening it up and reading it, and you're going to want an interesting cover. That's my kind of woman; she's pretty secure."

Norma isn't a militant women's-righter, but she isn't a closet feminist either: "I'm not one for going out in a crowd to try to change things. But individually, in whatever way I can, I do. I believe women are a very strong group of people who are finally coming into the light . . . into a world where they're valued."

About six years ago, Norma was divorced. She had been married for ten years: "We were both nineteen when

"I'm not alone; I am on my own!"

Even her so-called signature looks can't be counted on to be around forever. Most people, for instance, expect that On My Own, her West 56th Street shop, must be floating in parachute jumpsuits—after all, she's famous for them. But she hasn't done them for years. The one thing she has done and done (and will probably continue to do and do) are the exaggerated shoulders, which is chiefly because "I haven't got any of my own; I have the absolutely smallest shoulders in the whole world. When I was sixteen, I would Scotch-tape pads to my shoulders and then put on my clothes . . . by exaggerating the shoulders, you create a proportion with the hips; my hips aren't that big, but with no shoulders to balance them they can look big."

Another myth is that the typical Norma Kamali customer is tall, skinny, and dripping glamour—models, performers, publicity saints. Many are. Many are not: "I do clothes for me first, and I, who am practically a midget, feel very comfortable in them. They don't overpower me, and they happen also to look good on women who are tall and thin." Who wears Norma Kamali are women of any size,

you're a capable lady who can do your job as well as anybody (you probably have to prove that you can do it a little bit better), you can wear what you want. I'm not talking about low cut, with tits and ass; I'm talking about any style, any color. If your performance commands respect, why shouldn't you wear bright red if that's what you like?"

There is at least one characteristic common to Norma Kamali wearers: "They feel comfortable about expressing themselves. It's like a book cover. If there's not too much going on inside the book, or you can't express what's going on inside, or you haven't explored what's going on inside, then you may not want your book cover to be too eye-catching or too exciting; you

we got married. And being nineteen then was completely different from being nineteen now. I couldn't just go live with someone. I was a good Catholic girl; I couldn't possibly hurt my mother that way. One didn't do these things. So we got married. Two kids—we literally grew up together. And of course, we changed together, each in our own way, as growing people do. . . . Just as I hit my thirties, I began to know who I was. And I see that happening to a lot of my friends. That's why I think that if you want to get married, you should do it in your thirties. . . . I was so young. I allowed myself to be very dependent—to be given money when I needed it instead of asking for a salary [Norma and her husband were business partners for almost as long as they were married]. I can't blame him; I wanted it that way. It was that old thing of 'The man has got to take care of me,' even though I was working, I was hustling, I was holding up my end. . . .

"Still I felt that I had to be protected by the male. And that is a terrible burden to put on any man. How dare we do that to men? It's just not right. But I think it's a different world now. And

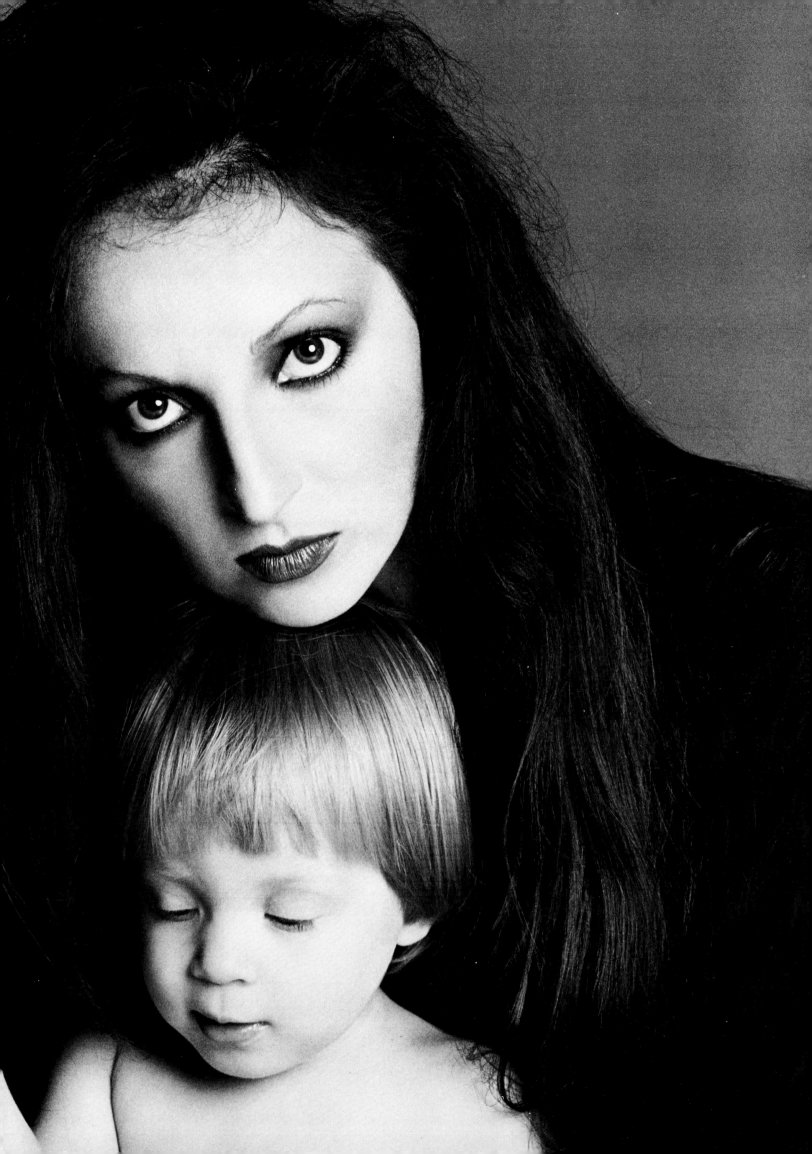

Joy Land

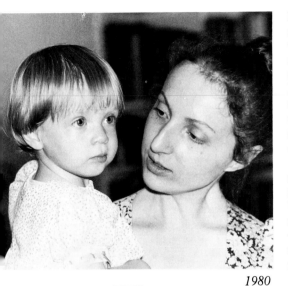

1980

both ways. Joy is an exception. Unmade-up, she is gentle, almost ethereal; with those pale, full-lidded eyes, she reminds me of a Flemish painting. ("People tell me that all the time. I have an anachronistic face; you don't see too many like it.") In the other picture, with an all-out Way Bandy makeup, she is a ripe peach—a ripe cherry. Makeup makes her blossom.

Working at the studio and watching such artists as Way taught her a lot of makeup technique: "It would have been unthinkable not to learn something, and I have built on that. I do a very stylized makeup. I don't do it with the intention of looking natural, hoping that people will say, You don't have

self; no one else has this dress, no one else does with it what I do. . . . I feel better if I have a very pulled-together look. I also feel that it is appreciated if you look special when you go somewhere; you honor your host if you get yourself together in a special way. It appeals to my sense of romance. . . . I love silks and other beautiful fabrics. I adore very expensive, very high-heeled shoes."

I wasn't at all surprised when Joy told me she had worn four-inch heels when she went to the hospital in labor. Or that she had shaved her legs before she left the house. Or that she had gained only four pounds and didn't have to wear maternity clothes. Or

—

"I eat next to nothing. More and more, I incline to vegetarianism, although I am not a vegetarian."

—

Joy Land is one of the most together women I know. Until she got pregnant, she was my studio manager. She handled the bookings, the billings, the correspondence, the temperament. She is fluent in Italian and French, which she once taught (when we began to get European clients, she spoke French with the French-speaking ones, Italian with the Italians). She is a Cordon Bleu cook, who has free-lanced for restaurants and caterers; I have never eaten so well as I did when she was here and used to fix us all lunch. No fuss, no kitchen hysterics. . . . In a crackpot world, she is an island of calm—efficient, collected, always groomed to the teeth (she says she has gone to the supermarket in her bathrobe; I can't even imagine it—unless her bathrobe is a Saint Laurent dressing gown, perfectly tailored and made of cashmere).

These photographs with her daughter Dawn were done a week before Joy's thirtieth birthday ("The camera froze me in time forever at twenty-nine"), and they point up something quite unusual: In nine cases out of ten, women who look marvelous with makeup don't without it. And vice versa: A woman who can go around with a naked face rarely looks as well with makeup. Seldom is anyone good

any makeup on. I don't want to look outlandish, but I definitely do like to paint my face. I henna my hair so that it has an auburn cast—I hate when people don't admit to coloring their hair. My natural color is a pale brown. I think the reddish color is more appealing. And I like the look of fair skin, so I paint myself fairly white. I do a tawny or violet eye, with browns and pinks blended together to get a shadowy effect. I would never put just a color—blue or green or anything like that—on my eyes. And I do a fairly defined mouth."

She is not the kind of woman who feels that to not give attention to one's appearance—or to pretend not to—is somehow an indication of high-mindedness: "Personal style interests me, developing something that is uniquely my own—perhaps something that might have a bit of timelessness about it. I don't mind looking the same all the time, as long as it works for me."

Joy's style is not punked-out, ratty-skatty, or bits-and-pieces: "I love extravagant clothes. My great weaknesses are Chlöe and Saint Laurent. I spend an awful lot of money on clothes, and I have a good wardrobe. It's important to me, because it's something I do for myself. It is privately and exactly for me, one of my expressions of

that, although her husband drove her to the hospital, she sent him off to his office almost as soon as they got there —as had been planned: "I think sitting downstairs in the hospital is the lowest; if you are not participating, best just get out. We had discussed it all, and it didn't bother me that he didn't want to be present in the delivery room. I think it would have destroyed forever his romantic image of me."

Joy exercised throughout her pregnancy; before that, she ran as well. Now, there never seems to be time; so, mainly, "I just diet. Stringently. I eat next to nothing. More and more, I incline to vegetarianism, although I am not a vegetarian. I would certainly eat meat if I were a guest at someone's house, and I serve meat to my husband. But I find that a vegetarian diet makes me feel more alert. And it's good for the skin; my skin has better tone." Her skin is lovely: "Mostly, I just try to keep it clean. And I drink a lot of water; I do think that makes a difference. Also, I frequently have a fast day. A fast day does miracles for everything. If you have an inclination toward a double chin, just fast for a day, and you'll get this nice tight chin. It really helps a lot . . . it makes the whites of your eyes clearer, for instance.

"My very favorite skin treatment is

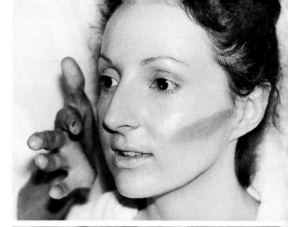

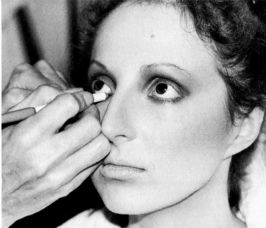

1. Dark contour to slenderize face
2. Pencil full length of eye for deep effect
3. Beige eyebrow pencil to arch brow
4. Use pencil to build mouth shape
5. Bright color to balance mouth and eyes

a mask that I learned from Way Bandy. It's made from yogurt—about one quarter of a cup—and about a teaspoon of honey, blended together with the yolk of an egg. The recipe is enough for five masks—you need only the tiniest portion at a time—but it keeps in the refrigerator. You let it harden on your face, and after it's been on a while, you wash it off with tepid water. I like to follow it with a citrus- or cucumber-based astringent. Afterwards, your skin is very, very tight and silky. It's not greasy, but it shines—it has a glow. Mind you, I don't use this mask every day; I wish I did. But if I know a week in advance that I've got something important coming up, I use it religiously. . . . I don't go for facials. I have never been to a skin-care center. As far as I am concerned, all those seventy-dollar bottles from Dior and Estée Lauder are absolutely no better than this yogurt mask, which breaks down to about nineteen cents a treatment."

Joy was twenty-eight when Dawn was born and had been married for nine years. A baby wasn't on the agenda, "out of selfishness. I adored being free. At times, I would travel by myself. And I enjoyed the life we had in New York. We used to go out almost every night. We went to the opera. We went to the ballet. We went to the most divine restaurants. We really weren't accountable to anyone. A baby changes that so much. The thought of what it involved was just staggering to me. Some women seem to have a very carefree attitude about bringing up children, but I felt that if I were going to do this thing, I would try to do it right.

I think that the responsibility for all the phases of rearing a child and seeing the whole thing out for as long as you have to is almost a lifetime project. I felt, and I continue to feel very strongly, the responsibility of having a child, and I assume willingly the responsibility for my child's life. No matter what else I might go on to do, I think that what I do with Dawn now

could possibly be the most important thing I do in my life."

As mothers have wished from time immemorial, Joy would like her child "to grow up in flowers . . . never to feel pain, never to be hurt." More realistically: "If I could instill one thing in her, it would be a sense of the dignity of all people. I try to treat her with dignity; I would no more hit her than I would shoot her. Treating people well is incredibly important to me. . . . My secret fantasy for her is that she will grow up to be very, very beautiful. And I hope that what I'm trying to do with her now will teach her that being beautiful is not a license to act without conscience, as I've seen so many beautiful people do.

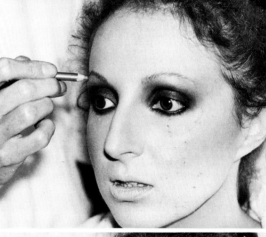

"I have an anachronistic face; you don't see too many like it."

"People adore beautiful people. We all gravitate to them. And people who are exceptionally good-looking often take advantage of that and treat other people shabbily. They get away with it, because the others want to bask in that aura of beauty and so they keep coming back for more. If you are beautiful, I think you have an extra responsibility to behave with conscience and kindness to others."

While she would not go so far as to dismiss any link between physical beauty and beauty of the spirit—"my Catholic education makes the concept of a good person or a living saint extremely appealing to me"—she does not buy the idea that good is automatically beautiful and attractive. She quotes a friend who was told this bromide, and who replied, "If you really believe that—well, you know, Eleanor Roosevelt was a widow for more than twenty years. Why didn't you call her up and ask her to go out with you?" To Joy, it is a simple, non-negotiable fact: "Beauty is one of the most tremendous graces a person could have. If you have even a little bit of it, you should nurture it . . . and be proud of it . . . and be enormously happy that you've got it."

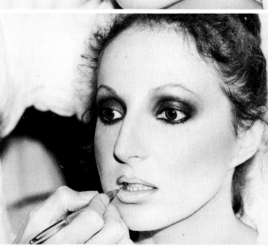

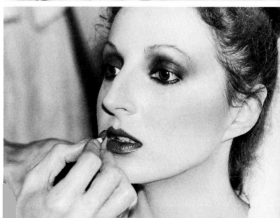

A glamorous, sultry look that works for a professional woman

Janet Langhart

Whenever I watched Janet Langhart on television—she was co-anchor on *A.M. New York* and *Sunday Night New York* and interviewer/reporter on *America Alive!*, and she had her own show, *Good Day!*, in Boston, and a new one there called *Sunday Night Open House*—one thing about her always bugged me: Here was a stunningly good-looking woman masquerading as a merely pretty one.

To me, it seemed typical TV-think: women journalists and talk-show hosts must be neat, attractive, and wholesome; glamour makes female viewers feel insecure and male viewers faintly uneasy. Not me; as far as I'm concerned, the Janet I'd like to see coming into my living room is the one with the come-hither eyes and the Egyptian-princess hair.

It isn't that her hair is hideous the other way, just ordinary and sort of cutesy—it makes her look like the girl next door. And why settle for the girl next door when you can be the Queen of Sheba? I wanted her to look the way the girl next door would sell her soul to look—drop-dead glamorous, like Dolores Del Rio.

I wanted to see her with hair that would finally let that beautiful forehead and fine bone structure come through. Not only did Andre Douglas's sleek-to-the-head, wet-looking waves do the trick, it showed Janet that she didn't really need that mass of hair

around her face: "One of the big things this sitting taught me was to wear my hair more naturally. Now, a lot of the time, I just pull it all back and off the face, and maybe allow some of my ear to show."

Janet is makeup-smart, but she had been making one crucial error: Because she felt—mistakenly—that "my eyes are drab; they don't jump out," she rarely went anywhere, and not ever on television, without fake lashes, which —never mind that they didn't look quite believable—were actually distorting the shape of her eyes.

As John Richardson, who did her makeup, pointed out, "The bands on these lashes are so strong that they can do weird things to the eyes. In Janet's case, they were bending the lid in such a way as to make her eyes look rectangular. What you have to do is to grip the band between your thumb and index finger and with your free hand take a little tiny manicure scissors—closed—and scrape the non-cutting edge over it. This way, you reinforce the curve of the band so that it doesn't form odd shapes of its own."

Then, having shown her the right way to do fake lashes, he proceeded to show her how to do without them forever. First—not to be visible, but to give a sheen and definition to the eye—he outlined in blue. And on top of the blue—in the lash and over the lash and inside the eye, on the lower rim—he put a smudge of kohl liner all around. Plus mascara on the lashes, tops and bottoms. . . . What a difference! People don't always put their finger on it, but they know something has changed: "I was with some friends who had never seen me without fake lashes, and one of them said, 'What did you do to your face? You look different.' I was kind of embarrassed, so I just said I hadn't put on my makeup. And she said, 'I wasn't

complaining; I meant good-different. You look so much softer and younger.' Everybody has been saying that."

Actually, it takes more makeup (and more skill!) to do Janet's eyes without fake lashes than with. It just looks like less: "A key thing I learned from this is that you have to put on a lot of makeup to look as if you don't have any on. That is, you start with what seems like a lot, and then keep toning it down and blending it out . . . and toning and blending . . . and toning and blending. It's a switch on 'Less is more.'"

Janet is as quick on the pickup as anyone I know; she can take what she learns from a pro like John and turn it her own way. For instance, because he feels that foundations made for black women often tend to go gray on the skin, he likes to liven them up by mixing in a little red or orange or yellow, even white or black. With Janet, he used a bronze-y foundation, and first—to get rid of her under-eye shadows, as well as to give a lift to the whole eye area—he mixed it with a dab of pearlized yellow powder and blended it all around her eyes. To highlight the lids, he mixed the foundation with white pearlized powder and with a dab of red cream to liven up the color for the rest of her face.

"You have to put on a lot of makeup to look as if you don't have any on."

The Janet Langhart version: "For daytime and evening, when I call myself 'dressed,' what I do is to put moisturizer on first, to give my face a little sheen; then I put Erase all around the eye—up to the eyebrow, out to the cheekbone, into the inner corner. Next, I use something called Indian Earth, which I get at Bloomingdale's. It comes in a clay pot with a little puff and a cork. And you take the color—it's a sort of earthy, ruddy, henna color—right off the cork with the puff and spread it over your face. There are flecks in it, and these seem to work like natural highlights; the standout areas of your face, like the cheekbones, just glisten. So I don't have to wear all that much rouge anymore, which I always thought looked a little phony. I mean, here I was trying to look as though I had a natural blush. And black women rarely do.

"Occasionally, when I'm *really* dressing—when I'm judging the Miss

Janet Langhart

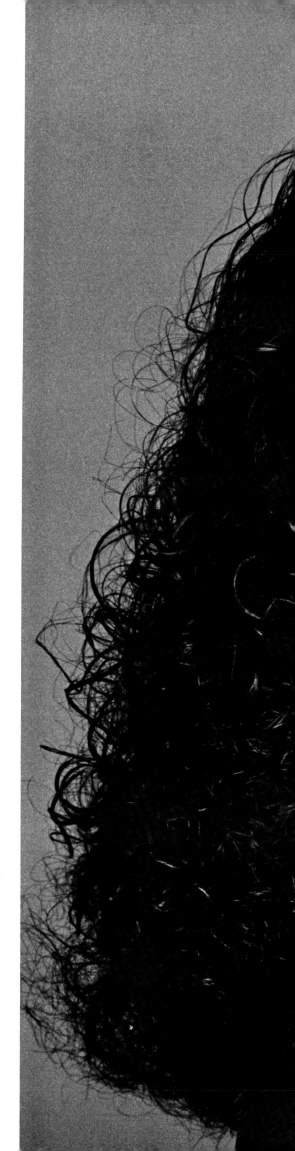

America Pageant, for example—I'll use a foundation. For one thing, even though I have fairly good skin, foundation gives a look of perfection. For another, the Indian Earth is easier to smooth on over foundation. The one I like is Revlon's Natural Wonder—the water-based kind seems to cover most evenly—in a shade called Honey Bronze. Also for something major, like the pageant, I put yellow eye shadow in the crease of my eye, and I rub it and rub it and rub it, so that it's all very subtle and natural-looking. There's just enough—along with the kohl liner—to bring out the brown of my eyes."

Janet has been a Miss America judge three years in a row. If you ask her for a general profile of the contestants, she'll tell you, "They all have wonderful posture, great skin, terrific smiles, average IQs, extraordinary ambition, and they're heavily into ultrasuede." It isn't meant as a put-down. "Initially, I felt that the pageant was racist, sexist, and corny. But when I got in there, I became an instant convert. I thought, Where else can a young woman get this much money? I looked at their backgrounds, and they're not kinkies that come out of rural areas and just want to show off in center spreads. These young women are proud of themselves; they don't see anything wrong with competing in a swimsuit. What they see is that other young women who have done it have gone on to do things in medicine and in show business. And what other outlet do they have?"

That there are so few black contestants doesn't especially disturb her—or rather, it disturbs her less than the conflicting emotions she has had when black girls have been up for the prize, wanting desperately to vote for them and equally determined not to compromise her own integrity. "I remember asking Miss Connecticut, 'When you saw me, did you feel that you had an easy shot, that I would be more lenient?' And she said, 'No; as a matter of fact, I thought you'd be harder on me.' She was absolutely right. I *am*

more critical. Because the young woman that I would want to be the first Miss America who just happened to be black would be so outstanding as to be almost flawless. At least up to the standards of the best white girls."

Janet has a double perspective on beauty contests, having, in the sixties, picked up a few titles of her own—Miss Chicago and Miss Sepia, among others: "I was constantly entering, because, one, it was a way to get attention if you wanted to be a model and, two, it was a way to get additional revenue, which I needed, because I was intending to go back to college. I did go back for one more year, but the modeling got so good in Chicago, I thought, Gee, I can make a lot more money as a model than as a schoolteacher. . . ." (P.S.: She has gone back to school; in New York, where she keeps a small apartment, she is taking courses in economics and speech dynamics.)

Her permanent residence is in Milton, a suburb of Boston, where she lives with her husband, Robert Kistner, a gynecological surgeon, writer, and professor, who was one of the team of doctors responsible for the development of the contraceptive pill. They met as doctor and patient. He was a recent widower, with grown children and young grandchildren. She, divorced, childless, and planning to stay that way, was on the first solid rung of her career with the *Good Day!* show in Boston.

Three years ago, when they were married, she was working and living in New York, which, in a part-time way, she has continued to do—an arrangement that is less estranging than it might appear, when you consider their separate careers and individual time clocks. He keeps surgeon's hours, early to bed and up at five. She can't sleep if she goes to bed before one or two. (To relax, "I just kind of wear myself out. If I'm lying in bed trying to sleep, I can see all the dust accumulating in the room. So I get up and clean. I scrub the floors, polish the furniture, Windex the glass.")

Still, at least on the surface, they might seem an odd couple: the prominent-physician son of a prominent physician, and the Baptist minister's daughter, whose father abandoned the family when she was seven, and whose mother went to work as a domestic to support Janet and her younger sister and brother. Not to mention that Janet is thirty-eight and black, Bob sixty-five and white. . . . To ask how come such a marriage of opposites works like a dream is about the same as asking, How can a marriage fall apart when the partners are of matching backgrounds, matching ages, and matching colors? It sometimes just happens that way.

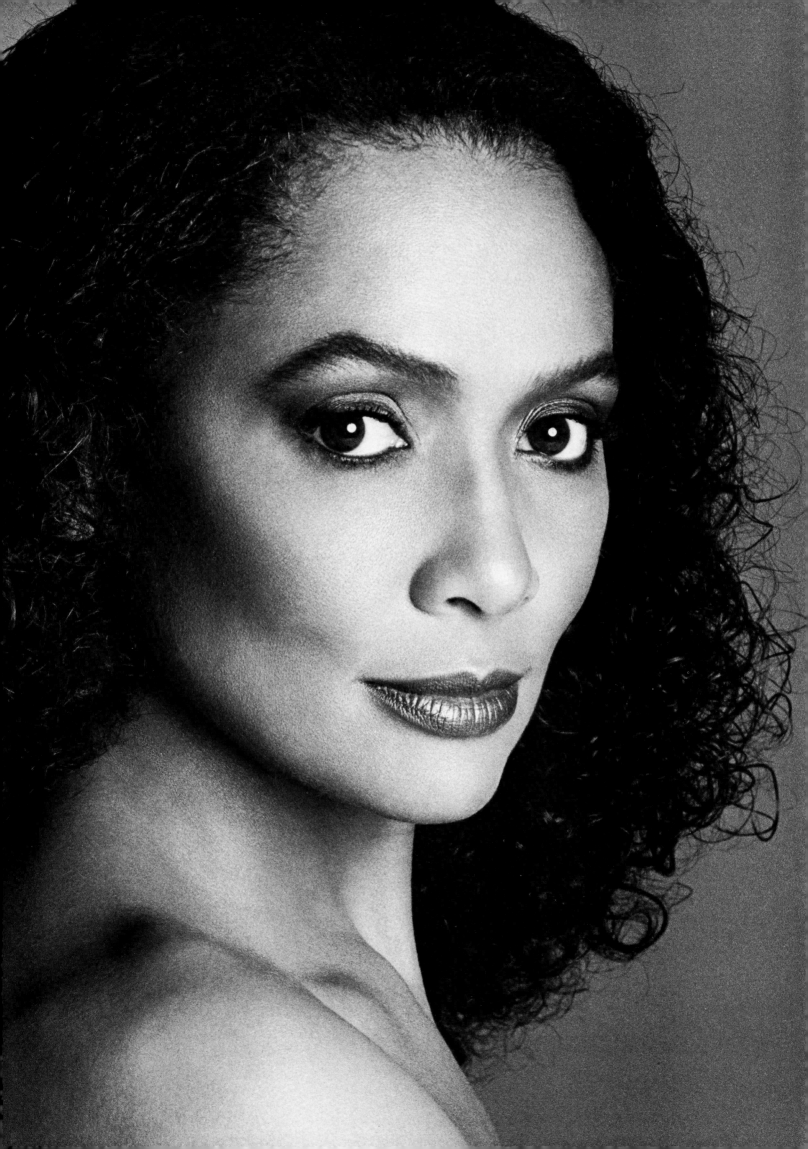

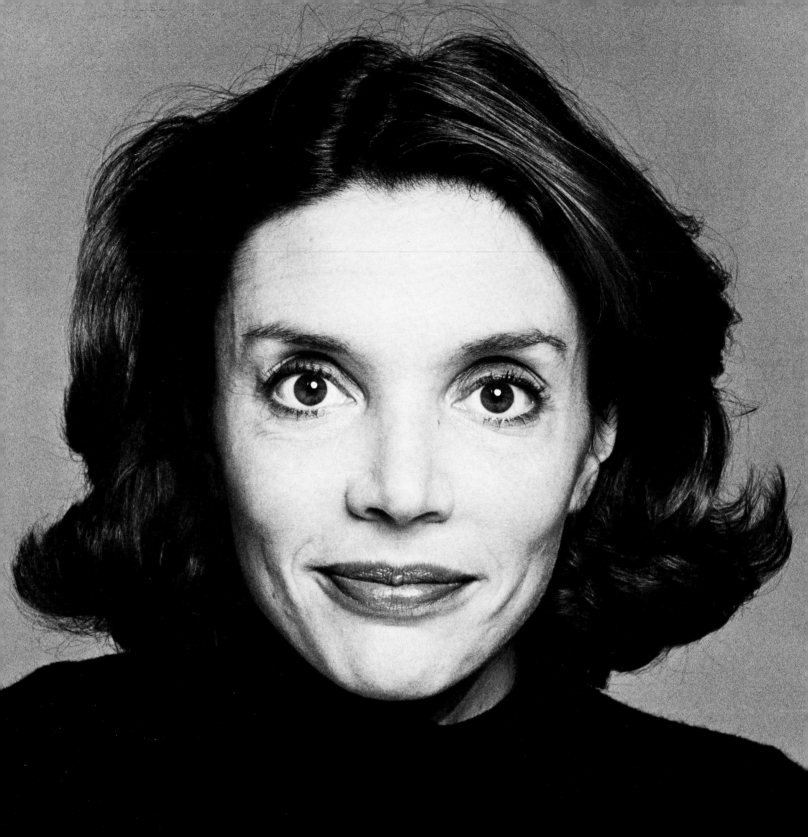

Judy Licht

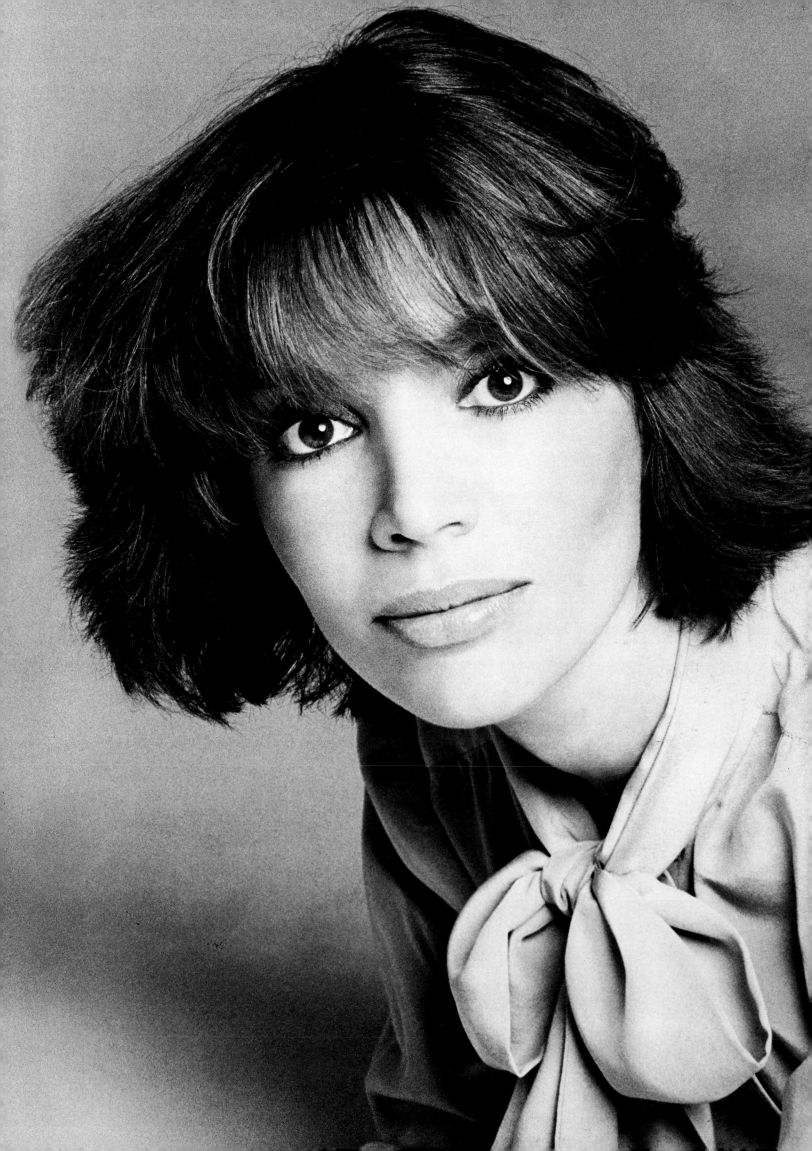

Judy Licht

"My eyes are good, but I really love my mouth. It's big, but I love that it's big. . . . I don't believe in blandness. I believe, if you have something, go with it. I'd like a big chest but I don't have it. I have a mouth!"

Judy Licht, the Brenda Starr of the Channel 5 ten o'clock news, is a five-foot-four-inch firecracker, smart, feisty, and fast on her feet. Standing still, she seems to be running. She writes, edits, produces, reports. She covers Senate hearings, strikes ("when you've covered one labor confrontation, you've covered them all"), murders, elections, fires (ditto), actors ("my least favorite interviews—self-absorption makes you intolerably boring to talk to"), fashion ("I don't see it as back-of-the-book fluff stuff. To me, if I'm going to spend eight or ten hours on the job, I'd rather do it with things that are beautiful, that really distill the essence of a time. I think you can tell as much about a time from fashion—from style—as you can from hard news. It's part of history . . . the history of pleasure")—she covers everything.

▬

"Laughing and sex are in a tied position for things I like."

▬

She has covered a dancing bear: "The trainer thought it would be cute if I danced with the bear; 'All you have to do,' he said, 'is to give him some soda pop and Frito-Lays.' Well, the bear just grabs the Frito-Lays, lies down on the floor, and starts rubbing the damn things all over himself. . . . I hate animal acts!" She has covered me doing a fashion sitting . . . out of which came this portrait.

What I wanted most of all to do with Judy was to relax her. Plus, she needed a good haircut and a soft, soft makeup. So we gave her an easy-breezy Harry King Special. And Way Bandy did a lovely moist, natural-looking makeup, paling out her mouth to bring up her eyes—her best feature, I think. She doesn't: "My eyes are good, but I really love my mouth. It's big, but I love that it's big. My news director used to say, 'Wear lighter lipstick; your mouth fills up the entire screen!' And I said, 'I know, isn't it terrific?' . . . I don't believe in balance. I believe, if you have something, go with it. I'd like a big chest but I don't have it. I have a mouth!''

In a spoofy beauty article for the *Daily News,* Judy listed as the ultimate beauty tip: "Start saving for a face lift." She wasn't joking. "I've thought about whether I would do it when I get older. I think I'm gonna. It's funny. People have these incredibly strong principles about not. . . . Bette Davis was doing a show, and she was adamant about not having any cosmetic surgery or hair coloring. But she flew in this makeup artist just to apply those tape lifts all over. Then she put on a blond wig, so that when she appeared, it was as if she had the face lift and the hair coloring. . . . I don't understand why faking it is better than doing it."

At thirty-three, however ("your typical urban career woman, in her thirties, neurotic, the type everyone is writing a book about"), Judy is just beginning to enjoy the face she has: "My ex-husband once told me—and I think it's absolutely true—people don't have faces until they're in their thirties. You don't grow into your face till then . . . it begins to take on definition, and your character starts showing. I suppose people who don't have a lot going on in their lives don't like the way they start to look. But if you're happy with yourself and with what you're doing, you're going to look better than you did in your twenties. I think I do."

"People don't have faces until they're in their thirties."

She is reasonably concerned with conventional beauty care: She watches her weight ("When you're little and gain three pounds, it's like a bigger person gaining twenty"), she has started to exercise ("I have a lady who comes to me, which sounds fantastically indulgent, but it works out to about the same as the better gym classes. . . . I would always find an excuse for not going to classes, even if I had paid in advance. I don't have that kind of discipline"), and she has taken makeup lessons ("Way taught me enough so that I could do it, sort of . . . basically, I'm just terrible with makeup").

All these efforts help, but they are only scratching the surface; to Judy,

the real secret of looking good—looking better than good, looking downright sensational!—is: "Falling in love. Now, making love is one thing, falling in love is another. Making love is merely related to circulation and muscle tone. Falling in love, however, gives you a twinkle in your eye. Optimally, if you're lucky, you can do both. And that is the best. . . . What else is terrific is to have around you the kinds of people who really get off on you. I have a friend, a male friend who is really just

a friend, who I know likes the way I look and the way I am. And when I spend time with him, I know I look prettier. It's a stimulus/response kind of thing. Most men don't understand how important compliments are. . . . When somebody praises you, when it's sincere and not just BS, you almost live up to the praise. You glow from inside because it makes you happy, and your muscles relax. I know I have looked really terrific on nights when I haven't had enough sleep or haven't been eating well. . . . If I'm surrounded by people who I know really like me or like the way I look, or who I sense care about me and have a good time with me, my muscles relax, I feel vibrant, and I look better.

"Conversely, you can do everything right in the world—get the right amount of sleep, the right amount of sun, the right amount of food—and if you're insecure about the way someone feels about you, you're tense. Your muscles are tense, and your reactions are hyper; you're *trying.* And you never look as good with that person as you do with other people."

Her other major—crucial—beauty aid is: "Laughter. If I can't laugh hard twice a day, I look crummy. Laughing and sex are in a tied position for things I like. . . . I went through a few years when I really didn't laugh a lot. Things weren't terrible; they just weren't terrific. And one day it hit me: 'I haven't been laughing very hard lately.' That's when I got separated, and that's when I changed jobs—I did big things about

it. And I had been successful. I had a good job that paid good money. I had a marriage to a man who was respected and who loved me and who was wonderful and terrific. I just wasn't laughing a lot; obviously, my life was not giving me enough pleasure. The year after that was just incredibly crummy. Now I'm sort of back. But I know that if it's been a week when I haven't laughed a couple of times a day, it's no good. And I'm not going to look good."

"Making love is merely related to circulation and muscle tone. Falling in love, however, gives you a twinkle in your eye."

What makes Judy laugh is "almost anything. Mainly, it's the company of people that I enjoy talking to. Because life is such fun, anyway. Life provides the laughter. Life provides the jokes. It's just somebody to share them with."

For the moment, Judy lives alone in a sleek, modern, hotel-efficient West Side flat, which suits her sense of being at a transition in her life. An "old funky apartment" would be more her style. And her distant dream is "a big house in the country, with lots of kids and dogs and cats"—the classic fantasy of a city child (Judy is from Brooklyn) who grew up without brothers, sisters, or pets. Once, when she was very young, she brought home a cat; her mother "was absolutely phobic." Suddenly, remembering the incident, Judy has a flash of insight—it dawns on her that she knows why Jewish mothers don't like cats: "Because you can't make a cat feel guilty!" And she goes right up and over her hard-laugh daily quota . . . her muscles relax . . . her face glows . . . her eyes twinkle. She looks great.

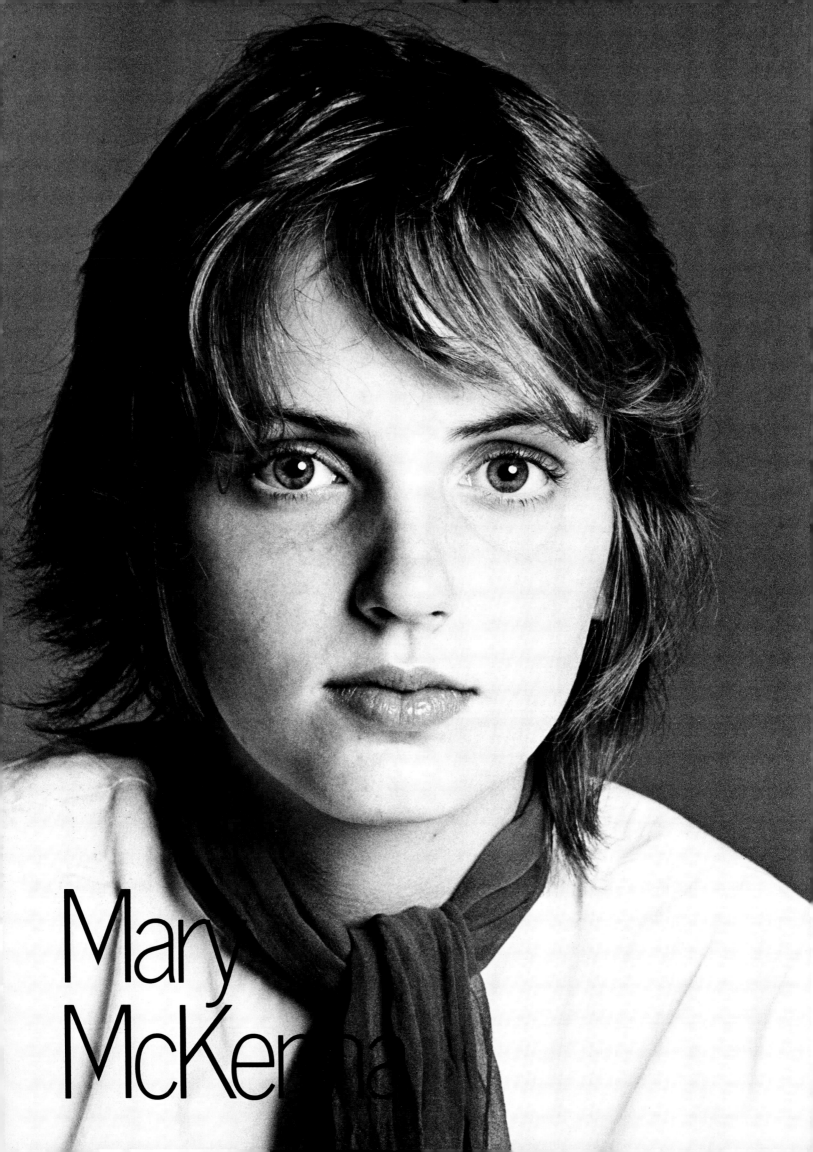

Mary
McKenna

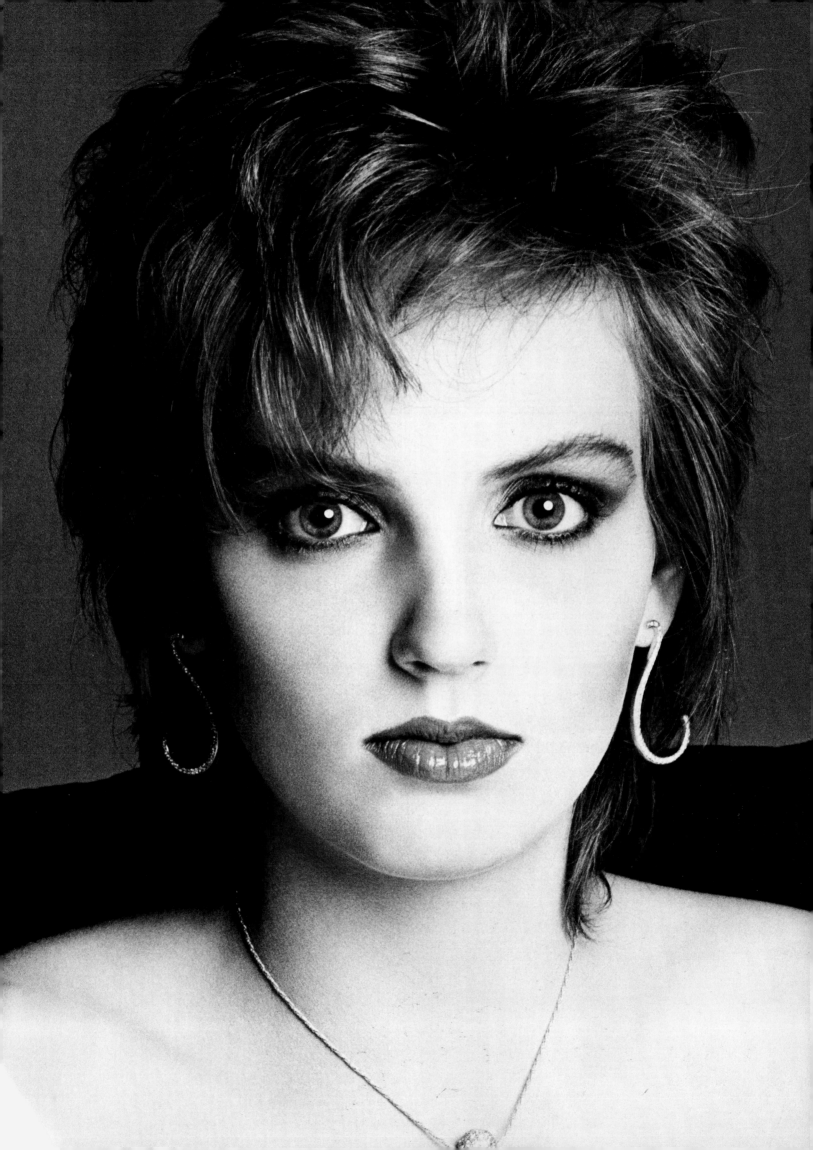

Mary McKenna

"I enjoy wearing makeup. And when I wear it, I *wear* it. I don't like sneaky makeup. I don't like to pretend that I don't have anything on when I'm really wearing ten pounds of foundation. I wonder about people who do wear sneaky makeup. Maybe they feel that wearing makeup is cheating."

f I've said it once, I've said it a thousand times: Hot new modeling prospects don't just come off the street, off the public transit, or over the transom. It just ain't gonna happen that way.... So here is Mary McKenna, age fifteen, whipped off the steps of the Metropolitan Museum of Art, into the studio, and onto the cover of German *Vogue.*

Mary, at the time a high school sophomore at the Marymount School, was on her lunch hour. And here is how this properly Catholic-educated, first-generation Irish-American girl was dressed: bright purple silk pants and black cashmere sweater, over the neck of which spilled layers of purple chiffon ruffles; her mouth was purple, her nails were purple, her eyes were outlined in purple, and her hair looked as though she shook it out every morning and just rumpled it around with her fingers. Don't ask how this went down with the nuns (a clue: the year Mary graduated, uniforms were reinstated at Marymount), but she knocked me out. At fifteen, she had more style in her little purple-tipped finger than a lot of women grasp in a lifetime. Also she was—as she is now, at seventeen—a beautiful girl, with huge green eyes and white translucent skin like the inside of a camellia petal. Put this together with a luscious little Marilyn Monroe mouth, and you've got quite a dish.

"I'm not just another face in the crowd. My looks are dramatic."

There was nothing I wanted to change in her makeup; the idea was to make the most of everything. Even her hair was basically right. All it really needed—and got, from Harry King—was a good shaping. And there were no flaws to correct or camouflage with makeup; maybe a little shading down the sides of the nose to give it a tiny bit more definition, but that was it. As makeup man John Richardson said, "With this one, you want to show off everything."

He did. To make her skin even whiter and more luminous, he mixed in a smidge of pearlized white powder with the lightest foundation and dusted it with Johnson's Baby Powder. Then he went to lavenders—lavender being a natural undertone of very white skin— adding lots of pearlized colors for sheen. On the lids, he used pinky lavender tones; to outline the eyes, a mix of lavender and black, which gives a deep, blackish-purple effect but softer than if you used either color alone. The mouth is outlined and filled in with shiny, pinky lavender. And right in the middle of the lower lip, he put a voluptuous little "dimple"—actually a dab of lavender-red, just touched on.

"I tend to be suspicious of people's feelings about me, especially men: Is it really me they like, or the way I look?"

This was the first year Mary had worn makeup, and she jumped on new ideas. Before the sitting, for instance, she hadn't used eye shadow: "I'd wear a heavy purple liner, but no shadow; since my eyes are so deep-set, I felt I didn't need it. But when I saw myself! Now I wear purple eyeliner, plus purple eye shadow with some pink blended in, and pink cheeks and pink lipstick—bright pink. . . . I enjoy wearing makeup. And when I wear it, I *wear* it. I don't like sneaky makeup. I don't like to pretend that I don't have any-

thing on when I'm really wearing like ten pounds of foundation. I wonder about people who do wear sneaky makeup. Maybe they feel that wearing makeup is cheating. It's like if you tell someone she looks lovely, she doesn't want to say, 'Oh, well, it's only because of this nice, wonderful jar of gook.' They want you to think they don't need makeup, but it's usually pretty obvious that they've got it on."

In the sixties, Marymount switched from a policy of uniforms to dress code. But at the parochial school Mary attended for the first eight grades, uniforms were the rule. Now, there's something to be said for uniforms. Some people (as the Chinese have reason to know) consider them a great leveler. And some people find them a blessing—no agonizing over when to shop, what to buy, what to wear. But with others, you put them in a uniform, and it's like corking champagne; when you finally pull that cork, everything goes *whoosh!* Mary is a *whoosh*er. "When I dress I like to have fun with it. I like to inspire with it. Any form of art should be an inspiration. And my art—my personal art—is my life, how I live. Being me means to express myself, and to enjoy myself through what I do. And if I enjoy dressing in bright colors, I find it restricting to have to wear gray. Why shouldn't I be allowed to wear purple or fuchsia or wine or black? Occasionally, I would go to school completely in black. The nuns didn't go for that very much; my English teacher called me the Lady in Black. . . . The way I feel is this: If I look good, I feel good. Sometimes, if it's just not my day, I'll get out of bed, shake myself up, put on clothes that I like, put on some makeup, tousle my hair. And that cheers me up!"

On the whole, Mary likes the way

she looks. "I think I look good. I'm not just another face in the crowd. My looks are dramatic—the big eyes, and the bone structure is rather elegant in that it's pure. My nose doesn't have a whole lot of definition, which is nice, because I don't particularly care for noses. . . . Very often, the way I look causes problems; I'll be walking home, just wanting to be left alone, and a bunch of men will hoot at me. That sort of thing drives me up the wall. . . . I tend to be suspicious of people's feelings about me, especially men: Is it really me they like, or the way I look? Also the other way around; I think some people will dislike me because of how I look."

It happens. Three years ago, when she was visiting relatives in Ireland, she walked into a wall of teenage resentment. "They were still wearing pants that came up to *here* and were *this* wide, and I showed up in tight, straight-legged jeans. And I smoked. I'd go into a phone booth to make a call, and this whole pack of boys, ranging in age from about seven to seventeen, would march around in a clump outside, saying, 'Who's the girl with the cancer stick?' over and over. They used to follow me around the town on bicycles, and come by the house where we were staying, and scream things in the window to embarrass me. And it wasn't as if I were being really outrageous, the way I can be here; they should have seen me walking down the street in New York, in my black satin baseball jacket that says, in big red letters on the back, PANTHERS!"

Mary strikes a lot of people as outrageous: She smokes; she drinks a little wine and beer; she has been going to underground punk-rock clubs since the age of thirteen; and she may be the only high-school senior in America with a yearbook picture by Scavullo. On the other hand, she draws seriously; she pulled top grades in calculus; her idea of a good read is Baudelaire; and her record at Marymount was impressive enough to get her accepted by every college she applied to. With an eye to a career at a magazine, she chose the Fashion Institute of Technology. I say, give her ten years or so, and she'll own *Vogue*!

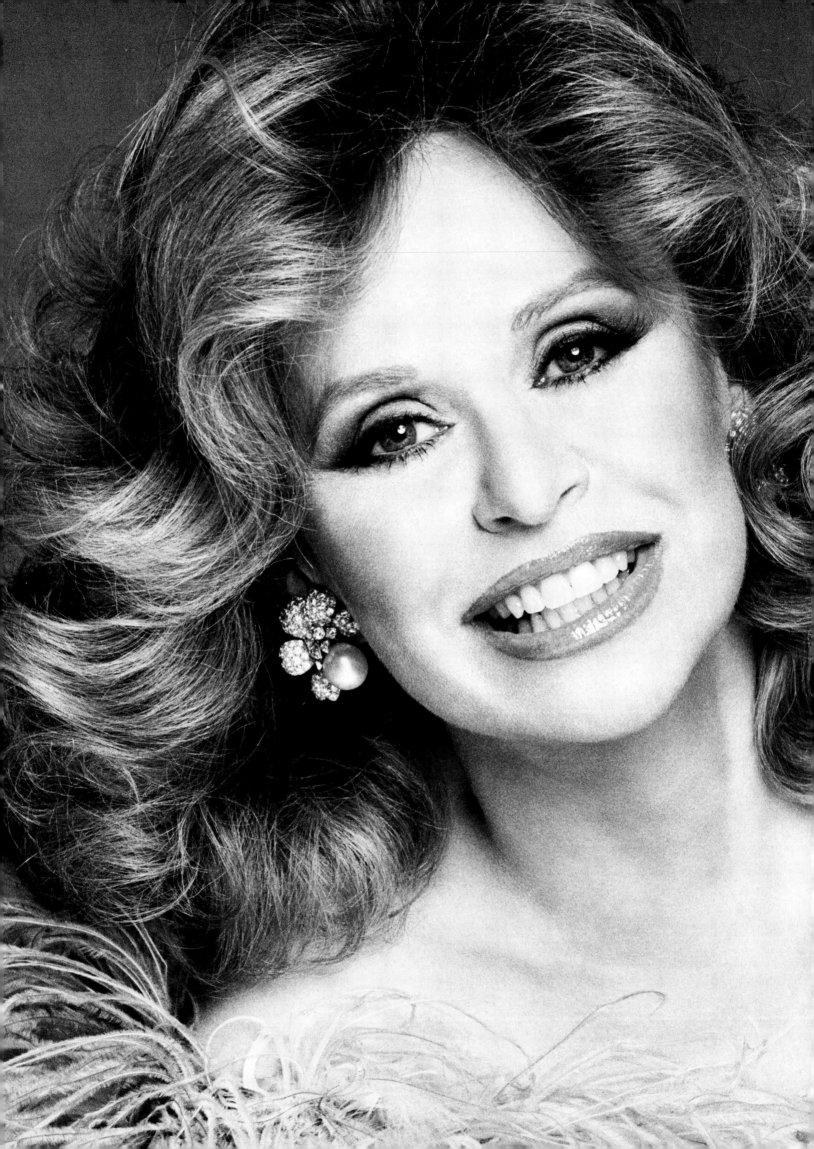

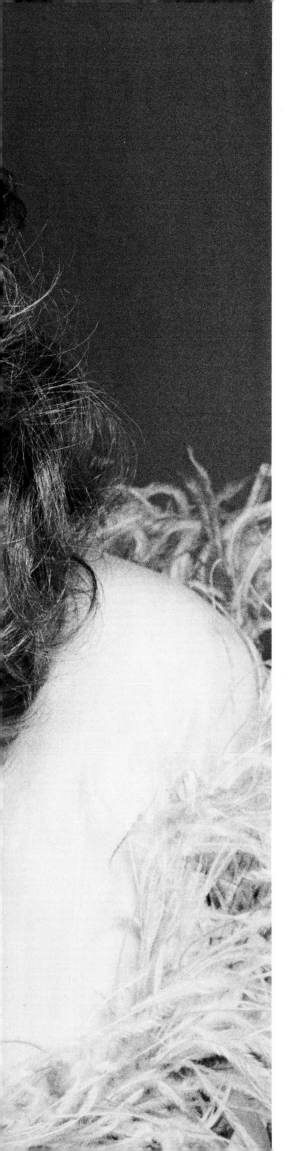

Warmth and spirit that start with a smile

Aileen Mehle

"The idea that beauty comes from within is just another dumb cliché. Only two things that have anything to do with beauty come from within. One is health ... and two is being happy.... If you want to talk about where beauty *really* comes from, let's talk about brains and discipline. Because a woman with these qualities can do a lot toward making herself very, *very* attractive."

Aileen Mehle

Aileen Mehle—alias Suzy Knickerbocker of the *New York Daily News*—is a small, fluffy, adorable dynamo of a woman, absolutely boiling with zip and charm. She is also a brainy, large-spirited, thoroughly nice human being who has managed, without a drop of malice, to create the liveliest gossip column in town ("I stick in the needle, but I pull it out fast . . . and then I rub the sore spot").

She is a dream to photograph; all she has to do is smile and the camera falls in love with her—it is *the* most gorgeous smile. Every time I see it, I want to pull out that jaw and put it in my own mouth. It's Aileen's single great vanity: "Look," she says, like a kid in a Crest commercial, "only one cavity!" (Which is, anyway, too far back and too tiny to see.) And she likes to tell about the time she was being photographed for *Vogue* and Diana Vreeland, then editor, said to Cecil Beaton, "Now, Cecil, you have *got* to take a picture of those teeth and those gums!" And Beaton, clenching on every word, said, "I am not a dentist, Diana; I am a photographer."

Aileen is one of those rare women who understand their faces perfectly. And she is always open to knowing more; she draws on the expertise of such makeup artists as Way Bandy, who did her makeup for this photograph, and John Richardson. Equally, she can be instructive; John remembers the first time he worked with Aileen: "I wanted to emphasize her warmth and outgoingness, so I did a very warm makeup—all apricots and sunny yellows—and it was dead wrong. When I did it her way, with a very, very pale foundation—I think she used Chanel— it gave her a sort of translucent glow and just seemed to lift her whole face. Her eye makeup was a light-blue and brownish mix that reflected light . . . the entire effect was right. Aileen knows more about makeup than any other woman I've met."

She knows a lot about a lot of things. About people: "People should be edited . . . all you have to do is see them two or three times. Or less. I can take a look at a person, and I like him immediately . . . or it's an instant distaste. And it lasts; I have never had a wrong first impression. I'm very good at sizing up people . . . except husbands. But I've only had two, and I liked them both instantly. . . . It's hard to dislike a big smile and a big hello. One of the nicest compliments, even better than saying 'You look marvelous' and meaning it, is to give someone the big hello and the great big smile. Maybe you put on just a little tiny bit, but it's really only to make that person feel good."

About sex appeal: "You put ten men in a room and you say to the ten, 'Do you think that woman has sex appeal?' And if eight men say she does, she does. But if two men say she does, she really doesn't—not to the degree that's meant when somebody is described as sexy. Ten or twelve years ago, I saw Brigitte Bardot at a couple of parties in Paris, and I thought: This is it. She had everything—the hair, the eyes were beautiful, the nose; the mouth was full-lipped and sensuous— she was the most ravishing creature! But Brigitte got a little bit coarse, and the coarseness sort of took over. It's wonderful to have a sexiness about you, but also to have a classiness so that you don't look like a hooker."

About being thin: "Women are hung up on thinness; they're crazed. They think it's chic or stunning—you know, 'You can't be too thin or too rich.' Well, that's half right; you can't be too rich, I don't think. But you certainly can be too thin! I see these women running around with spindle shanks and hideous skinny legs with no calves, just dreadful little sticks hanging out of their skirts—dreadful!—and funny little spindly arms, and no breasts. Some women's idea of heaven is getting into a size six. To me, that's all wrong. I think the woman who is supposed to weigh 115 and weighs 120 looks a lot better than the woman who should weigh 115 and instead weighs 110. I

■

"I don't do things for a man. If men like it, great; if women like it, great. But if I like it—hurray!"

■

---

know many women who should—*tomorrow*—gain twenty pounds. I know models are extremely thin, but they are also extremely young and they have beautiful faces. . . .

"I think that a face—a face plus a mind—can handle a body, but a body cannot handle a face. Meaning, you see someone with a fabulous body, the way you see them in Brazil left and right in a million bikinis, but if the face is not great it almost cancels out the body. If you have a beautiful face or an interesting face or a lively face or a face that draws people to you—and a mind that draws them, and humor and charm— then you can handle some imperfection of the body. . . . If I had my druthers, I'd rather have a lovely face than a lovely body. You can work on your body; you can make your waist smaller, and you can make your stomach flatter. But if you have a mouth that isn't pretty, you're not ever going to give yourself a pretty mouth."

About beauty: "The idea that beauty comes from within is just another dumb cliché. Only two things that have anything to do with beauty come from within. One is health, because if you're healthy you have got to have some kind of a glow. And two is being happy, because when you're happy everything is up, up, up; you're animated. No woman, no matter how beautiful, can just sit there like a lump and say, 'Well, admire me.' People don't do it. . . . A pretty woman can be sitting there, and you look at her, and you say, 'My, she's pretty.' And you look a second time, and you say, 'Yes, she is pretty.' And if that's all she is, you don't look again.

Pretty is not enough. If you're happy it won't change your nose, but it will keep you looking good.

"If you want to talk about where beauty *really* comes from, let's talk about brains and discipline. Because a woman with these qualities can do a lot toward making herself very, *very* attractive. But without them . . . I have seen the most incredibly beautiful women just throw it away: overeat,

---

"I have never had a wrong first impression."

---

overdrink. I suspect that lurking in the back of their minds is the thought that they can turn themselves around if they want to: 'I shouldn't drink this fifth glass of champagne. But when I want to, I can stop. I can go on a diet. I can exercise.' The discipline is to not sit

there and drink and eat like a pig. The discipline is to do the exercise, to take care of yourself. Just keeping clean is a tremendous job—keeping your hair clean, your body clean, your teeth clean, your nails and everything clean and done—never mind adorning yourself. And you have to keep at it and at it and at it.

"Discipline, however, does not mean that spartan thing, that business of streaking out of bed and getting on the floor and doing an hour of the most excruciating exercises in order to have a wretched, skinny belly, so that when a man puts his hand there it goes in instead of going up a little on soft, beautiful flesh like satin. Of course you exercise; discipline means exercise. It means being slender. But not skinny and dried up. And not fat. You want to get somewhere in the middle. If you go from a size eight to a size ten, don't worry about it; go there. But stop there. That's where the discipline comes in."

About her own discipline: "I use Nivea oil to take off my makeup. And I wash my face every day, once a day, with any good glycerine soap. If my skin looks as though it's getting a little dry, I don't use soap that day, just water. Then I put on moisturizer, and makeup on top of that. I'm a firm believer in makeup. I've worn it since the age of fourteen. Also, I think it protects your skin. . . . Maybe once a year I go to Heidi at Dr. Berman's, my dermatologist, and she steams my face and puts a little cream on it. And that is all I do about my skin. I have never, never had a facial, and I never, never would; all that skin-stretching stuff is awful for you.

"I am greatly in favor of plastic surgery, but I have never had anything done, not even my eyes. . . . I do think

you can go too far with face lifts; some women I know are getting to have a very weirdo look, very weirdo indeed. . . . This silicone thing I don't like at all. There's one doctor who has become famous for it; he's unbelievably busy ironing out everybody's wrinkles with silicones, but he'll never iron out mine. I think it looks terrible. . . . I streak my hair; otherwise it is my own natural ash-blond color. I have not one gray hair, not O-N-E. And everyone knows it, because they see me all the time and they see me at the hairdresser.

"Dr. Berman got me out of the sun years ago. He said, 'Are you crazy? I hate brunettes in the sun, and you're a blue-eyed, fair-skinned blonde—*out!*' I used to get very tanned. I was very young, and my hair was very blond and down to my knees . . . all that tan and white dresses! I thought I was kind of wonderful. But I gave it up; anything is easy for me to give up. After your

---

" 'You can't be too thin or too rich.' Well, that's half right; you can't be too rich."

---

youth is over, you cannot go out there and bake and expect not have those wrinkledy-crinkledies. You have to take care . . . you don't have to turn into an ugh just because you turn forty or fifty or sixty."

Why, I asked, does she take the care, make the effort; is there a man in her life? "Certainly. There always has been. But I don't do these things for a man. If men like it, great; if women like it, great. But if I like it—hurray! That's who I do them for: myself. Every woman should. . . . Go with it as long as you can, and then be a lovely-looking old lady."

I haven't a clue how old Aileen is, except that Roger Mehle, her son by her first marriage, "is old enough to be a banker." Nothing more is forthcoming. "Can't you just say, 'She looks younger than she is'?" Right.

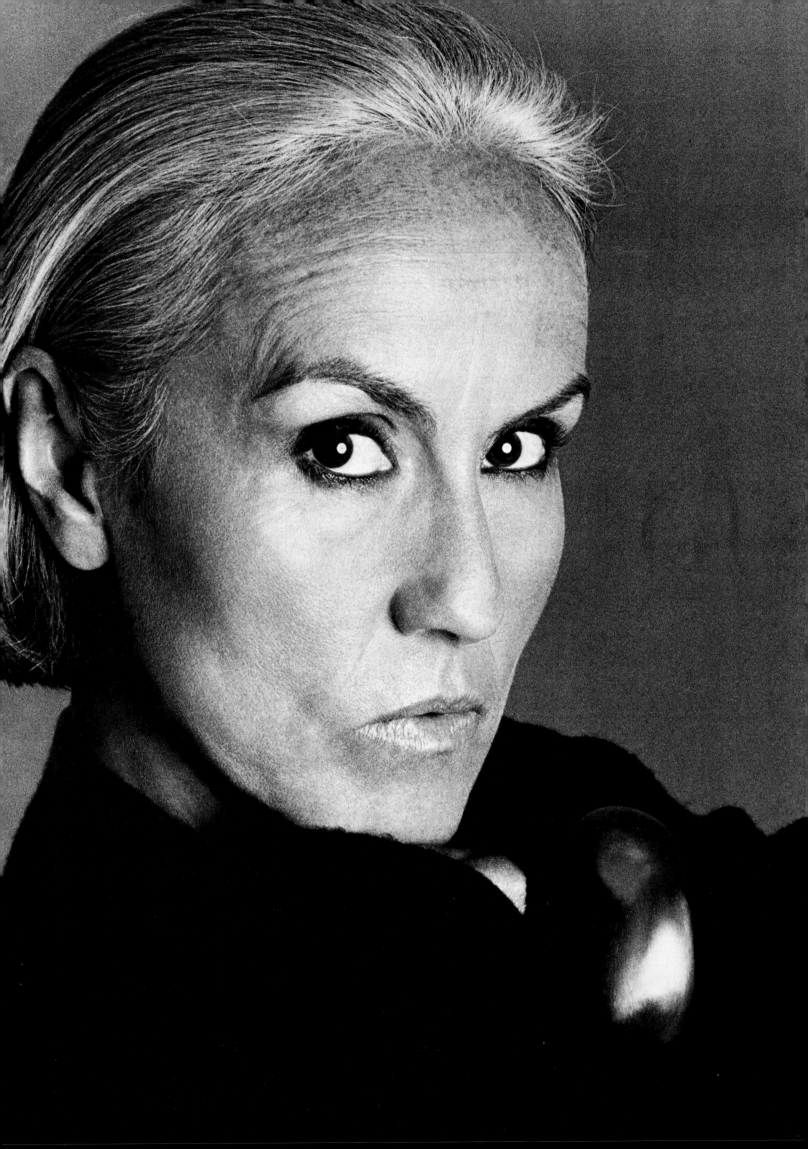

Beauty as presence and style

Polly Mellen

A fashion editor is the heart and mind of a sitting—mother figure /cheerleader /psychologist /psychic all rolled into one. A good editor, by definition, knows to the last split second what's happening in fashion. A great editor is tuned to a higher frequency; she's picking up the next vibration, the thing that could, with a little twist, a little turn, a little tiny bit of a push, just possibly happen. So she gives that little push. I have seen Polly Mellen take a scrap of cotton scarf and fold it in a certain way and tie it in a certain way in a certain neckline . . . and a minute after *Vogue* hits the stands, I see women walking around New York looking as though they'd been grabbed by the neck by Polly Mellen.

Polly Mellen of *Vogue* is a great fashion editor; with over thirty years of twisting, turning, tying behind her, she is the *doyenne* of fashion editors. She is also a superduper lady; she walks into the studio, this strong-boned, spare-featured, Indian-looking woman in her Harris tweed jacket and turtleneck, her perfectly creased non-designer jeans and polished leather shoes, and the place crackles with her optimism and enthusiasm. I love being around her— I get high on her energy.

I have never known her to be bored. She approaches every sitting as though it were high adventure, armed with conviction and ready to do battle if she has to. "Fashion is what we're seen in, and it is the way we present ourselves. And that's important. I care deeply about fashion, but I must tell you the *way* I care. I care about fashion for the person who is wearing it. I care that that person knows *what* she can wear. *How* she should look. Because I honestly think that I can look at any woman and say, 'Gee, if she did it this way, she'd look so terrific.' I never

think, Is she beautiful-looking? *Style* can be a person who is not beautiful-looking. Beautiful-looking is a girl, who has been born beautiful. Brooke Shields is a beauty. Vivien Leigh was a beauty. Carole Lombard was my ideal, a woman with wit, glamour, *style.* . . .

"Style is a person who dares, who has the confidence of knowing what is right for her. I've said a lot of times that you should try out something first before you take it out. But I don't do that always. Sometimes I just put on my purple leather pumps, with the bright-green cocardes on the toes, and go out anyway."

> **"Style is a person who dares, who has the confidence of knowing what is right for her."**

It could be that a talent for fashion is like a talent for music or painting or any other art: It's born in the bone and begins to manifest itself in the nursery. At least, there is no time in Polly's life that she can remember not being interested in fashion. As a child (Polly is the youngest girl in a family of four girls and one boy), she recalls, "We lived in West Hartford, Connecticut, and my mother had a dress shop—it was sort of a whim she had—in Hartford. And Mummy would say to me—I was about five or six years old—'Do you like this or do you like that?' And I'd say, 'I like *that* one!' . . . Through Mother, we learned color, and we were always conscious of fashion, and we were dressed very beautifully . . . a little bit ahead of the time always. But our clothes always had a little twist to them; that was Mummy. She was really kind of an extraordinary woman who had an enormous influence on my life. And the second most important woman-influence was Diana Vreeland."

Diana Vreeland, whose position in

contemporary fashion is roughly equivalent to that of Elizabeth Tudor in sixteenth-century England, is special consultant to the Costume Institute at the Metropolitan Museum of Art in New York and former Editor in Chief of *Vogue.* She was fashion editor of *Harper's Bazaar* when Polly went to work for her, an event that was preceded by a long apprenticeship. Polly started in the training program at Lord & Taylor, where she worked as a salesgirl in the sweater department, ran the College Shop ("the closest I ever got to college"), and finally went into window display. She then went to work in advertising and promotion at Saks Fifth Avenue, and from there to *Mademoiselle,* as Millinery Editor. ("I didn't own a hat, except a beret. So I kept it in my pocket for every time I went into the millinery market.") Meanwhile, over at *Harper's Bazaar:* "Connie Woodworth, who was an editor, and a very glamorous lady, had just left, and Carmel Snow, the Editor in Chief, said to Sally Kirkland—my sister's best friend, who was an editor of *Life* at the time—'Do you know any young woman who . . . ?' And Sally said, 'Don't say another word. I've got the girl for you.' "

The girl was petrified. " 'I'm not ready, really I'm not ready,' I said. And Sally said, 'You're ready. Put on your white gloves.' I always wore little white gloves, with one little button and always with three little points and always hand-sewn and always cotton. And I went to my interview with Carmel Snow absolutely trembling. I didn't understand half the things she said because she talked 'thaaht waahy.' But she was adorable. I just loved her." Evidently, it was mutual, and soon Sally Kirkland was back with the next, most terrifying news of all: Polly was going to see Mrs. Vreeland. "Well, the end of it was, I met the *most* warm, wonderful, kind, brilliant, unique, eccentric woman, and I was hired. I took glamorous Connie Woodworth's job with my little white-gloved hands. And it was a training of a quality that . . . no question, it gave me a background.

"I think the most important thing I learned from Mrs. Vreeland is, 'When you think that's it—that's the nth, the

Polly Mellen

zenith of as far as you can go—before you do it, think again. And you will go farther. You have to go out to the end of the diving board to find your way back to the center. And the center is mediocrity; who needs it? That's not what we're here for, mediocrity. It's gray. You don't want to be gray. It's black or it's white. It can't be gray. Gray is indefinite. Gray is not positive. Gray will get you nowhere.' And there she is sitting in gray flannel from her head to her toes—Mainbocher. The best. I coveted it. A fitted gray flannel coat, fitted like something I never saw in my whole life. I went right out and got a gray flannel fitted coat and never wore it to work until I told her I had bought it, and she said, 'I want to see it.' Then I wore it. Because her point was, When you wear gray, be *able* to."

At fifty-six, with her children grown up and on their own (the Mellens each have a boy and a girl from an earlier marriage), Polly considers that she is "in a teaching time of life, and that's what I care most about. I am the *luckiest!* I have the best job in the world, and I am fortunate enough to have a working relationship with one of the most wonderful people I've ever known, Grace Mirabella [editor in chief of *Vogue*], who is the best listener. There isn't a fashion editor anywhere who has had the training I've had. It makes me feel that I have a responsibility. . . . I must do my exercises. I must keep up my diet. I must stay in shape because of my responsibility.

"I get up with a bounce, and I can't wait to start my day, and I run to work or I run to whatever it is that I'm doing that day. But first I do my exercises—in total silence. I don't even like to have music. I don't turn on the radio. I have never seen *The Today Show*! There are

two places I'm not satisfied with: the underbelly of the arm waves at me, and my thighs are not as firm as I'd like them to be; I can see the thigh starting to slip a little."

Polly has the kind of hair you can comb with your fingers and forget about. It's marvelous, thick and Indian-straight. It started going gray at the temples when she was twenty-four. In those days, she colored it every two weeks ("I'm so dark naturally, and the gray would come immediately"). The year she went to *Vogue,* she quit forever: "One, I couldn't sit still that long; two, it wasn't worth the money; and three, my husband, Henry, said he didn't mind it." . . . Once a month, she has a facial at Mario Badescu. She picked Badescu "because I saw people with skin I admired, and they went to him. So I went to him, and now I use his products, and I do everything he says. I clean my face with an orange-smelling lotion and take it off with a warm facecloth, massaging in the proper direction—up and out, and very gently—starting from the neck. Then I put on a tonic with a cotton ball, and if there's any dirt on the cotton, I do it again . . . then I do moisturizer and a little eye cream."

Like most no-makeup makeups, there's more to Polly's than meets the eye: "I do a teeny bit of Eve of Rome—it's like Erase—under my eyes. And I do a little bit of brown eyeshadow and a tiny, tiny bit of liner, both with the same brown pencil. And—same pencil—I outline my mouth a little and put some Elizabeth Arden Eight-Hour Cream on my lips. Then I take the brown pencil and just touch my lips to get a little color. And then a little blush—dark-brown sort of stuff. Finished. Any real color—any red, any orange, any pink—takes away from what I want to project, which is the American Indian look [there's no accounting for it, by the way; the look runs in the family, but not the blood]."

When someone whose business it is to look critically at other people throws out beauty tips, it pays to listen. Listen: "I think one should always take a look at one's eyes. And I think either you dye your eyelashes or you do a little mascara or you do the barest bit of brown pencil. But if there is one thing that you ought to do, it's mascara. I dye my eyelashes so I don't use mascara. I love to do everything else, but I don't like to do that. It gives me the willies; it bores me. But the eyes—the emphasis on the eyes—is the most important thing. . . . Nails are important. I think people are all wrong about nails. All wrong. I think much more interesting is the hand with a nail that is not too long, that is not too bright,

because I love people's hands. Hands are fabulous. I love the way people use their hands. A man who is enormously masculine—Zubin Mehta—suddenly, he'll use his hands, and he'll use them like a woman, in the most delicate, beautiful, gentle way.

"After mascara, I think the most important beauty tip is: Never, never overdo it. If you're ever in doubt, don't do it. That's a beauty tip, and that's a fashion tip: If you have to ask where would you wear it; if it's that everybody's talking about this terrific new length, but you're not so sure you look too hot in it; if you think you don't quite understand it—leave it, don't buy it, *forget* it! Nothing looks as well as a navy-blue sweater and gray flannel pants. Nothing. I mean, *boom!*—perfect. Glamorous classics are *forever*. And you can take a turn to them; you can wear two shirts at once."

Extravagance isn't Polly's idea of chic. What is might surprise you: "Chic is my father sitting on the beach in his terry-cloth double-breasted jacket. He had two; one was white and had a sapphire-blue monogram on the pocket, and the other was sapphire blue with a white monogram. And he always had a beautiful, oversized white handkerchief tucked in the pocket, and a small hand towel tucked in the neck. The jacket had a notched collar and fastened with pearl buttons, and it just covered his bathing suit, which was three inches above his knee. I got a lot from my father. He was very chic. Super chic. . . . When I was at school, my greatest distinction was that I had the oldest father in the graduating class. He was eighteen years older than my mother—when she was born, he was a freshman at Yale.

"I have a lot of feelings about getting older. But I have never, never been 'age conscious.' What I have been always conscious of is people's capacity, their energy level, their attitude. The second thing that interests me when it comes to age is the obvious deterioration of the human body. I think it's fascinating. . . . The thing is, I do have the energy and I feel younger than my face looks. But I'm not, and that's it. And if it bothers me enough, I have to have a face lift—I've tried; I've stood in front of natural light and held the skin up, and, oh, I'd be *fabulous!* But I'm not going to do it. And the reason I say that is because at age fifty-six, in my fifty-seventh year, a man who is famous for his photographs of the most beautiful women, asked me to be in his book."

You bet I did; not to have had Polly Mellen in this book would be like throwing a party and not inviting the life of it!

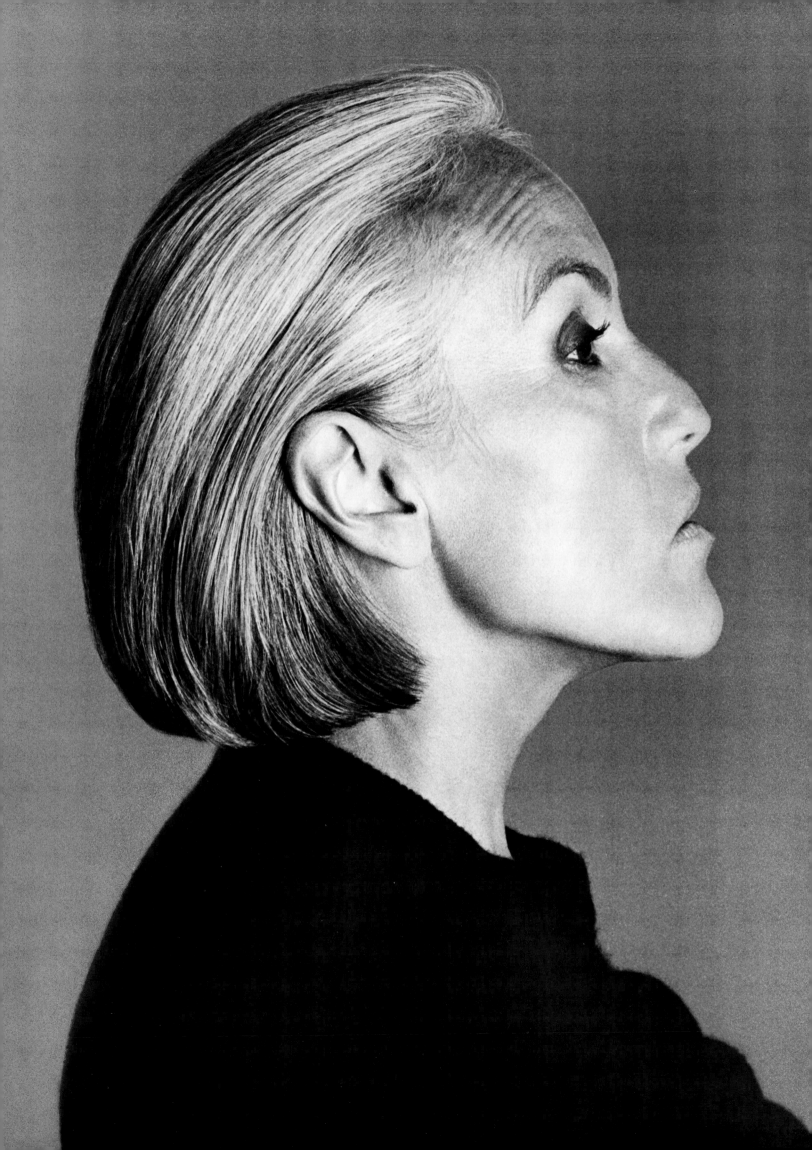

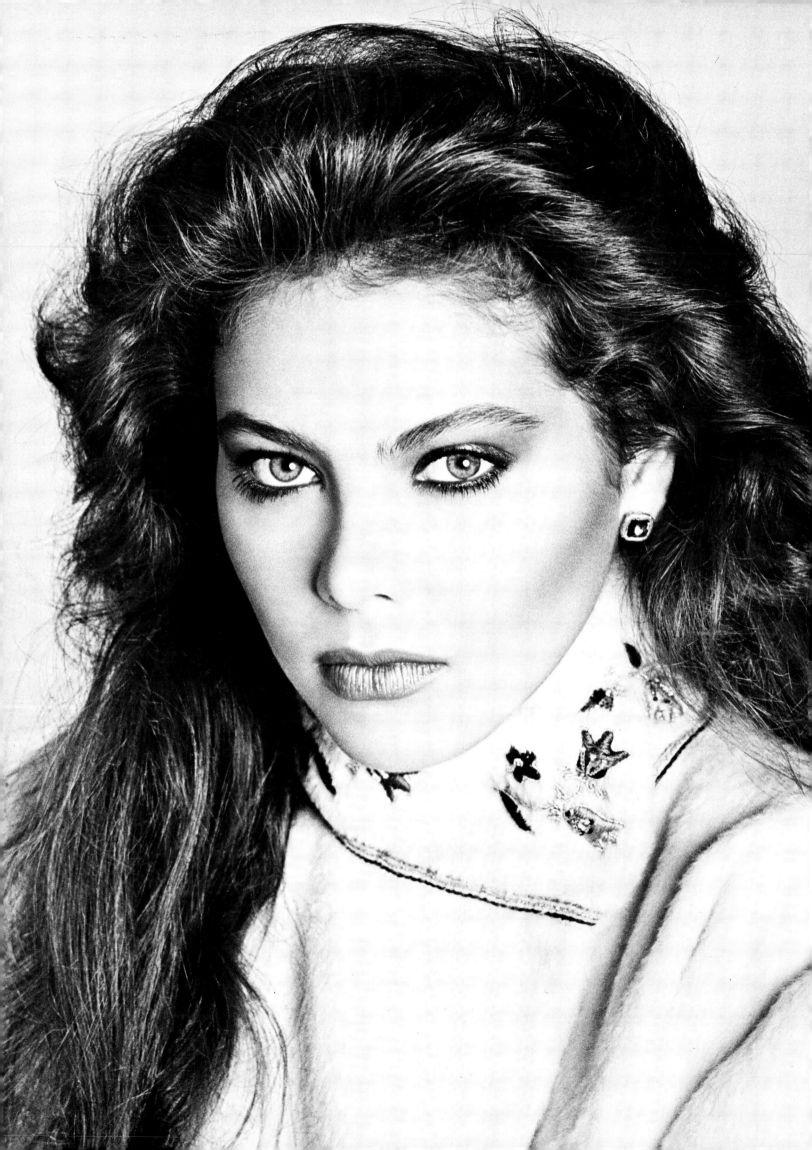

A sexy makeup that is also soft

Ornella Muti

Every woman is sexy for somebody. But some few are sexy for everybody. And Ornella Muti is one of them. When she first appears on screen —positively breathing lechery—as Princess Aura in *Flash Gordon,* you can feel the vibrations in the audience, and you can almost see an invisible comic-strip balloon above the hero's head: WOW!

She is just succulent, all slender curves, smooth olive skin, a kissy mouth, and gray-green eyes that turn up at the corners. I happen to be crazy about tip-tilted eyes. And I love the way John Richardson brought out the shape without exaggerating it, simply giving her eye shadow a quick swing at each corner and following the natural slant up to the eyebrow. (Another nice trick for eyes: Instead of putting just a line of black in the lower rim of her eyes, John first put a mix of shadows in Ornella's own eye color—gray and green, plus a touch of blue—then the black. Much softer than black alone, and it picks up the color of the eyes.)

Like many actresses who are their own makeup artists, Ornella saves the glamour routine for the camera. "If I'm working, then I put the foundation and all this stuff. I like to do it once in a while. But this big glamour, it's not really my type. Many days, when I'm not working, I'm not even made up, but if I am it's just the eyes and a little blush. . . . I never use the eye shadows or powders. I do everything with a pencil and a brush. It makes the look very natural.

"Every day, every morning and every night, I clean my face. And I put cream on. Most of my creams are made at home by a woman in northern Italy. She makes a normal cream, which is for every day. And then she makes a nutrition cream that's like a food for your face, very heavy, very rich. You put it on only three times a week—depending on your age, of course. I also do some masks for my face. And I do work out my body. I swim a lot, play tennis. I do gym. I jog.

This latest sex *gattina* from Italy may be fairly new to America (*Viva Italia!* was one of her few films shown here), but she is an established star abroad; as she says, "I am very famous in Europe." When Dino De Laurentis called her for *Flash Gordon,* she had already done twenty-eight films. Her first was at the age of fourteen. She is now only twenty-four. She has a six-year-old daughter, Naike: "It's an American Indian name; my husband had always an obsession with Indians."

Ornella's husband, from whom she is separated, is not Naike's father; that was "someone who didn't want the child and left me. I was eighteen. And I had to take a position: I would take care of my child myself or I would give it up. I didn't want to give it up. So, I had my troubles . . . You know, working and all—when you're very young, it's tough. The movie business is not easy. It becomes easy when you are a star; then everything goes along. But when you're not, you are fighting every day. Actually, I was lucky with my work. But still, you have humiliations. Because you are young, they say you don't understand anything. And sometimes—again, because you are very young—they treat you without respect. But now, everything has changed. Now I'm happy."

Happiness has a lot to do with her boyfriend—a stockbroker in Rome—whom she will marry in two years, when her divorce is final, and whom her daughter adores.

Happiness has also to do, of course, with her career, which is now cooking on both sides of the Atlantic; her next film here is "a weird story about adventure and love," called *Love and Money,* and this time her name goes above the title. After that, who knows? "I never make plans, because I don't like to be upset later. I just go on with what I have to do. . . . My dreams, they change all the time. I don't want this anymore, I want that. I don't have really big dreams, because I don't like illusions. . . . I mean, I have dreams for a long time to be a dancer, a ballet dancer. And my father never wanted me to study ballet—my Italian father, you understand—he was always saying, 'A dancer! A woman dancer! And you have to travel! And, and, and!' It was my biggest dream, and from the moment I saw that what I wanted so much —what I have put my whole heart into —was not coming out, I stopped really to have big dreams. Finally, he allowed me to have classes, but I was twelve. It was too late."

"I never make plans because I don't like to be upset later."

This, of course, was the Italy of over a decade ago. "Today it's changing, everything. The children just walk out— many, many young people run away from home. We have a lot of drugs. You open the newspapers in Italy, and you read—eighteen, fourteen, fifteen, sixteen—they die. They just die. I worry very much about Naike growing up in such a time. It is my only fear." Not that drugs didn't exist in Ornella's childhood. "Grass was going on, and LSD. But I grew up in a different way, and I think this has a lot to do with what happened to our family. My father died when I was thirteen, and my mother was in a lot of troubles; all of a sudden she was alone with two children, two women children [Ornella has a younger sister, a successful model in Paris and Rome], and she had to go to work. We would never have done this drug thing to my mother. She was needing help, not needing to be worried about us. So we both also started to work." Ornella, of course, went to work in the movies, which her father "never would have allowed—no, no, no!" . . . On the other hand, "if he could come back and see me now, I think he would be very, very happy." I think she is very, very right.

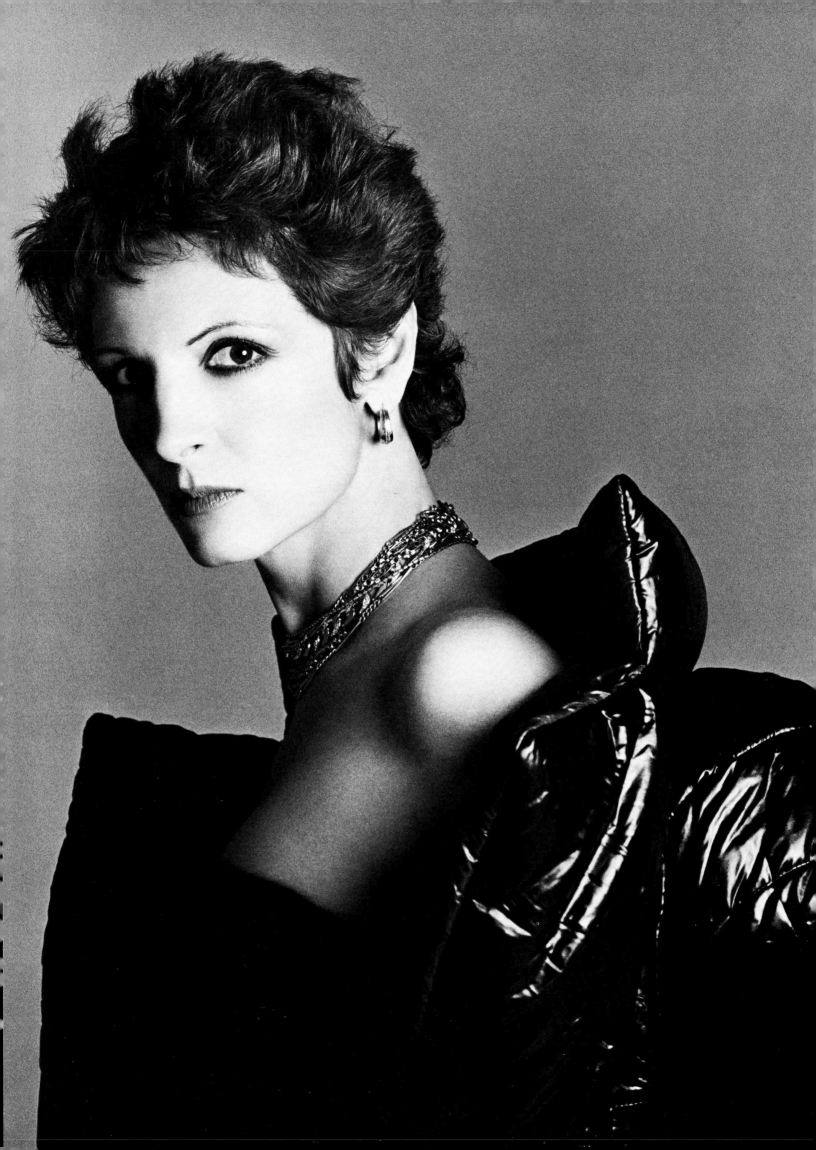

Beauty that flows from grace

Mirella Petteni

"I am a great believer in the power of the woman — not the greedy aggressive power, the *inner* power of the woman, of having man and family."

Most beauty, I think, is as subject to the whims of fashion as the clothes we wear or the way we furnish our houses. What one age perceives as beautiful is likely to draw a blank in another. What would Praxiteles have made of Brigitte Bardot, for instance? How would an Edwardian have rated Lauren Hutton? How would Lillian Russell go over in the 1980s—or, for that matter, Twiggy? The point is, every age applies its own yardstick. And in every age, certain women transcend it—I can't imagine a time in history when Garbo, say, would not be considered a great beauty, or Elizabeth Taylor, or Vivien Leigh. Or Mirella Petteni.

Fine-boned, with a delicately arched nose, deep-lidded eyes, and a marvelous long neck, Mirella is in the classic tradition of northern Italian beauties. She is, in fact, from the north—a country girl from the region around Bergamo. And to know just this about her is to know more than mere statistics: "The Bergamo people, they have great

willpower. They are very organized. They are achievers. In Italy, if you say to someone, 'I am from Bergamo,' they say, 'Oh, God, *strong!*' There is some kind of strength coming from there. I think they are good people—my parents, my grandparents—really good country people, down to earth, like only *paisan* can be. I am very glad I come from that part of Italy. It is the only thing that keeps me to reality."

Her Bergamo blood manifested itself early. At fourteen, when her father died, she began working by day as a secretary and going to school at night. Before long, she had a double flash of insight: "I realized that through that I was going to go nowhere. Also I realized I was good-looking, because the people are looking at me in the street." Where an American girl in a similar situation might pack her bags and head for a big-time modeling agency in New York, a Bergamo girl proceeds more cautiously. Mirella moved to Milan, got herself a daytime job as a secretary, and at night went to modeling school,

where, in about a minute and a half, she was discovered and at nineteen began one of the most successful all-around fashion careers in the history of the business.

Mirella is now forty-two. She was a top photographers' model. She was editor of Italian *Vogue.* She has managed the European licensee for Cole of California, the American licensees for Valentino and Gianni Versace. The first phase of her career—modeling—lasted more than ten years, during which time she married, had a child (Jacopo, now twenty), divorced, remarried, and had another child (Simon, her younger son, is fifteen). "Modeling was very good—very good for the ego—but thank God I've also been able to have something else going on; that kept me in balance. Modeling by itself is very empty . . . you lose a lot of reality. Instead, I was having my children, having my love stories. Yes, I had some stories . . . after, between this one and the other one. Why not? Basically, life has been moving from love to love. I don't know, maybe this is the way in Italy. . . . In America you grow up thinking that work is very important. In Italy, no. I mean, now maybe —*maybe*—they're starting, but still what is important is 'the private life. The man with whom you're living, that is your success. I think it's good. As a matter of fact, every time I tried to be just an independent woman or a businesswoman, I felt a failure. I have an incredible need to achieve, but loving somebody, married or not married, it is very important for me. Just work—let men work. I can say that, because I've been working since I'm fourteen years old. I tried and I did it. I did it very well.

"When I reached thirty, I decided then I wanted to stop modeling, because it's much better if you to decide to stop than if somebody is asking you to stop. I always do that in my life. It's

Mirella Petteni

the same in a love affair; if I see that something does not work well, I am the one who leaves. Probably something does not work because I don't want to make it work . . . mostly it's the woman who makes it or doesn't make it. I am a great believer in the power of the woman—not the greedy aggressive power, the *inner* power of the woman, of having man and family. . . . I have a lot of conflicting feelings about being a woman and accepting myself as a woman. One part is independent, and the other part is the one whose life is only if her man is there and she is part of this man. . . . My ideal are those women in the country—in Italy there are many—the great matriarchal figures in the background. They don't do too much. They don't talk too much. They just look, they move, they are calm, they serve their men. And they have all in their hands: the men, the children, the houses—everything."

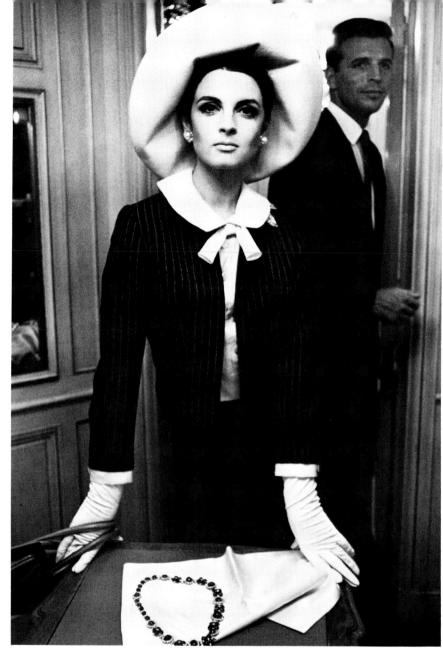

1960

Since coming to New York five years ago, Mirella has been separated from her husband. She lives alone (her older son is a student at the London School of Economics; the younger is at boarding school in New England) in one of those old East Side apartment buildings, in which even a three-room flat seems spacious. The once white-walled rooms were recently painted apricot, and there is lace at the windows. These changes have significance for her: "All my life I've been living in white. I always moved into beautiful places—the apartments of my husbands—and they were already decorated. Everything was very masculine, very chic, but very linear. And they were all white, all the time. Now, suddenly—I don't know if it's more confidence with myself, or maybe just a new aspect of me—but I love color. I'm accepting color. I'm accepting lace. It's

---

"Basically, life has been moving from love to love."

---

like I'm letting myself go and accepting to be a woman . . . accepting being feminine."

A more serious change was triggered by a spinal-disc injury almost two years ago, which damaged nerves and muscles in one leg. The recovery has been steady, but "the muscle in the calf has not fully rebuilt yet, and the foot does not come up." She's working on it: Three times a week she takes a regular exercise class; twice a week she has physical therapy; one day a week she has an all-over massage; one other day a week she has special foot massage; and every single day without fail, for two or three hours, she walks. There is no question that the leg will mend completely—or that it will take time. As a

result, she has decided not to work for a year. It was not a lightly made decision. "Work is my life. I come from a very Catholic family: you have to work. If I was not working, I felt guilty. Even when I did not have the necessity to work, I always made myself work because I was feeling guilty. Now I don't feel guilty anymore; I have my leg to take care of."

A funny thing I've found in talking with women for this book. Many of them—especially the very beautiful women—are curiously reluctant to talk about how they care for their looks, as though to admit that they took any care at all would somehow diminish their beauty in the eyes of the world. With Mirella, there is none of that. She shares all her secrets, happily shows you all her little jars and bottles: the Clinique eye cream and moisturizer; the things she brings from Italy: Mustela cream to cleanse her face ("they use it for children in Italy"); Aqua di Rosa to freshen it; a collagen concentrate ("I put it around my eyes and around my mouth every morning, and that is what makes my skin have good tone . . . elastic. My hairdresser in Rome sells it to me. When I'm here, I write to him, and with the next person who comes to New York, he's sending me my collagen. If I don't have it, I use Vitamin E oil. It is also good.").

Every three months or so, Mirella goes for a facial to a place on the West Side of town—"not elegant, not chic" —run by two East European women who do body massage and waxing as well. "They go from the leg of one lady to the arm of another to the neck of a third—it's an amazing scene, like a Fellini movie. But they do superb facials. They have a cream, too, that sometimes I buy. It smells very 'family.' As a matter of fact, when I'm wearing it my boyfriend says, 'You smell terrible!' But I've been using it for years on my face and on my body." She has also been using a bust-toning treatment oil by Clarins. "I had a lot of stretch marks from having my children, and I don't say they have disappeared but they got very, very, very close to each

I go to Bruno's Le Salon for my hair. Bruno is the owner. He's a very nice guy, and he cuts my hair in five minutes. . . . I learned to do my own color. Right now, my hair is very gray. But I always make the color, because it was very dark before, too dark for pictures. So since I start to be a model, I was making it lighter."

I have had many beautiful women tell me that beauty comes from inside, and for the most part I chalk it up to excessive modesty and/or a desire not to appear vain. But Mirella manages to put teeth into even this old cliché: "Of course, God gave me my face and my eyes. They are there, yes. But if they're not filled with something from inside. . . . I can be beautiful when I'm happy, but you have to see me on days when I am depressed—you don't see features of any beauty. I can see it in myself. There are days that my face gets in pieces, and the way I move, the way I talk to people, the way I'm aggressive —oh, I can be so ugly.

something you can make happen because it's a combination of many things. You can take better care of your skin, you can take better care of your hair, your body, your eating habits. You can make it happen. I'm a great believer that everything you want you can achieve.

"Some people are born stupid, and there's very little that they can do. But if you work with the minimum ingredients—just enough intelligence, just enough good looks, plus you have a good willpower—you can make things happen. You know, I come from the country, and I was maybe a nice-look-

"What is important is the private life."

ing girl. But there are many nice-looking girls like me in the country; they're still there. I made things happen. I got out, I did something else, I moved on, I worked on my face. My face was very round. My eyes were not so big and they were going lower down. My nose was much bigger, and I have done nothing to my nose, I assure you, or to my eyes. Of course, maybe it was also that I lost baby fat. But it was very much the willpower that I put into it. You really can achieve your face. Sometimes you see models do that. They come in and they look like nothing—empty, white, nothing. And then they make themselves look like Brigitte Bardot on one day and like Sophia Loren on another. It depends on the makeup, on the hair, on what you put on.

"There are many things you can become. . . . I haven't put energy into becoming more educated, but I'm a very curious person. I like to learn, I like to hear. I'm a good student. I didn't get a degree because I started to work when I was fourteen, but I continued to study in the evening. And I know that if I had been less good-looking I would have put all my will to becoming something very great in another field. But I had a nice figure; I was tall and skinny; I was feeling secure about myself as a model. So maybe I chose the easier path . . . with no competition. I hate competition. I have never done anything where it could be a possibility that I was going to lose." So speaks a winner.

"I hate competition. I have never done anything where it could be a possibility that I was going to lose."

other and not so deep. I don't just believe in things. I only believe when I see, and in this Clarins thing I believe very, very, very much." She also believes in Keri body lotion ("a doctor at the Mayo Clinic told me it was the best") and Sardo bath oil. She does not believe in using too much soap or in taking too many baths, as doctors have also told her, "You can keep yourself very clean without taking a bath every day; it dries up your skin."

To put a lot of makeup on skin like Mirella's (Way Bandy calls it "pasta skin") would be a sin against nature. She uses next to nothing: "Some Clinique foundation just around my nose. And I use Indian Earth all over, like a blush; that's what makes everything so glowy. On my eyelids, I put Vaseline first, then I put some brownish-goldish shadow from Dior and smudge it around with my finger . . . the Vaseline just makes it shine a little bit. Then the mascara. Sometimes, in the evening, I put black liner. But that's it: very simple. I do my makeup in one minute and a half. . . . I don't want to spend time.

remember when I started to be a model, I got to the point where I had the face that I wanted to have: I had the eyes that I wanted, I had the mouth that I wanted, I got thinner the way I wanted. I always believe this. Obviously, if you are terribly ugly—if God gives you a terrible nose or tiny little eyes—then no, but I think a normal woman who wants it can really put herself together to be good. Also, what you have inside can help a lot. And third, what helps is the approach you have to people: If you are kind and nice, people are kind and nice to you; if you are gentle, it comes back. I believe that everything comes back. As to beauty, it is

A simple, classic makeup for women over thirty-five

Claudia Rhodes

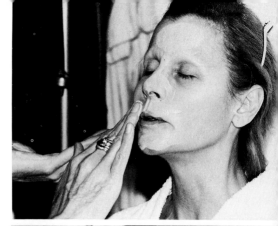

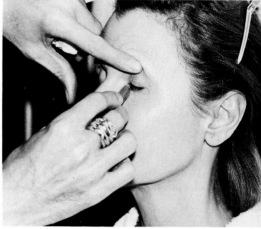

1. *Foundation to even skin tone*
2. *Eye pencil line to define shape*
3. *Dark shadow to elongate eye*
4. *Blush to emphasize cheekbone*
5. *Blow dry for softness and bounce*

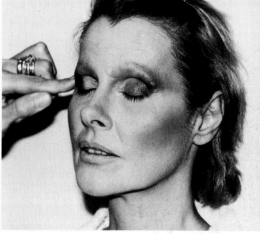

One of the givens of the business is that a model's life, professionally speaking, is as brief as a butterfly's. The girls who are now in their mid to late twenties and still in demand —the Janice Dickinsons, the Beverly Johnsons, the Patti Hansens, the Rene Russos, the Roseanne Velas—can be counted, literally, on the fingers of one hand. And Lauren Hutton, a decade older, is sufficiently unique to be practically a legend in her own time. The fact is, at any age when most young women would be on the threshold of a career, a model—unless she has landed herself a film contract—is just about ready to pack it in.

And then there is Claudia Rhodes, mother of nine, grandmother of three, in and out of modeling since the age of twelve and now, nearing fifty, in again.

Claudia's career goes back to the early forties, when successful models were either Powers Girls, who were famous for being at least five-feet-nine, or Conover Girls, who could squeak through at less. Claudia, who is five-feet-six, started as a catalogue model with Harry Conover and quickly moved up to magazine covers and beauty pages. When she was still in her teens, she married, quit modeling, had five children in a row, divorced, picked up her career again, dropped it nine years later to remarry, had four more children, and by 1980, with all her chil-

dren married or working or in school full-time, this comfortable New Jersey housewife, whose customary means of transportation is a chauffered Bentley with a license plate stamped HERS (as opposed to HIS Rolls Silver Cloud), was back in business, this time doing TV commercials.

"I'm a woman, not a girl, and of course my face has changed."

When I looked at Claudia, what I saw was: beautiful skin, cheekbones, good nose. And a God-awful haircut, with bangs that were almost closing her eyes, which are *fabulous*. She has that great distance between eyebrow and eyelid. Garbo has it, Dietrich has it. It's sensational for makeup, because you have tons of space for shadow—provided you can see it. So before we did anything else, I had Harry King give her a whole new haircut, which was mostly a question of getting the bangs out of the way and layering the rest.

Then Way Bandy got to work on her makeup, really concentrating on the eyes (if you've ever doubted the impor-

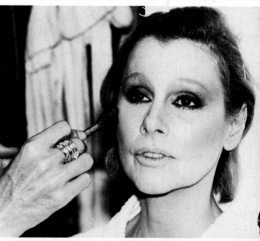

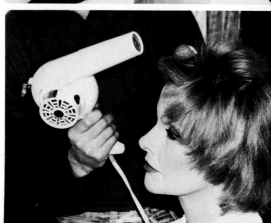

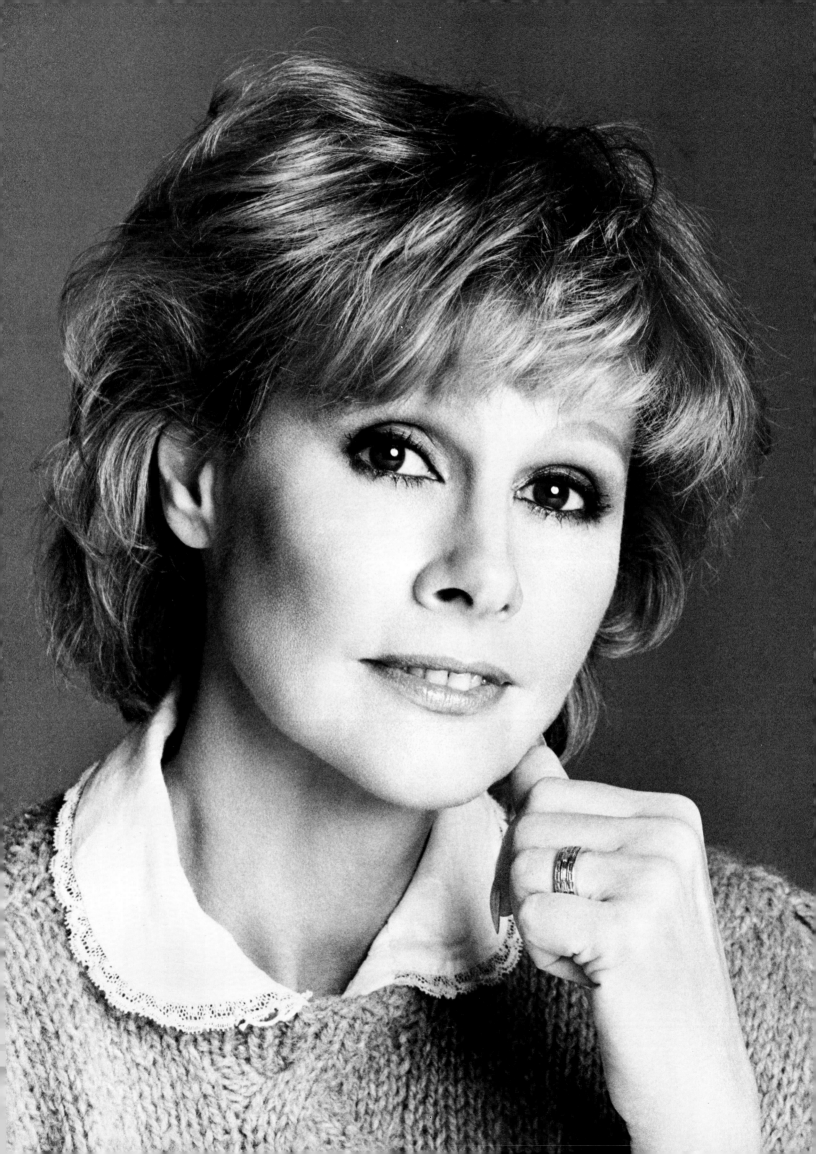

Claudia
Rhodes

tance of eye makeup, look at Claudia with and without—how much whiter the black makes the whites of her eyes, how much more alive and youthful her entire expression!). Way worked mainly in tones of black to gray to white, keeping black nearest the lashes and blending upward into grays, then finally into white just under the brow

and of course my face has changed. It's much thinner, much less broad, and places that used to be full have sunken slightly. This happens as you get older —they say the body shrinks; the face does too. But if you have good bones to hold you up, you're not going to shrink so much and you'll look younger longer. I'm lucky; I have good bones."

"People are too dirt-conscious. Your body functions clean you naturally. If you're healthy, if you eat well—if what you put inside is healthy— you'll be clean."

. . . lots of mascara, but no extra lashes . . . and soft gray pencil on her eyebrows (I prefer gray to brown for black-and-white photography, but just in general I think it's nicer for a blond. Since it's only with the very young that you want to emphasize hollows under the cheeks, contouring is minimal. And the base is very light, which tends to wash out lines (for the same reason, I like to use soft, full-face Paramount lighting; it's extremely flattering to any woman, whatever her age).

The point wasn't to do a Big Glamour Number on Claudia; that would go against her image now: "It would ruin me for the kind of television commercial I do—a housewife in a carpeting commercial, for instance. My type is fortyish middle-America nice. If I tried for something too much younger or more glamorous, I wouldn't get the job. Why should I, when there are so many girls out there who really are young and glamorous? I'd be a fool to risk it."

There is nothing foolish about Claudia; more than most women, she is objective about herself. She understands, in a matter-of-fact, unregretful way, that looks change: "When I was a young girl, people used to come up to me and say, 'You are gorgeous!' Now they say, 'You're such a pretty woman.' I love to hear that, but I know the difference. I'm a woman, not a girl,

To compensate for the changes, Claudia does a basic makeup for herself that I think any woman over thirty-five can learn a lot from. It's a simple, classic technique based, like all makeups, on light and shadow—except that where a full-faced twenty-year-old would be trying to create shadows by diminishing the fullness, Claudia does the opposite. What she wants is to make her face fuller—to plump up the recesses and even out the planes. Her trick is in two parts:

First, a cover-up: "Beauty Checkers at Bendel has a whitish-blue one that I like; it gives a nice clean look. I use it wherever there are lines or depressions —at the top of the chin, between the eyebrows, all around the eye, including over the lid (it looks fresher and more youthful than shadow), and at the corners of the eyes to open them up."

Second: "No color on the cheekbones. Even though my first claim to fame was my cheekbones, to highlight

them now would only call attention to the hollows underneath. And after thirty-five, that can be a little haggard-making. What you need to do is to fill in. The secret is to put color only where color comes naturally. Look in the mirror after you get off the tennis court or when you finish jogging and your circulation is really up. Wherever you see color is where you put your blusher, including up around your eyes and the middle of your earlobes." She prefers cake blusher ("the creamy kind sinks in"). So does liquid base; she doesn't use any. And no powder ("too stage-y").

Claudia is an anti-soap militant: "The only time I ever use soap is in the bathtub, and never on my face. I get my face clean the way I have forever: I wash it first with a washcloth and hot water—that opens up the pores right away—then I use cold water. Next, I cream it all off with unscented Albolene. After this, I use a washcloth and warm water and, finally, icy cold. I go through a lot of washcloths, but it's worth it. . . . In the daytime, I'll put on a moisturizer; at night, nothing. And nothing in the summer, because my skin has a lot of natural oil and more, it seems, in the summer. I don't usually have a breakout, but if I do, I put alcohol on it—pure alcohol. . . . I think people are too dirt-conscious. Your body functions clean you naturally. If you're healthy, if you eat well—if what you put inside is healthy—you'll be clean."

She is selective about her self-care: her diet is long on fresh vegetables and brown rice; short on such frowned-upon items as salt and eggs. On the other hand, she is one of a vanishing breed: She is an unregenerate sun worshiper (although she has cut down her exposure time from "all day" to "half an hour . . . well, maybe an hour").

Claudia's chief form of exercise is tennis, which she plays year round and at near-championship level. She adores the game; it's almost the only thing that ever causes her to fret about getting older: "It's not anything to do with my looks. Mainly, it's that I think, Oh, God! when I get to sixty or seventy, I'm not going to play great tennis anymore! But then I remember, that's how I thought ten years ago. . . ." And just look at her now.

If you're one-of-a-kind,
be original and creative with makeup.

Zandra Rhodes

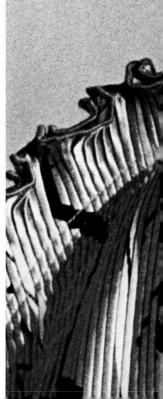

"I like myself made up all the time. I wear lots and lots around my eyes, and a whitener to go on the bags underneath.... I always use rouge.... I powder my face with talcum powder. I never take off my makeup. *Never.* I sleep in it. Of course, I wash it off in the morning. Then I put a whole new lot on."

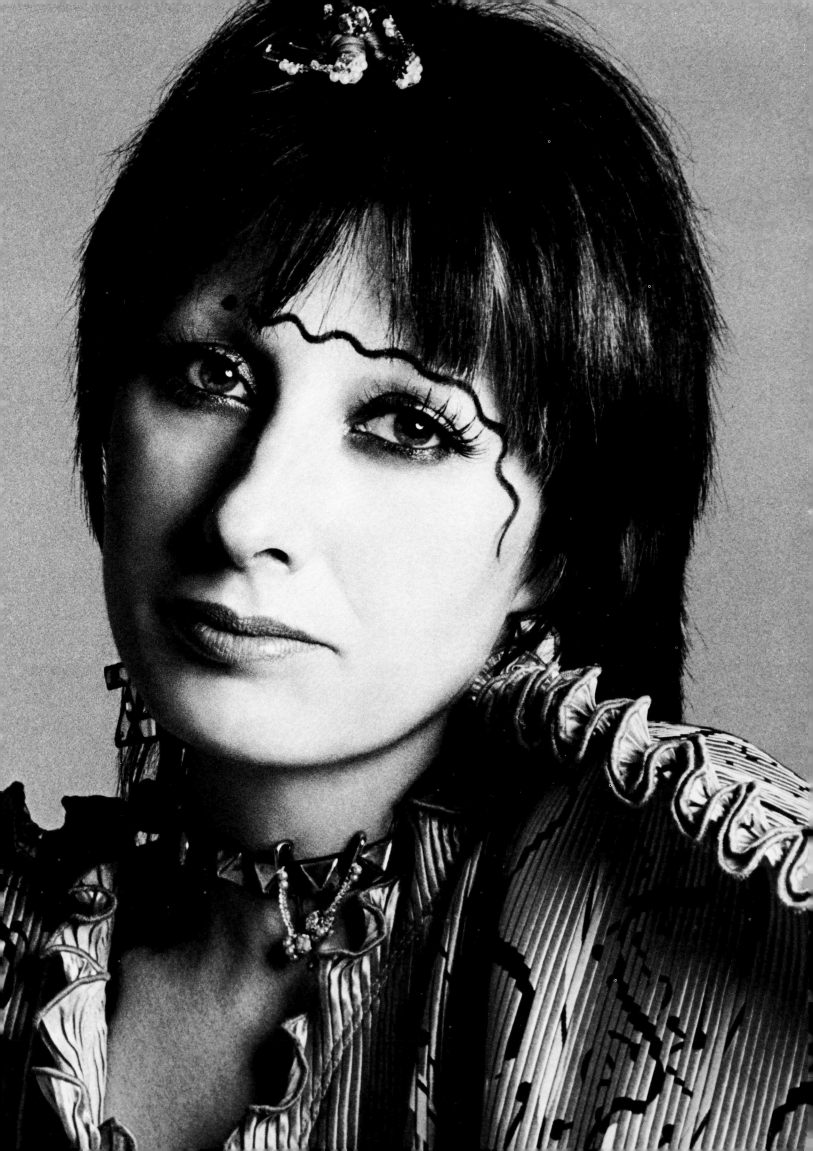

Zandra Rhodes

Everything about Zandra Rhodes is extraordinary. Her flamingo-pink hair is extraordinary. Her scalloped eyebrows are extraordinary. Her clothes most of all, her wonderful, wonky, fantastical, beautiful clothes, are extraordinary—every woman should own at least one Zandra Rhodes!

With most people, in my work, I like to give a new image or strengthen the existing image. Zandra I don't touch. She is an original, a one-of-a-kind. There isn't any way she can be edited; it's a matter of simply recording her: her makeup, her hair. On this particular day, her hair was two shades of pink, hemmed in black. (She had just come back from Kenya, where "the sun, together with whatever they put in the swimming pool, bleached the front whitish-pink, which everyone liked so I left it. I had the bottom dyed in a straight black row, because then, when the roots grow out at the top, you don't really notice . . . and I don't have to jeopardize my hair by having it done too often.") When I first met her, it was green, another time purple. Her eyebrows, which are painted-on pink scallops—for the moment—have been on other occasions "two pointed pagodas, three eyebrows in black. . . . I've got none of my own; I plucked them all away years ago, and they never grew back. . . . It doesn't make any difference; if I need an eyebrow I just draw it on."

She invents herself with powder and paint: "I like myself made up all the time. I wear lots and lots around my eyes, and a whitener to go on the bags underneath. . . . I always use rouge. . . . I powder my face with talcum powder. I never take off my makeup. *Never.* I sleep in it. Of course, I wash it off in the morning. Then I put a whole new lot on." Once on, "I never look at myself in the mirror."

Zandra has been called the Princess of Punk; actually, she was punking out before it had a name. Back in the sixties, when a punk was still a rotten kid and Zandra was just starting as a textile designer: "I suddenly thought, Well, hang about . . . if they can dye sheep's wool. . . . So I went to Leonard's and got him to dye it; I think we tried green first." Until then, Zandra Rhodes, late of Chatham, Kent; graduate—with a first-class honors degree in textile printing—of London's Royal College of Art ("the mecca of art colleges for the whole world"), was a closet brunette. "I used to wear turbans—*always*—and lots and lots and lots of jewelry. I didn't think I looked that extreme, but the girl I was in partnership with then said, 'You look so extraordinary, you frighten the customers.' "

1969, on her first trip to New York, she met Angelo Donghia, the interior decorator. "If you look as amazing as that," he said, "you must do wonderful work." He immediately bought a collection of her prints. Two other big boosts came out of that trip: *Women's Wear Daily* gave her a double-page spread, and *Vogue* did two color pages of Natalie Wood wearing Zandra Rhodes: "It has just built up from that."

She has also been called "the designer's designer, because I live for design and I'm prepared to stick my neck out for what I believe in." She has sometimes felt the ax uncomfortably close: "There was a period when I thought it would be intriguing to try beaded safety pins and do dresses that had sleeves pinned in and that looked as though they had holes in them. Why can't we have sleeves that pin in; are there always going to be sewing machines? If you don't question, you don't come up with something new. I christened this look Conceptual Chic. But it got labeled punk, and a whole lot of

> ## "I want to develop my character, to become so amazing that people don't notice what I look like."

One man's meat. . . . In ladies thought, My God, if she looks like that, I can't buy chiffon dresses from her. People were nervous, and for a while it badly affected my business. But I'm driven by being truthful to myself. And now people don't mind at all; they say, 'Oh, well, that's just Zandra.' "

All along, there have been women who collect Zandra Rhodes as they would a work of art; now that they have been joined by a whole new democracy of admirers, she is thrilled . . . and worried that she could "become establishment." It seems unlikely. Still, there is a sense one gets that the tide may be turning away from what she calls "high-chic look-alike

■

"If you don't question, you don't come up with something new."

■

fashion" and flowing in the direction of "the world's fantasy lady." Certainly more women than ever before are buying her offbeat, individualistic clothes —enough of them, even, to relieve her other fear: "One might become a cult figure." Since at least one common stripe of cult figures is that their followers tend to be a lot like each other, she might as well stop worrying: All kinds of people love Zandra Rhodes. Her clothes are worn by such seen-around types as Bianca Jagger and Cleo Lane, as well as by art critic Rosamund Bernier and best-dress-listee D. D. Ryan— not to mention the unsung wave of women who, with the introduction of her new starting-at-$100 line, will at last be able to afford the fun of being a Zandra Rhodes Lady.

To its creator, the Zandra Rhodes boom indicates that women are beginning to be a little more adventurous in their dressing: "I think people don't just want to know the dull facts of life all the time. Of course you need practical clothes, though I don't happen to be the world's most practical person—I wear things for daytime that other people would only consider for evening. But why not? You shouldn't be afraid to wear what you would like to wear when you want to wear it. . . . Dressing up is great for one's morale. Even if you don't know that it's going to be something dressy, dress up. It's a compliment to the host, and it makes you feel terrific. So what if you're very dressed up? People tend to want me to be. . . . I'm in the rather strange position now of belonging to my public in the matter of how I look and how I dress."

How she looks and how she dresses rarely go unremarked. "If I walk down 58th Street, I get stopped by tourists who want to take my photograph, as if I were a freak; if it weren't for the fact that I have built up within myself the confidence of knowing who I am and how I am, that could be quite defeating. But I feel very strongly that people shouldn't be defeated by these things, and I don't let myself be. I don't think about it."

What she does think about is: her work (in addition to the new American ready-to-wear line, she has been asked by Kenneth Macmillan to design a ballet in Covent Garden); holidays (which is "when most of my dreams start. I do a drawing every single day; in Kenya, for instance, I drew zebras in the grass, natives with their earrings. When I get back to London, I take these and my Instamatic photographs and I piece together ideas that gradually take shape and become, first of all, the textile designs, and then the textiles, and eventually the whole thing."). Sometimes, she thinks about marriage; there is a man in her life now, and she lived with one man for twelve years. "Though I think men can often exist without women, I don't think we can exist without them. Except for the ones that have been turned round by the Women's Movement—which I think has de-balled men and, in general, done more harm than good—women still dress for men, still mind what men say. . . .

"I don't necessarily want to be beautiful. What I want is to develop my character, to become so amazing that people don't notice what I look like— that I'm only five-feet-two or that I'm normally in such a hurry that I've got ladders in my stockings." . . . To me, she has always been six feet tall.

■

"I've got no eyebrows of my own. . . . It doesn't make any difference; if I need an eyebrow, I just draw it on."

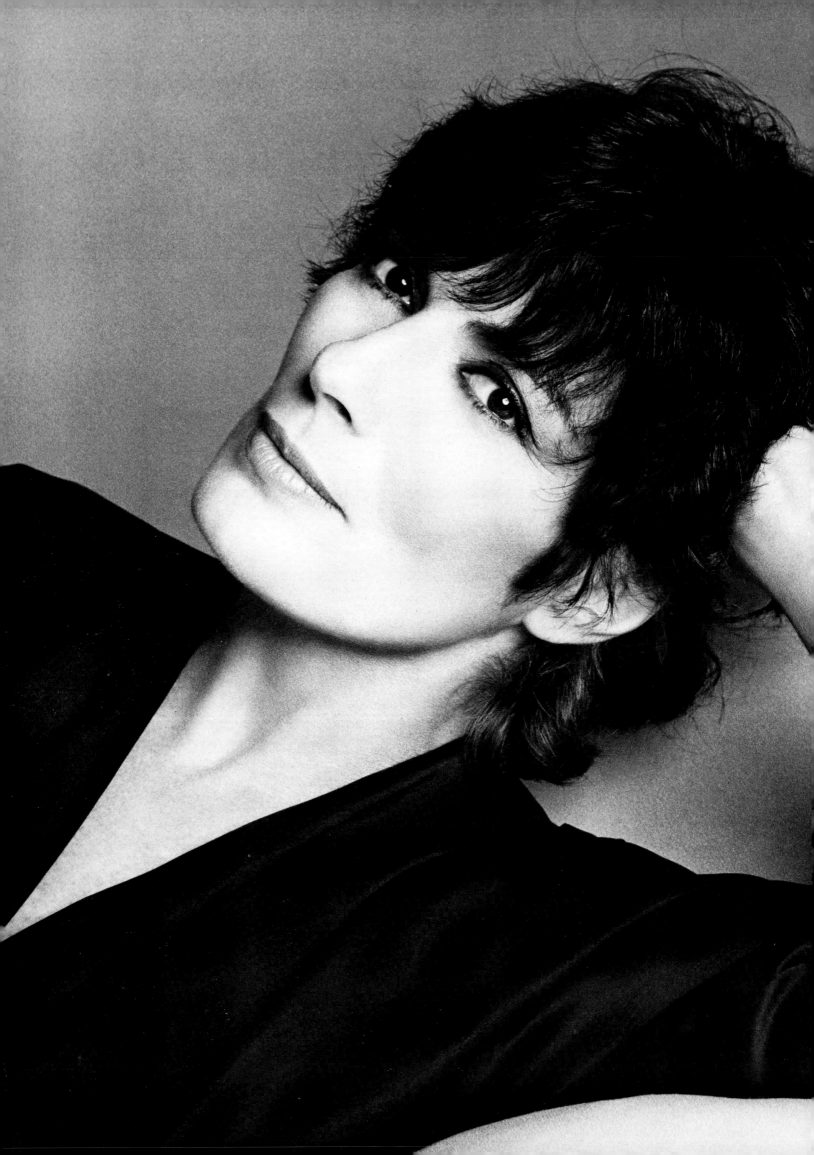

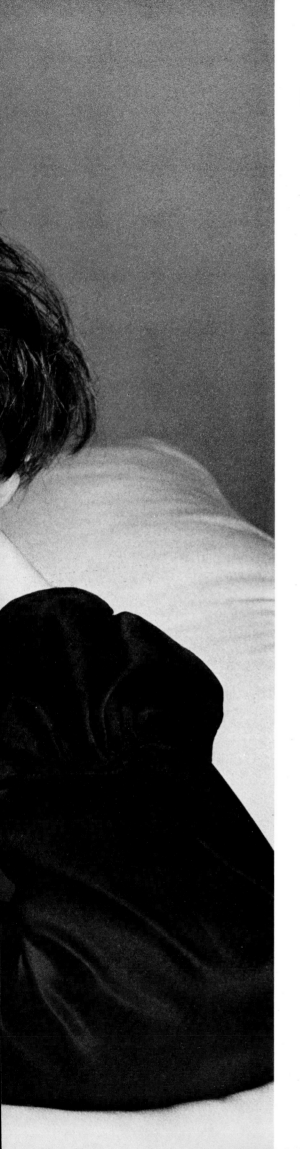

Femininity means intelligence, independence, and a sense of humor.

Jackie Rogers

"Never, never overdo it. If you're ever in doubt, don't do it. That's a beauty tip, and that's a fashion tip. . . . Nothing looks as good as a navy-blue sweater and gray flannel pants. Nothing. I mean, *boom!* — perfect. Glamorous classics are *forever.*"

Jackie Rogers

Jackie Rogers, the fashion designer, grew up (chubby) in Boston; came (thinner) to New York and worked as a fashion-show runway model; went to Rome, did some modeling, and acted in Italian films (among them, Fellini's *8½*); went to Paris in the early sixties, got a job modeling for Chanel, threatened to quit unless she could also work on the clothes, stayed (on her terms) two years; returned to New York, worked in television commercials, and opened the first hairdressing salon for men, in a Madison Avenue brownstone ("very elegant, very crazy"), which led her to try her hand at designing men's clothing. ("No one had ever really designed clothes for men. There was a good reason: no necessity. After all, men should just be wearing nice sedate clothes.") Her luck changed in a big way when she started designing for women—extraordinary beautiful clothes that she sells at her shop on Madison Avenue to such stylish dressers as Jacqueline Onassis and Diana Ross.

"New York is the only place where there is energy, true energy."

I adore Jackie. She is a marvelous woman—intelligent, independent, sophisticated, funny, irreverent. And more opinionated than anyone I know; there is almost nothing and nobody she doesn't feel strongly about.

Here is Jackie on marriage: "I was married . . . for twenty minutes. I was nineteen. This guy was in love with the Red Sox; he cried whenever they lost a game. He was a nice, simple boy, very rich, very cute. My father came to get me when the marriage broke up. I ate and ate and ate and got fat. He [her former husband] was going to kill himself when I left; he's been married twice since. I never have again. . . . When I first went to Venice in around '59, I was at a huge party—everybody looked so happy—and everybody was with everybody else's wife or husband. They were very sophisticated, very out-front. In those days (and I don't know that it's changed all that much), nobody ever got divorced, especially in Italy. In this country, it's absurd, a money game more than anything: women marrying men for money and power. Then they divorce them—or they kill 'em off because they've worked them to death—and marry someone richer."

"There used to be a lot of men that I respected, but less and less as I get older."

On places to live: "You go to California to live and you lie by your pool and you wake up and you're sixty-five. . . . Europe used to be exciting. It's boring now; I think they're all moving to America. . . . New York is the only place where there is energy, true energy."

On men: "There used to be a lot of men that I respected, but less and less as I get older. I admire Solzhenitsyn. And let's not forget Bobby Kennedy. When he was assassinated, it was the end of the great leaders. . . . I like to be with gay men. They have a sense of abandonment. They're fun, simpatico. Black men have abandonment too; they're also simpatico. Harlem was fabulous to go to in the fifties. . . . All straight white men are dull; they don't seem to have a good time. Straight is boring."

On drugs: "People take anything to get their heads somewhere else. It's a dull society, that's why they do it. Drugs destroy a society. They give people a false sense of joy and a false sense of creativeness. We have drug movies. They are bad movies, made by people who go off on location and think they've shot a great movie. Then they come back and it's missing and pieced together badly, and they want to kill themselves in the morning."

On the media in America: "Solzhenitsyn, when he spoke at the Harvard commencement exercises a couple of years ago, said it: Who elects them to office? To whom are they responsible? Meaning the press. It's true. Their irresponsibility in reporting the news is disgraceful. The way they destroy people, destroy a career—it's frightening. I mean, the *New York Post* is disgusting. . . . The way news is reported on television is flip. The approach isn't serious. It's all, Let's entertain, let's be controversial, like Mike Wallace and *60 Minutes*. It's gotten to be a joke, a circus—offensive. There's nothing intrinsically wrong with a light hand. But I mean, my God! . . .''

On how she designs: "I work from line. To me, it's all proportion. I'm obsessed with it: If the line is not right the whole thing is wrong. The proportions have got to be all together, and once I see them all come together, then, no matter what I'm designing, it works. And it has to work for everybody. When it does, I know it's right. . . . My clothes are very personal, very

meanor is much more feminine than if you were going to wear those heavy knit sweaters and a pair of freakin' clogs!''

On Women's Liberation: "I think it's all just a destructive element that is very confusing to a lot of people, men and women. They don't understand it. . . . I don't understand it, and I'm not exactly stupid. If you want to be liberated, then you should be. But if you shouldn't, you shouldn't. I mean, it wasn't in the cards for me to live at home with a husband and a couple of kids. But it is for some women; instead, they force themselves to think they must do it—must be liberated. And they wind up in the shithouse. I blame Gloria Steinem. She's made a great career for herself, and I think she's full of shit; anyone who gets on television and says 'et cetera, et cetera, et cetera' is not very articulate. I would not become a liberated woman listening to Gloria Steinem. But I think a lot of warped souls are listening to this woman . . . and they come home and either kill their children or leave their husbands.

we pay for that equal wage? I still want a man to open the door for me. I still like a man to call me up and ask me to dinner. At what price is it really worth the price? I hear women saying they can't find a man, that all the men are screwed up or they're gay. I don't blame the men. These women frighten me too. They're not feminine. . . . I haven't seen anyone come forward from any Women's Liberation organization who's a great beauty. Frustrated women are not very attractive.''

On keeping in shape: "If you want to feel good about yourself, you have got to have a good figure, you've got to keep yourself trim. . . . I'm always try-

"Clothes should make you feel good— and feel good about yourself.''

"Drugs destroy a society. They give people a false sense of joy and a false sense of creativeness.''

sensuous; they're cut on the bias, so that when you put them on and feel them on your body, you feel good. The whole point is that clothes should make you feel good—and feel good about yourself.''

On fashion hates: "These sacks that women go around in—they're not sensuous; you can't tell what's underneath. I think sensuality is the most vital thing in dressing . . . it makes you act differently . . . you wear high heels and you walk differently from the way you walk in flat shoes. Your whole de-

'm not saying women shouldn't have equal wages with men. But I also say, Well, hey, what's the other price

ing to lose ten pounds. I eat too much on the weekend and work it off during the week. . . . I go to the Sports Training Institute two or three times a week. I work on the Nautilus machines, and I do pull-ups and push-ups; I can do a hundred and fifty push-ups in a row. . . . I've never been one for massage, but I love pedicures. They make you feel marvelously relaxed—it's because of all those nerve endings in your feet.''

On what's important: "We must nourish creativeness—that's basic. We must preserve any kind of talent at any cost. It's easy not to give a shit, but you come on this earth only once. No returns. Life is short. The most important thing is to be at peace with yourself, or you're in trouble. I'm very demanding of myself, but I don't take myself too seriously. . . . I just love life. And it's getting better!''

Rosemary Rogers

"I'm very much my own person. I've learned to be. I like being with myself. I like being alone. . . . There's a difference between loneliness and solitude; I don't think I'll ever really be all alone. It's what it means to be self-sufficient. I have friends, and I like to talk with my friends and be with them, but at the same time I like to do what I feel like doing when I feel like doing it."

A curious phenomenon of the literary universe is the world of the original paperback novel: the Western, the sci-fi, the romances: Gothic, modern, historical. In a way, these books are to publishing what successful daytime soap operas are to television: scorned by the highbrows, relatively unsung, and loved only by an audience so large and so loyal it boggles the mind. And makes their creators rich beyond your wildest dreams.

All of which applies to paperback fiction. Especially, it applies to Rosemary Rogers. Just in case you thought Judith Krantz was *the* hot lady writer on the best-seller lists, listen to this: Between 1974 and 1980, Rosemary published seven romances—five historical, two contemporary—and sold 25 million copies, give or take a million. If you have a pragmatic turn of mind, these are some of the things that such magical numbers have brought her way: college and/or private school educations for her two daughters by her first marriage, for her two sons by her second, and for her niece, whom she has adopted; two houses in California, one in Carmel and one on Big Sur, with a hot tub, overlooking the ocean; an apartment in New York; a Mercedes SL with a sun-roof back. And, most prized of all, total independence.

Rosemary Rogers, who looks like a Rosemary Rogers heroine—tall, narrow-waisted, with a lovely full mouth and limpid eyes—was born in Sri Lanka in 1933, when the country was still known as Ceylon. Her parents were well-to-do, strict, conservative. "I was always a free-thinker. I always read a lot. My father used to bring back all kinds of books from Europe and stash them away. I found out where, and that's how I came to read *Lady Chatterley's Lover* and Henry Miller. I kept abreast of what was happening in the rest of the world. . . . I got married just to be able to leave home, because my parents wouldn't let me date; at eighteen I wasn't permitted to go out alone, even with a girl friend. And naturally, no makeup. . . . Finally, I went to college; it was my first break from home."

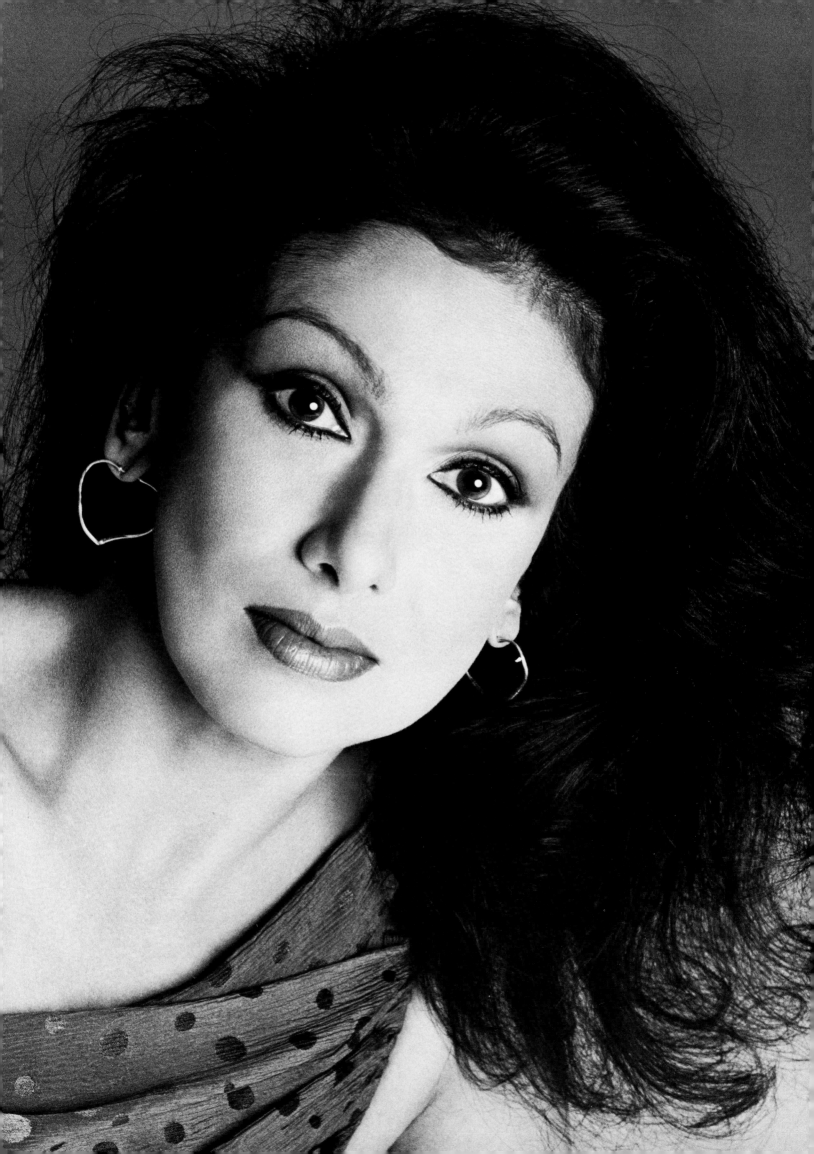

Rosemary Rogers

At the University of Ceylon, Rosemary made her second break. She married her first husband, a track star known as "the fastest man in Asia." The marriage produced two children and eventually broke up. Today, she and her ex-husband are good friends. "Once the anger and the bitterness of the conflict die down and you aren't arguing anymore, you find you still have a lot in common: the same background, the children. And I like him. Much more than I did when we were married. Then I was very constricted. I was supposed to conform to what was expected of a wife and a mother, and I've never been a conformist."

In 1962, with her two daughters, Rosemary moved to London, married an American serviceman, came with him to California, had two sons, worked as a secretary. In 1964, she divorced, switched jobs, and became a closet writer. Ten years later, *Sweet Savage Love* was published. You would have thought books were going out of style; it didn't walk off the shelves, it flew. It soared. It made her independent.

'm very much my own person. I've learned to be. I like being with myself. I like being alone. Lots of people ask me how I stand it out at the beach—it's very isolated, and I live there all by myself, with a dog who keeps me company. With the children grown up and away, or ready to move away, I discovered I like being alone. It's not that I'm antisocial. When I am out with friends, I enjoy that too. But I do enjoy it alone.

"I've been married and divorced twice. After that, I all of a sudden discovered—whilst eating a lot—that I was still thinking I had to have a man or a lover or something. But we're brought up that way; it's a form of brainwashing. Then I realized, I don't really need it. I don't really want it. . . . I lived with a man once, for about four years. That was the last occasion. He was in the air force, and he got stationed somewhere else. And when he went I thought to myself, It is such a relief not to have to depend on somebody else's time clock to have meals ready, to wake up, to go to bed, to plan my days and hours around somebody else's schedule. I don't have to depend on anybody. I know it's selfish, but so what?

"There's a difference between loneliness and solitude; I don't think I'll ever really be all alone. It's what it means to be self-sufficient. I have friends, and I like to talk with my friends and be with them, but at the same time I like to do what I feel like doing when I feel like doing it. It's great to know that I can pick up and leave at a moment's notice. Last month I was in New York, and a friend who was in Marbella, in Spain, said, 'Why don't you come over?' And just like that, I bought a ticket and off I went.

"There's somebody who's pestering me to get married, but I don't know if I will. It's very doubtful . . . I have too much fun as I am. I don't want to be tied down to one man, one person." This isn't how it goes in a Rosemary Rogers novel. There, the path of true love is anything but smooth but its ultimate destination is clearly eternal; in *Lost Love, Last Love,* the final line reads, "It was the beginning of forever." Though you never know with this couple, who, through three novels so far, keep coming together and falling away like shutters in a hurricane. The trouble (we should all have such troubles!) is: "The characters are so popular that I've had to write other books about them. They end up in each other's arms and then they split, and then back again, and then they split again."

The readers who make these demands range in age from girls in their teens to eighty- and ninety-year-olds. They write letters. They write to get more details about the characters' lives, backgrounds, what they call their children. They write when a book has given them special pleasure: "I remember a letter from one girl who said that since reading *Wicked Loving Lies*— and having her husband read it too— she realized there were other uses for champagne besides just drinking it. You know, we can always pour it all over. . . ." They also let Rosemary know when they're displeased, as many, particularly her older readers, were when she published her first contemporary romance, which ventured into fairly graphic sexual detail. It isn't her usual style. "I don't like pornographic sex, though I think you can be a little more explicit than writers used to be—you know, where he carried her into the bedroom and kicked the door shut. I go into a bit more detail but not too much, not clinical—I *sneak* into the bedroom."

"My skin is better now than it was twenty years ago!"

Rosemary writes at her beach house, usually right through the night. "Sometimes I work until about noon or three or four in the afternoon. Then I go to sleep. I can sleep at any time, anywhere. I can sleep in automobiles. I can sleep in airplanes. If I tell myself I'm going to sleep, I sleep. And I'm very good at catnapping. You have to learn to do that, especially on tour. It's a killer. Absolutely crazy. You live out of suitcases for weeks on end, and then your whole day is organized for you: interviews, autograph sessions, television, radio, usually a dinner with book buyers or booksellers. And then you fall into bed, get up and catch a plane, and go to the next place. And it starts all over."

No matter where and come what may, she has never been known to look less than smashing. The trick, she says, is "keeping calm." Meditation is one way she does it. "Usually, after I wake up, I do a few of the hatha yoga exercises, where I concentrate more on meditation and the mind, the taking in of light and moving it out. It has nothing to do with transcendental meditation, which is almost a form of self-hypnosis. TM relies on the mantra the way a hypnotist relies on a trigger word for post-hypnotic suggestions. With hatha yoga, *you* have to do it—through the exercises and the stretching of the body. All the time I'm doing the exercises I'm concentrating on the breathing and the opening of the *chakras* in the body, which are the nerve centers, and the taking in of light. And you can meditate on anything: something you can visualize, something you want to happen. You don't have to clear your mind. They say if you try to, consciously, it gets even harder to unclutter. What you do is relax and let every thought come into your mind, and gradually you find them all going away as you concentrate on the light and the breathing.

"I was always a free thinker. . . . I've never been a conformist."

"Also, my house on Big Sur, where I spend most of my time, has got ocean on three sides and the mountains behind, so it's very relaxing to be there. I can gaze at the ocean for hours; that's another form of meditation. . . . And I'm a hot-tub addict. I have my own, set into the deck, which overlooks a little cove that comes in from the sea. There are benches right around; the thing about a hot tub is, it's common; everybody gets in. You take off your clothes and you get in. Mostly, I do it by myself. But if I have friends there, they come in. And my children love to come. It's very nice . . . social."

Another guaranteed calmer for Rosemary is the commonplace ritual of removing her makeup, "always; it makes a great difference in how I feel.

No matter how tired I am, if I put makeup on, I take it off. Then I put a night cream on—something with collagen. I know it helps. Definitely—my skin is better now than it was twenty years ago!"

Like a lot of women who've put their faces in the hands of Way Bandy, her makeup routine has not been the same since. "After the sitting, I went to my favorite restaurant and a disco later, and everyone said, *What* did you do with yourself? You look fantastic!" So she stayed with it; who wouldn't? "I keep my eyebrows plucked and shaped the way he did them; they used to be thicker and closer together. . . . I used to color my eyelids one color and take it up a little bit; Way showed me how much better it was to use a darker eye shadow, shading it all the way onto the bone and into the socket, and then taking it out at the corners a little bit by sort of blending the pencil into the shadow."

Following Way's advice, she uses a *lot* of moisturizer, "two different kinds, plus one that's tinted. First I put on Aloe Vera with Vitamin E, which I've always done, and it sinks into the skin right away. Then, as Way suggested, I use a moisturizer by Stendhal. And over it, I put their tinted moisturizer, in a browny beige color—it just looks as though I've been out in the sun. Sometimes I don't use anything else, but if I'm doing a real makeup, I put two bases on top of it: a porcelain-beige one, by Clinique, and a Stendhal, which is golden tan. Finally, Way said, always spritz the face with Evian water, and I adore that. I think all these things are keeping my skin very soft. . . . What I love for cheek color is Indian Earth— you put it on with a little sponge, and you have a lovely natural glow. You can even do it on your nails; it gives a

shine, like buffing, and just a touch of color. It doesn't stay on for ages and ages, but it lasts for an evening."

A slim woman with the body of a sixteen-year-old, who turns out to be fifty and to have four grown children, attracts attention for a reason. Rosemary's is simple: She eats once a day. And she eats vegetarian. "I don't eat meat at all. I don't drink coffee or tea, because they're not good for the body. I don't eat fruits that are packaged or canned or have artificial additives. I'm a health nut. Most of the stuff I eat is from the health-food store; even my pasta is from organically grown grains. I take vitamins by the handful—B complex, B-15, B-12, E, lecithin. . . . I love to cook; I love to create. I cook everything, anything— Ceylonese food, Italian food, French, Greek, Mexican. I cook a very quick marinara kind of sauce, with fresh tomatoes and green peppers, onions, and little tiny bay scallops. Delicious! . . . Cooking is my therapy."

She would swim and play tennis if her schedule didn't mean that she's usually asleep when most people do these things. Her sport is the night people's sport: "I love to disco. I love dancing. Sometimes I disco all by myself. I put on some music and just dance with the beat." The music goes all the time, especially when she's writing. Only then it's "classical music, always. . . . With this new book, I've been playing Wagner over and over and over again." I can see it now: Siegfried crushes Brünhilde to his chest "and somewhere behind them the fire sputtered into oblivion . . . the sun forced itself between carelessly drawn draperies . . . it was the beginning of forever."

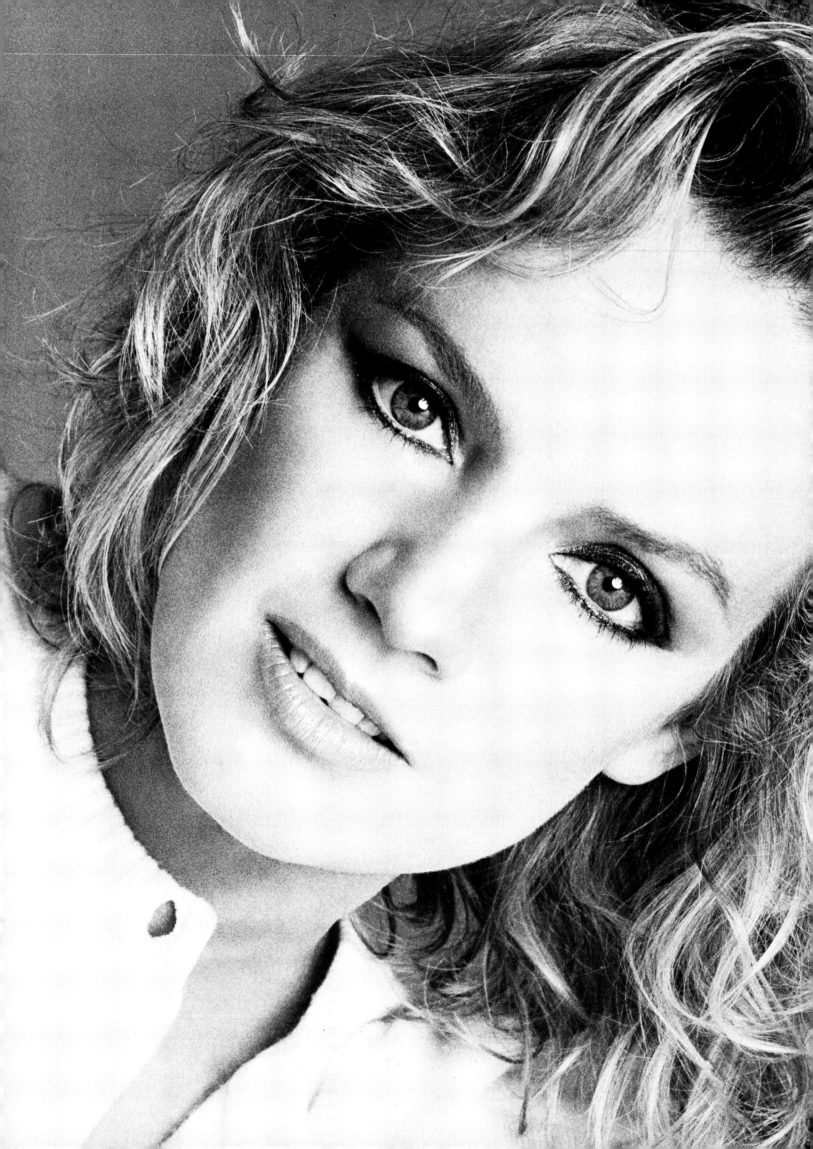

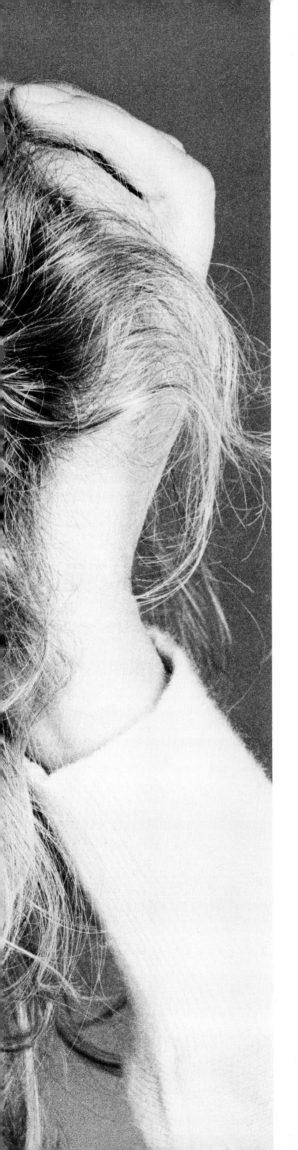

Feeling good about yourself—
inside and out

Jil Sander

"I learned early that I had to become strong in order to do what I wanted. Every woman in the eighties needs a strong personality. It's much more valuable than beauty."

Jil Sander

The thing that really gets me about this woman is an extraordinary cleanness. In the evening, when you know she's wearing makeup, you aren't afraid to get close. You know nothing's going to rub off. Too many women use so much makeup they become like those beautiful oriental lilies—fabulous to see but dangerous to touch, unless you want a sleeve full of pollen. You see those women and stay away. You

ing for anyone's OK. She's a modern woman, definitely liberated. She's out there competing, living her life the way she wants to live it, doing the work she wants to do—and she's fabulously successful at it. A thirty-eight-year-old fashion designer with the dash of a latter-day Chanel, she has two shops of her own and over a hundred franchise outlets all over Europe, a line of cosmetics, perfume, and, coming soon, a treatment line which promises to carry out her spare, crisp style. She is, in a word, contemporary.

We tend to think American women have an exclusive on this kind of look and life. Jil happens to be German. And though things are changing today even in that bastion of the *kinder, kirche, küche* tradition, in 1966, when Jil started her business, German women were still pretty firmly tied to the

"If you make your life unhappy, you look old."

learn to fight. Because it was difficult, I was lucky. I learned early that I had to become strong in order to do what I wanted. I think every woman in the eighties needs a strong personality. It's much more valuable than beauty. Flat beauty—someone beautiful without personality—is perhaps OK for certain cases, but it's boring and short-lived. The appeal of a strong personality continues all your life. . . . I don't want to cover the personality when I design for women. I want the strength to show. I want to see her face. If you cover too much, if you dress a woman with all this *chi-chi,* then you see only the body. It's possible to be body-minded, but I am face-minded. I'm interested in personality, and you see that in the expression, in the eyes, when a woman is not overwhelmed by her clothes. I want people to be themselves, to feel well in their clothes. If you have clothes with a simple style, of good quality, that will happen.

"I am face-minded. I'm interested in personality and you see that in the expression, in the eyes, when a woman is not overwhelmed by her clothes."

know you'll be a mess if you get too close. Jil's makeup for day or evening is actually a no-makeup makeup. Way Bandy got the same effect for the photograph with a suntan color base. He diluted it with Evian water to a very thin and watery state. It's hardly there, but is enough to lift and even the texture and color of the skin—something everybody needs, Way says.

Jil Sander almost epitomizes the American ideal in her looks—fresh-scrubbed and glowing, classic clothes in beautiful fabrics—and in her style: doing just as she pleases without wait-

home. Even in America, equality of the sexes wasn't much discussed then. For Jil it wasn't even an issue. "In my work I never found being a woman to be a problem, just because my competitors are men. I always worked with men, had good contacts with men. I don't think those concerns are there anymore. If you know your business you do it, whether you are a man or a woman. You deal with other women or with men on a human level, and it's so easy. Simple and pure.

"I was just twenty-four when I started. Because I was young I had to

You can't design for every woman. You must say, 'This is my way, this is how I see women!' I am very egoistic. I think first of how I like to dress, how I feel easy and comfortable, what I want to wear. I wear my own clothes and use my own products. I would be very disappointed if I couldn't. Of course, there must be not only things I like to wear, but for women of different needs. The collections are quite big, from evening to sportswear."

"When I was building my business I almost destroyed myself. I was working, running, I was trying to move the world. I didn't think about taking care of my body or how to train myself to be in good form. I was smoking like an idiot. I partied. I didn't drink so much, but I just wasn't careful what I put into my system.

"So I became sick. It took a terrible

you start thinking about health. Better to think before ruining your health. I was a little late on that. The real problem of bad eating is that so many people really don't know about food. But you must learn. You have to clean your insides. If you don't, nothing can help you, not even the best cosmetics or treatments. I see it all from the point of how you feed yourself. If you eat well, if you rest and exercise, and if you try to be happy it will contribute so much energy and excitement to life. Positive thinking is very good for your life and your looks. Even if you have problems, say, 'OK, if I worry more it will not help, it will only make me more unhappy.' If you make your life unhappy, you look old.

"If you have security within yourself, you can do whatever you want. You are free."

Actually, I've always seen her in pants—and she's great in them. "I really love pants. It's partly habit. I always wore pants in school. Jeans. My father hated it. On the few times I wore a skirt my teacher, a real lady, would say, 'Oh, you look so sweet,' but I never gave up pants. It's easy and casual. In the last two years, though, I have been designing skirts. Everyone was saying about me, 'She can't do skirts,' so I felt I must prove that I could."

Taking the dare, proving herself, is instinctive with Jil. It doesn't make for an easy life for her or any other workaholic. With all that competitiveness and drive, something has to give:

scare for me to turn around my way of living. I was having trouble breathing and went to a doctor. He said I had some tumors on my throat and said, 'Listen, we have to take that out.' I thought, When they start to cut you know it will be the end. I went to a lot of other doctors. They all said, Operate, if you wait it will be worse. Then I went to a homeopath and an acupuncturist. They were able to get rid of the growths without surgery. These things I had were benign, not cancerous, so it was OK. But they said they don't know how these things develop; it may be from bad food, pollution, stress.

"I began to eat and drink only things that help the body. If you become ill

It's nice to have money to travel or to buy a painting. But I could give it up. I feel I am following my own line, but I'm not stuck. I could go to another country and start again. I think if you have security within yourself you can do whatever you want. You are free." . . . That's what I call liberated!

"The real problem of bad eating is that so many people really don't know about food."

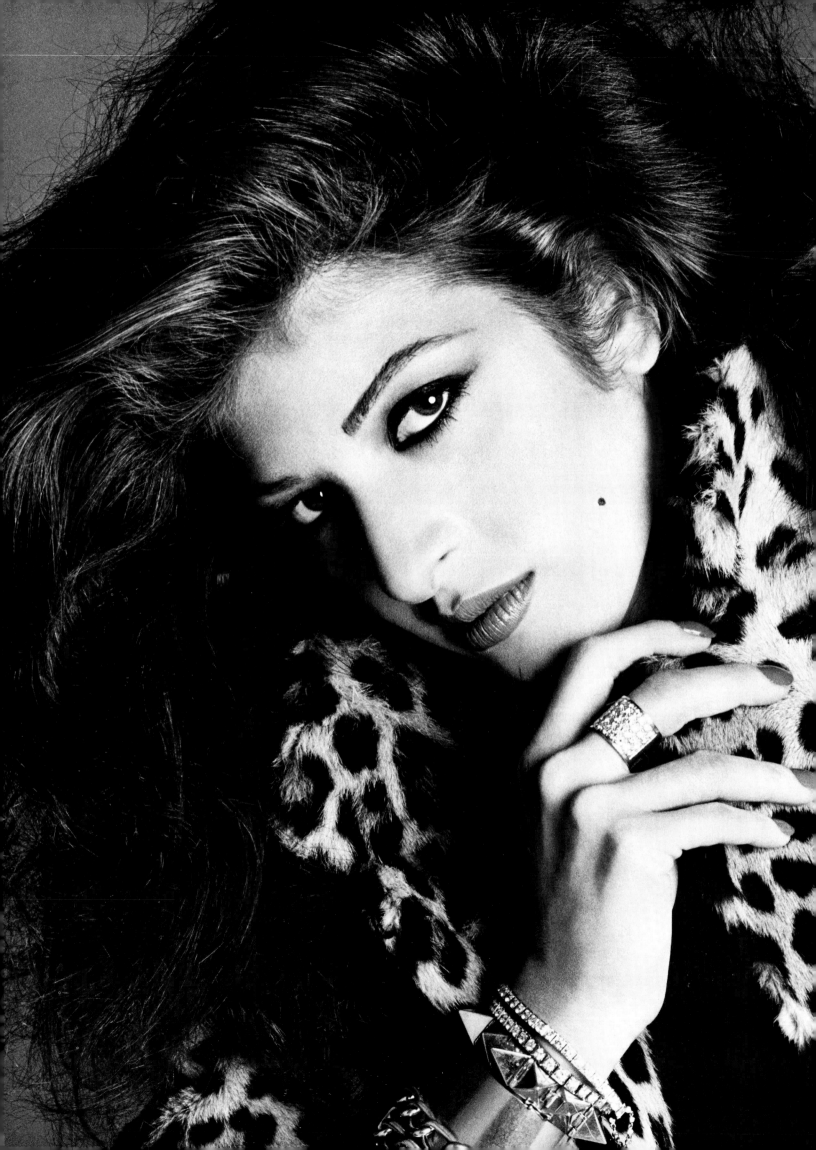

Janis Savitt

"I like to experiment. And I love it when someone else puts my makeup on because then I can learn a professional's technique and try to imitate what he's done."

Where Janis Savitt works, you don't throw anything away. When you wash your hands, you save the water; when you clean off the tables, you save the dust; when you sweep the floor, you save the sweepings. You'd have to be crazy not to . . . because where Janis Savitt works, there's gold in them thar sweepings: gold dust, silver dust, all sorts of specks and flecks from whatever precious metals and stones Janis and her staff may be working with on any given day. Eventually, the carats will all be separated out from the junk, turned back into their pure state, and used to create some of the best-looking contemporary jewelry being made anywhere in the world today.

Janis is the designing lady of the three-sister team of M & J Savitt. At twenty-six, she is the baby of the family and an old jewelry hand, having started at twelve making jewelry for friends. Four years later, she sold to Bloomingdale's the now-famous "elephant-hair" bangles and rings and earrings that were made of silver—which nobody took seriously in those days—with little gold wrappings. Overnight, silver was big-time. And so was M & J Savitt.

As creative spark of the company, Janis is into everything from original concept to final sketch, from stringing beads to overseeing everybody else's stringing and setting and cutting and polishing. "It's extremely important for me to be here, to be where everyone is actually making the things. Not only because everything is handmade or made to order, and I have to be sure it's all being done right, but if I'm not here there's a different spirit among the people working together." She's usually in the workroom (the Savitt offices are on 47th Street and Fifth Avenue, the eastern boundary of New York's wholesale jewelry district) by eight thirty or nine,

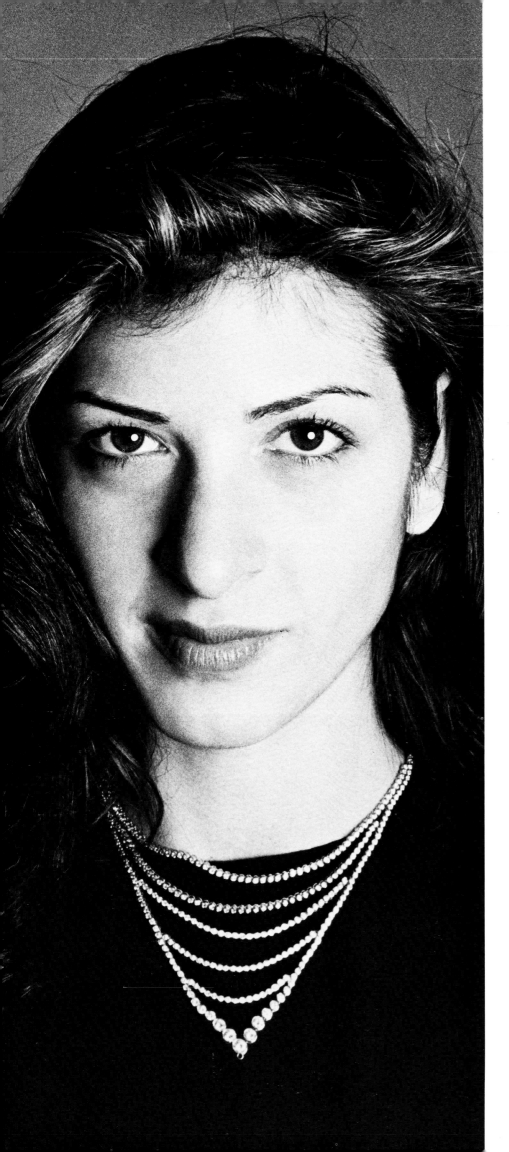

Janis Savitt

and leaves at seven, eight, ten—whenever, she is invariably the last to wash the gold dust off her hands.

"It's difficult these days. I've been like working, working, working, and then escaping for four days—I went to London for a long weekend recently. . . . I love working, but I don't like working to the point where I feel totally, physically a mess. I used to have a better balance of health, exercise, and work. Health is the most important thing. I'm more relaxed when I'm in good health. I'm happier, because I'm pleased with the way I look. And that means a lot to me, to feel good about my body and my looks. Even though I slave at my work, I want to compensate for it somehow—it's like going on a vacation for some people.

"My whole family has always been very health, weight, and beauty conscious. But it wasn't until around six years ago that I started seriously to exercise and enjoy it. I did yoga first, which is like an introduction to exercising without really straining yourself, and to learning how good you can feel. It doesn't build muscles but it does tone you and, like ballet, it gives you a little grace and an awareness of posture. . . . I like girls with muscles. I don't mean female body builders; I don't like big thighs and arms that bulge, but I like definition . . . I like dancers' bodies."

Janis has a fabulous body, slim, tall, and her legs go on forever. She works at it. "I used to go to the Sports Training Institute, and I belong to the New York Health and Racquet Club. But for the past several months I've been too busy to get there more than once a week. I call that not exercising. And it shows in your body—your thighs move on their own! Before, I was going all the time, taking yoga and calisthenics classes and working out on the Nautilus machines three times a week. The machines are very good for your upper body and the backs and fronts of your legs, but I don't think they're so good for working the inner thighs or your rear end. So I do all kinds of floor exercises as well; the ones you do on your hands and knees, like donkey kicks, are great for the rear end. And anything related to ballet has got to be good for the thighs.

Recently, because I wasn't getting to the club regularly, I decided to buy some equipment to use at home—little barbells, which are good for exercising the upper arms, and plastic-covered ankle weights for the legs; it's sort of like using the machines. . . . Exercise makes a big difference to me—not just for my body but for my head too. That's just as important as the physical thing. I exercise the way some people go home after work and have a drink or smoke a joint—to release the tension. And it's so much better a release!"

way your body reacts. Like, for years I was always going out in winter with no stockings and open-toed shoes—I remember going to parties where people would carry me over snowdrifts. But now if I'm not covered up I really feel it."

So now in winter she goes out at night with her stockings on, and—*wham!*—whole rooms light up on her energy. I know. I've taken her out and seen every man in the place turn to her as though he were being pulled by an irresistible force. He is; Janis is a great-looking girl any time, but at night she is an absolute knockout: a slinky, sizzling dynamo, with her thick dark hair, which is often just pulled back with a rubber band by day, loose and swinging and sexy as hell. It's how she keeps her life in balance: "Because I work very hard, I feel I need a release. And going out at night—changing myself totally from the way I am in the day—is one. It's a kind of variation of Janis. Work

walking up and down stairs—especially for the backs of your legs—but you have to wear flats with them." Otherwise, she is "strictly high heels," even with jeans—which, for Janis, are black, not blue, and fitted like skin.

"My taste has always been finding things and throwing them together rather than going out and buying a whole look. Even when I find something really beautiful by, say, Karl Lagerfeld, I'd rather take the inspiration and put it together my own way. Because with clothes like that, you can go out at night and see other women wearing the exact same thing. . . . I don't like to be seen in things that you can see on someone else. So I have a seamstress making things for me, with unusual fabrics. Or I'll find old things and have them copied or restored." She has cleaned out her closet "many times," and what that's about is "bored. Bored about looking at it, and wanting to start all over. Sometimes I regret the things I've given away . . . but on the other hand, I like to see change."

She is equally restless—and creative—about makeup. She can do more marvelous things with her face than any civilian I know. One time it might resemble what Way Bandy did for her here, another time it might be Audrey Hepburn. "I like to experiment. And I love it when someone else puts my makeup on, because then I can learn a professional's technique and try to imitate what he's done. I have a very good friend who's a makeup artist, and the first time he did it for me, I couldn't believe how it transformed my face . . . it was like being a different person. So I would try to copy him. Then I would clip pictures from magazines and try to imitate them. . . . My latest is the Maria Callas makeup from the Diana Vreeland book *Allure*. It's the way I do the eyebrows—strong and dark—and the eyeliner. I really love doe eyes . . . the 1950s makeup . . . the eyebrows, the liner, and the pale lips—nothing too much, not many colors or layers or contours, just flat. The other night, in a restaurant, three people I didn't even know said to me, 'You look like Maria Callas.' " . . . Or they'd have used some other excuse to talk to her, no matter what makeup or jewel or dress; when Janis gets it all together she attracts like a magnet . . . and, as she says, "That's the main idea."

"I don't like to be seen in things that you can see on someone else."

When she finishes working out at the club, Janis heads for the showers. "I usually take a sauna or a steam. If you do it the right way, your skin feels incredible. But it's a question of having the patience—you go in for maybe ten minutes, take a cold shower, rest for around thirty or forty minutes, then go in again for ten minutes, and finish with another cold shower. It makes such a difference, and afterward I put on Lancôme body lotion—the smell of it reminds me of the first time I went to Europe, but it also happens to be fantastic!

"Personally, I think the steam room is better for you than the sauna, because even though they're both taking water out of your body, the steam is also adding it, and water is the most important thing in moisturizing. Most people don't realize that it's not the cream that does it, it's the water; the cream just holds it in.

"I think beauty is a lifetime program. The older you get, the things you used to do a few years back might be showing up a little bit differently in the

is one way I am; going to the gym and trying to make myself feel good is another; and going out at night is another.

"If I were just daytime Janis or just nighttime Janis, I wouldn't be happy; I'd be compulsive. . . . You know the old saying, 'All work and no play'—you need the change. The night is almost like Hollywood fantasy—complete change. Sometimes I'm very conservative in dressing, and at other times it's all *va-va-voom*. . . . I just like change. I definitely like to be feminine. Even in the day, when I'm working, I feel dressed if I have high heels and lipstick on; with flats and no lipstick I feel as though I'm still sleeping. I just cannot get into wearing flat shoes, no matter what the fashion. I think they're for the tennis court. I've tried flats, but I just can't feel like a girl in them. It's terrible." Actually, she does wear them now and then. The reason is, she's discovered that those sensational legs of hers are in even better shape if she goes around the office in her ankle weights: "They're great to have on when you're

Being more attractive means getting back to the basics.

Terri Schwartz

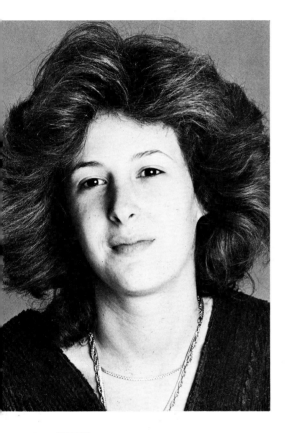

with. In other words, she didn't really know what she looked like.

You'd be surprised how few women do. Apart from models and actresses, there aren't many women I know who can look in the mirror and see themselves objectively—see what's good, not just what's bad (most women underrate themselves; they're usually a lot better-looking than they think they are). And this is what I try to show them in their photograph. It's the classic story: One picture is worth a thousand words.

First of all, I wanted Terri to see how attractive she could be with her own dark-brown hair coloring as opposed to frosting (which I hate for anyone; it's ordinary-looking, blatant, and it dries out the hair. If you're going to go that route, go all the way: have it subtly streaked all over by a first-rate colorist,

a better idea; a good old-fashioned coconut-oil treatment—working the oil into the hair and scalp, wrapping it up in a shower cap, and leaving it on overnight—works wonders.

Of course, we couldn't grow out the frosting on the spot, but by wetting her hair, hairdresser Deborah Tomasino could make it *look* dark. And by cutting it in a simple, rather gamine shape that could be just combed through with the fingers, she jumped Terri's hair from dowdy and old-looking to young and chic.

The other big, big eye-opener for Terri was to see herself thin, an illusion (and an incentive!) Way Bandy created for her by contouring. With a soft brownish rouge, and blending away madly, he went under the chin . . . under the cheeks . . . down the sides of the nose . . . around the eyes (a tremen-

> "I couldn't believe it was me—that I could look like that. But it *was* me! It made me see what I really was, what I could be."

It sometimes happens that a woman's whole look—her whole attitude about herself—is turned around by one good photograph. Terri Schwartz, for instance, arrived at the studio for a portrait sitting, a tall, shy nineteen-year-old, about twenty pounds overweight, with frosted hair, a cut with no shape to it, and a nowhere makeup. Hidden away in all this—and not very far away, either—was a pretty girl who wasn't giving herself a chance because she didn't realize what she had to work

or don't lighten it at all). For Terri, to lighten her hair—whatever the method —is the worst thing she could do: she loses all her drama. . . . Also, because it's a drier-outer, the constant frosting was making Terri's naturally coarse-textured hair even more so. Typically —and wrongly—Terri grabbed for cream conditioners, which coat rather than penetrate the hair and have, in the long run, the reverse effect of further coarsening the texture. Any kind of oil —coconut, olive, even mayonnaise—is

dous amount around the eyes, really bringing them up).

The "new" Terri was fabulous. More important, she thought so: "It was like a dream come true! It was incredible . . . gorgeous. I couldn't believe it was me—that I could look like that. But it *was* me! It made me see what I really was, what I could be." . . . Today, she *is:* slim, de-frosted, sure of herself—a look-alike for the girl we dreamed up in the studio. All she needed was to be shown.

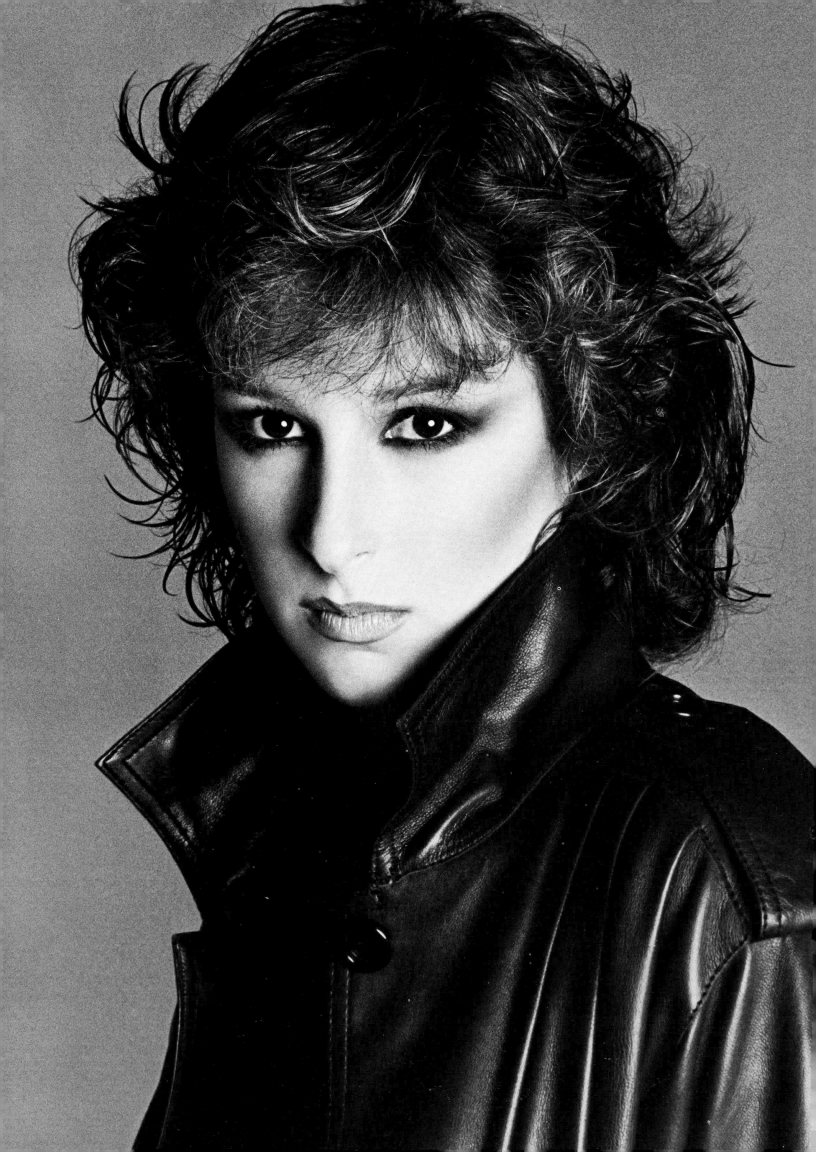

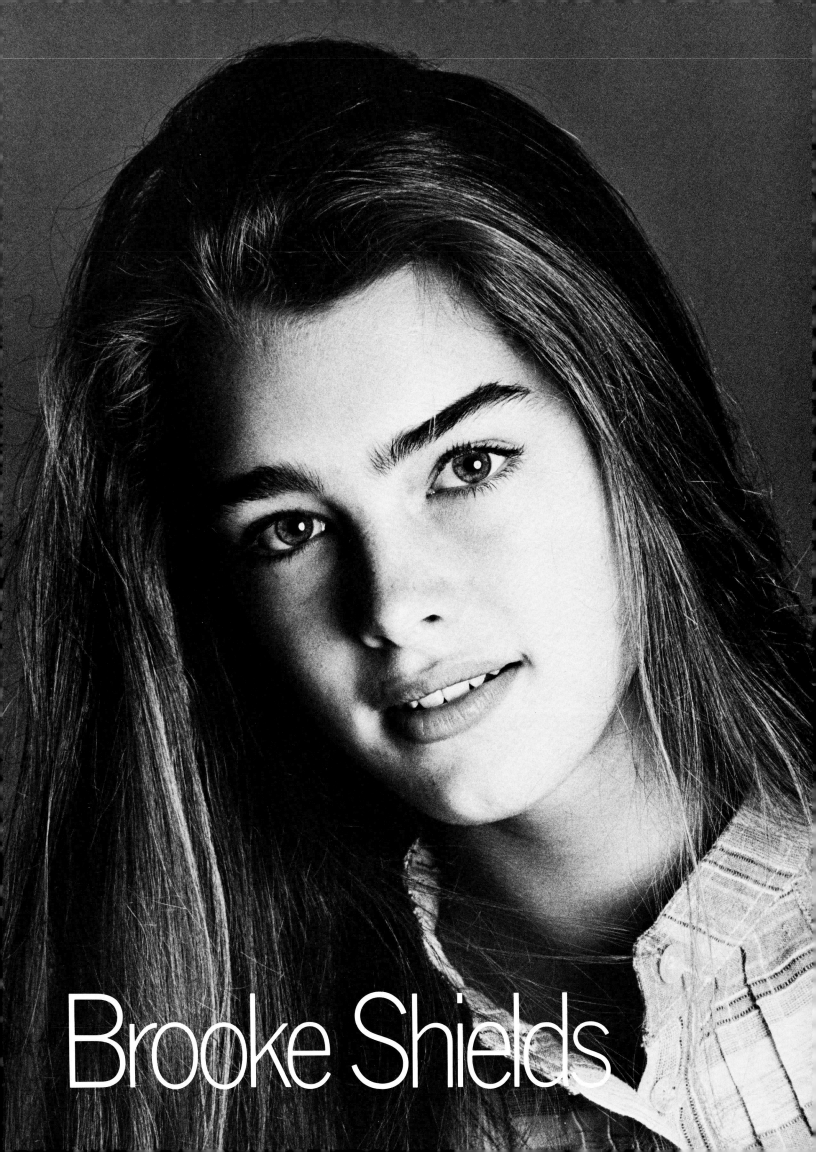

Brooke Shields

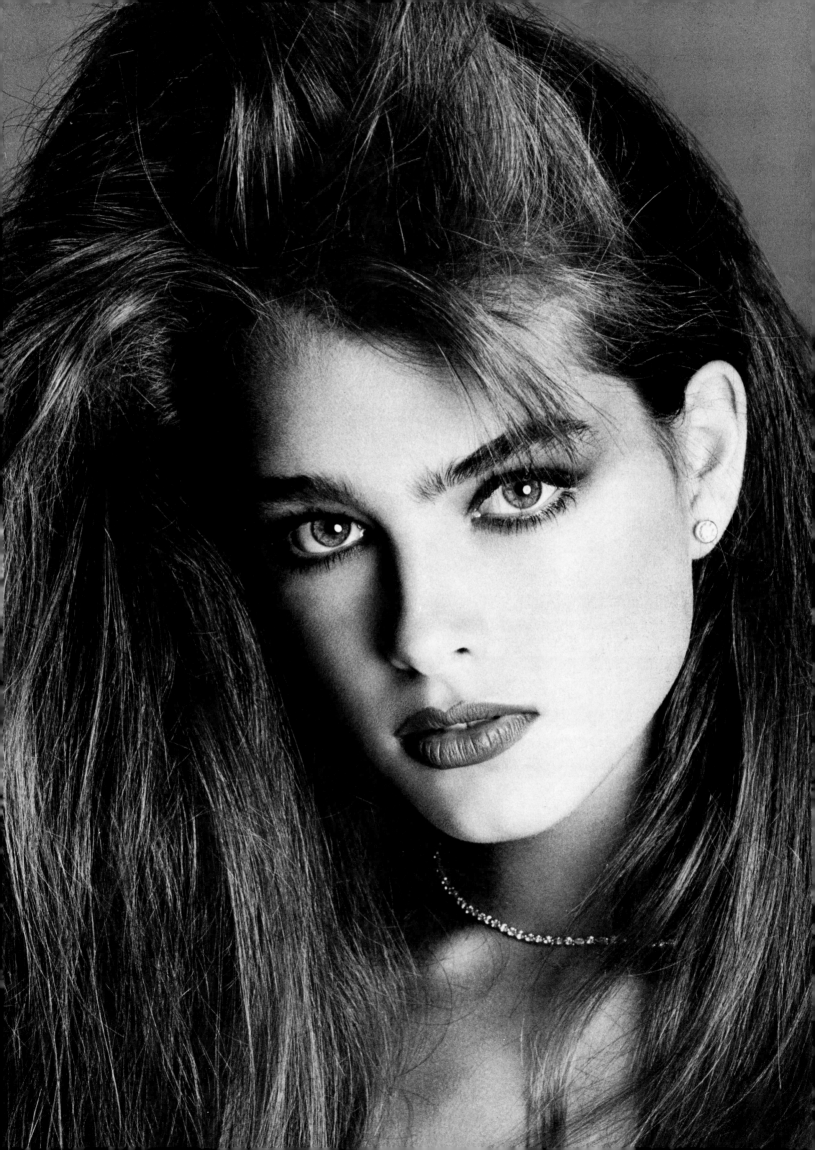

Brooke
Shields

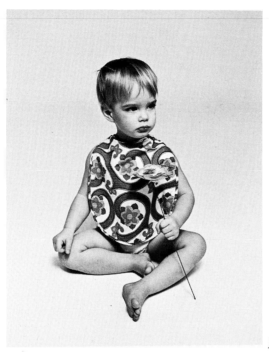

1967

Brooke wears very little makeup in civilian life. Rouge sometimes ("when I get up in the morning and I'm all pale") and petroleum jelly in her eyelashes when she's going out—at night, mascara on her lashes, and lip gloss.

rooke Shields is an absolute miracle—a beautiful, unspoiled, untemperamental, unaffected, unprecocious, uncomplicated, un-Goody-Two-Shoes miracle. She has made eight movies, always as a star, beginning with *Pretty Baby* at age eleven. She has been modeling all her life, always as a star. I have been right there with her, photographing her from her first booking for Ivory Soap, when she was eleven months old, through pages of fashion and magazine covers. She was an adorable baby, an enchanting child; at sixteen, she is a lovely young girl. She has lived, and is living, each of these stages as fully as any parent would hope for any child; she hasn't been rushed through her life. Teri Shields has made sure of it.

Between them, they almost demolish the myth of the baby-doll star and the ambitious stage mother who pulls the strings. Of course Teri wants things for Brooke, big things. As Brooke has said, "Every mother, whether her child is a little dancer or whatever, wants the child to be the best. My mother wants the best for me. And it's not that she's trying to have through me what she didn't have herself. She doesn't push me. She doesn't say, 'Now you will do this; never mind whether you want to or not.' We talk it all out. I trust her judgment on everything."

That's all very well, you may say, but a working child is a working child; you can't be all of one without cheating the other. Brooke apparently can. As anyone who has ever worked with her will tell you—editors, directors, fellow actors/models, photographers—she is a worker, a perfectionist, a professional. And as anyone—especially Brooke—will also tell you, she has not been robbed of her childhood: "There's never been a time when I've said I just want to be a kid, because all along I *have* been just a kid. I have never been deprived of anything. Actually, I think I may have gotten more out of being a kid than most. . . . I get to go to more places and see more things. . . . I've never really thought of what I do as work. I have jobs to do, but they're not hard-working jobs, because I have a good time doing them. I have fun."

Even a Paris Collections, which she did for *Vogue* in about a week of twelve-hour days, was fun: "We worked from around five in the afternoon till five in the morning, then went back to the hotel and slept until three or four, and then we'd go to work again. The hours were strange, but the thing that kept me going was that I was having fun, and, you know, you think of the result."

As she always is, Teri was with Brooke in Paris: "She came to the studio every day. She was on our schedule." They are extremely close—the most important people in each other's lives. Which possibly has less to do with Brooke's career than with their domestic situation: divorced mother/only child/remarried father with a new family. Brooke sees her father regularly, and she gets on well with her two half-sisters, her step-brother, and her step-sister, with whom she has become good friends. But Teri is the center of her universe. Both are aware of potential disruptions. Brooke, for instance, understands that her mother might remarry: "I'd probably dislike the person instinctively . . . just rebelling against the idea. I think I'd get over it . . . I want her to be happy. But . . . when I was a very little girl, I used to say to her, 'You're not getting married until I'm married.' "

On the other hand, the day is surely coming when Brooke will leave home,

and she worries that "it might be harder for my mother than for me. It's easier to go off when you're young and excited about things. . . . My mom and I joke about it. I'll say, 'I'm going to school in California.' And she'll say, 'What about that nice such-and-such college in New York?' She's always told me she could handle it, so I'm sure she can. . . . What's good is that she has a lot of friends. Everybody I know, everybody I work with—they all love my mom. . . . I think both of us will hurt some. But it's got to happen . . . it's going to happen."

But not in the next twenty minutes. When she isn't modeling or making movies or stalling on the rent to buy another pair of Calvin Klein jeans, she is in high school—a second-year first-class student (average A—) and cheerleader. She has been allowed to date since she turned fifteen. So far, this has meant dating in bunches and dancing to records at somebody's house. No drinking. No drugs: "I'm totally against all kinds of drugs. Even cigarettes. I get my quote-unquote highs from other things: babies, guitar music, animals." She has four of-unknown-origin cats, a four-year-old chestnut mare, and a nine-year-old hunter-jumper dapple-gray gelding. That many of her contemporaries are more sexually adventurous neither shocks nor tempts her, but "I think it's crazy —you don't know anything about anything at that age! Why mess things up for yourself? I was brought up to wait until I was married; I think it's right for me."

Brooke wears her celebrity easily. She is unfailingly pleasant with fans. They don't always respond in kind; one of the few things that makes her angry is to be dining in a restaurant, the fork

halfway to her mouth, "and people walk up and just sort of poke at me. . . . Right in the middle of eating, they'll start asking how I got started and how can they do it. When people don't have any cool about how they ask questions . . . or if they're snotty to me, or to my mother, that gets me angry." It passes quickly and rarely shows. "I try to control it. I don't let go of my feelings a lot, except with my mom." Brooke occasionally fights with her mother—"Name me one kid that doesn't—sometimes I yell. Mostly, I go into my room and mumble, or I'd get in a lot of trouble."

It's only when I look in the lens that I forget she's still a kid. Then, she doesn't look like one. And it's more than her beauty; she has—and has had from early on (don't forget who started the present trend to very young models!)—a unique ability to take a child's natural gift for fantasy and dressing-up and project it to the ultimate degree. It doesn't mean that nothing is too old for her; I think, for example, couture clothes are. I like her in younger, more contemporary-looking things—Kenzo and Stephen Burrows are great on her —or jeans and a shirt, the way she goes around most of the time.

"When I look at myself, I like what I see."

Like most models who are up to their ears in makeup every working day, Brooke wears very little in civilian life. Rouge sometimes ("when I get up in the morning and I'm all pale") and petroleum jelly in her eyelashes. When she's going out at night, mascara on her lashes, and lip gloss.

I've been trying to get her to let me lighten her eyebrows, just sort of clean them up a little. She won't let me touch them: "I'm happy with the way I look . . . it isn't that I pay all that much attention, but when I look at myself I like what I see." So do I. A lot.

"There's never been a time when I've said I just want to be a kid, because all along I *have* been just a kid."

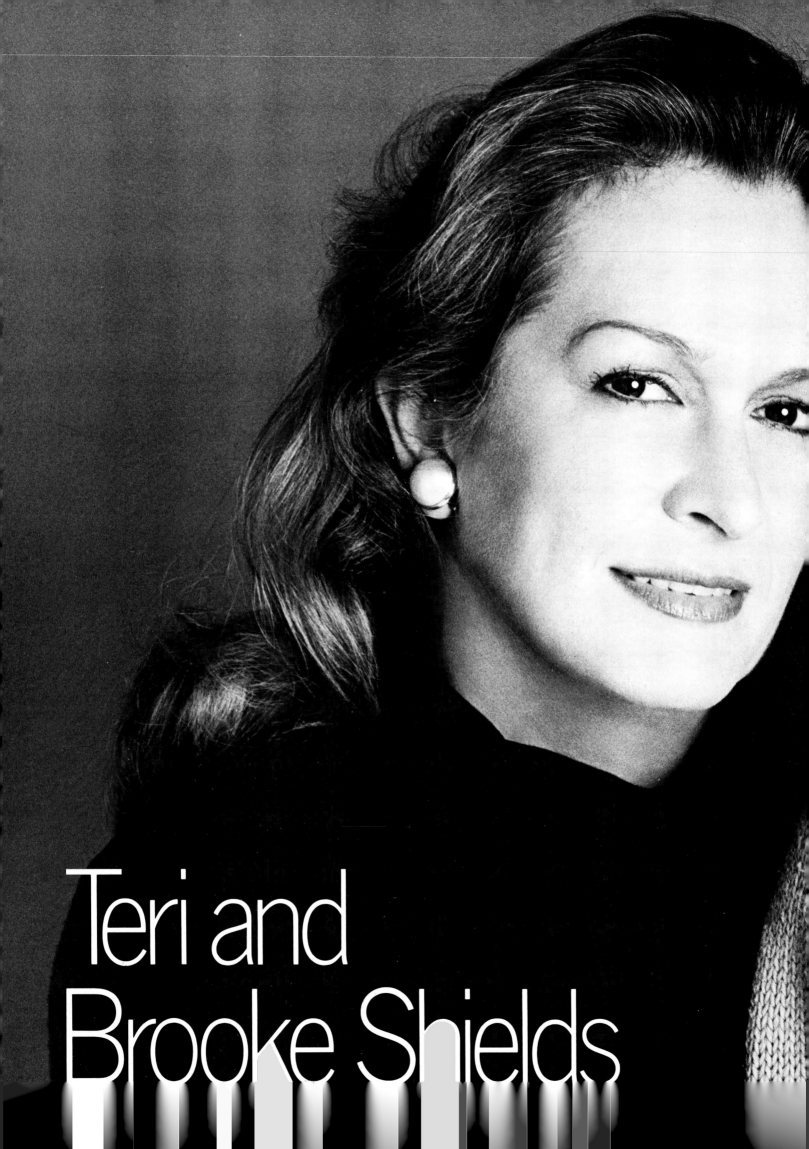

Teri and
Brooke Shields

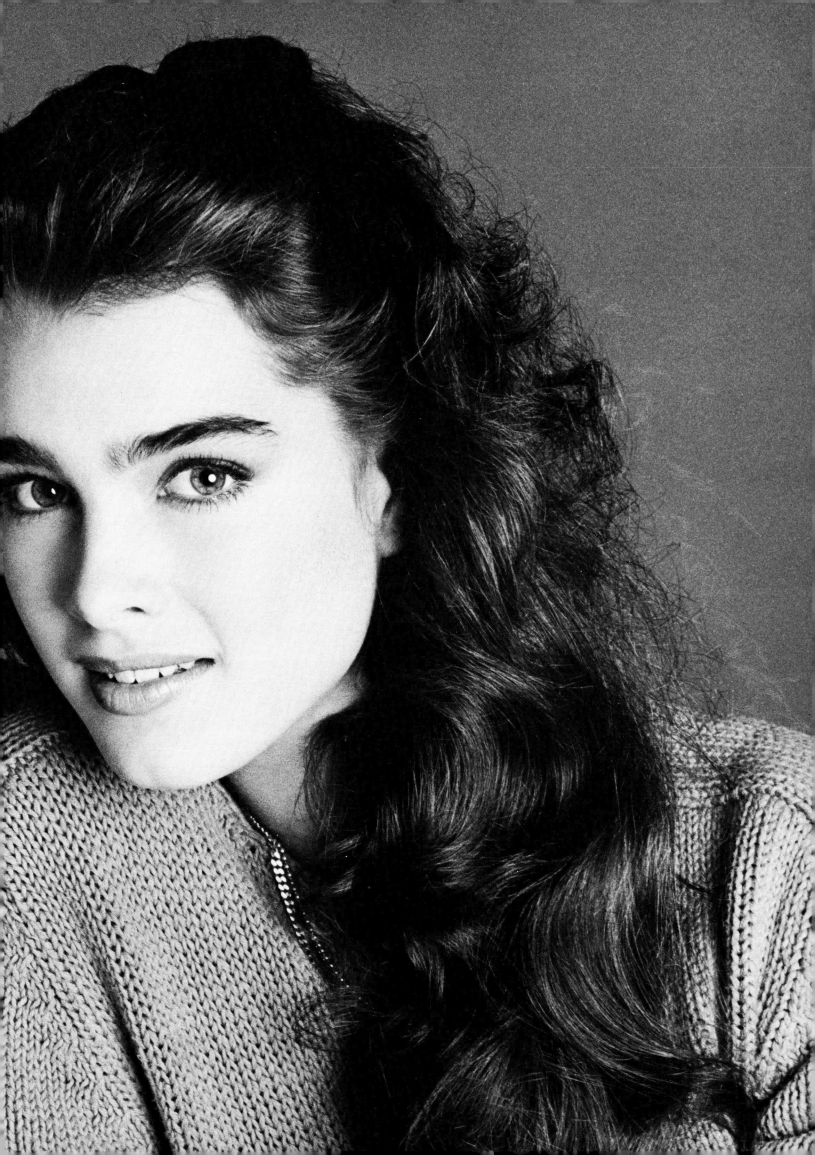

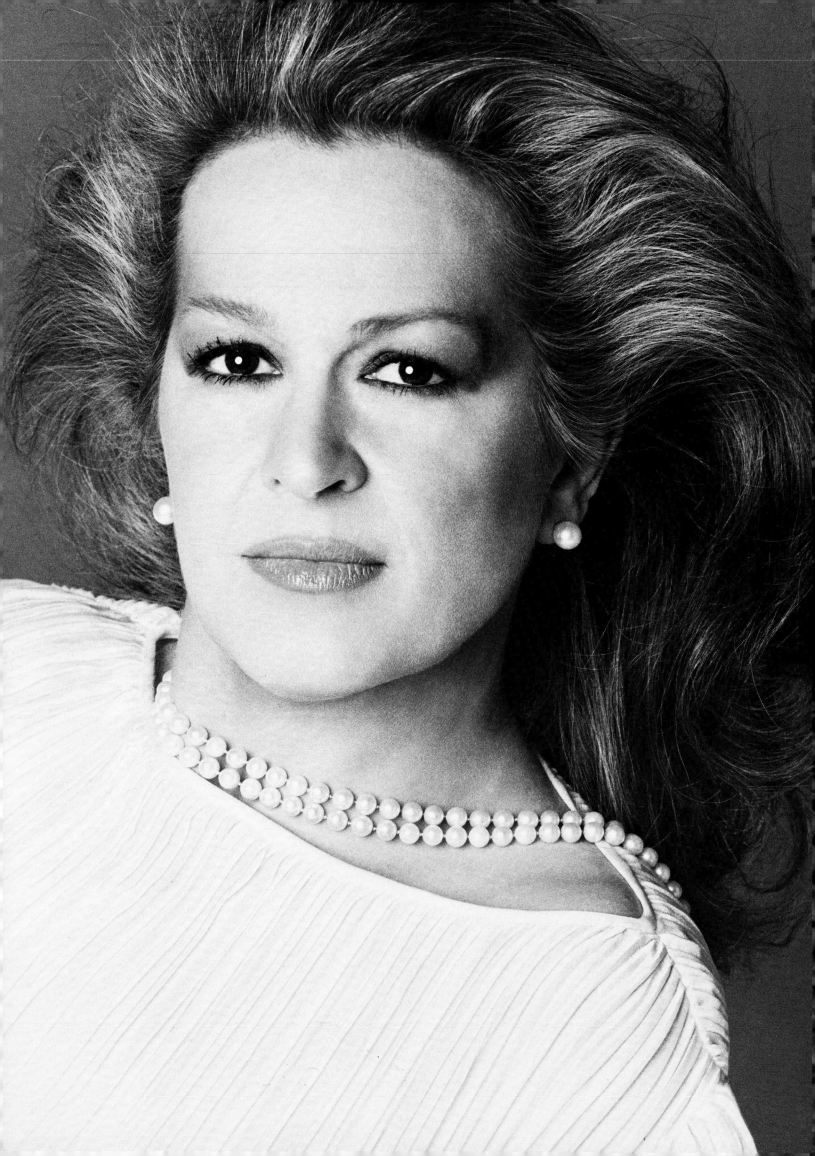

A foolproof beauty secret: liking yourself

Teri Shields

It's always puzzled me that there should be so much misunderstanding about Teri Shields; to get it right, all you have to do is look at her daughter. As *Vogue* Fashion Editor Polly Mellen says, "Brooke Shields is unique in the modeling business and should not be confused with this sudden rush of babies dressing up in big people's clothes. She is a beautiful young woman—and young she is: a sixteen-year-old girl who acts like a sixteen-year-old girl . . . a beauty inside as well as outside. And why is because of that great woman behind her. Teri Shields is really something—a nice, good, straight lady. I'm crazy about her! Brooke is her whole life; she manages her, mothers her, loves her. Once in a while, someone will make a crack, and I'll say, 'You don't know Teri; if you did you wouldn't say that.' "

So I am crazy about Teri, and not least of all for her grace under that fire of "cracks," which, predictably, gets hotter as Brooke's star rises higher. To charges that she was pushing Brooke too hard, robbing her of her childhood, and exploiting her sexuality, Teri's response has been that of a woman whose proof is in the pudding and whose conscience is clear. The onus of stage-momism "didn't bother me one bit; I knew I wasn't. I knew that if Brooke had wanted to do anything else it wouldn't have made any difference to me. The thing that is first in our relationship is total love, and we're able to work everything around it."

She has been known, when she felt Brooke was being hassled, to pull her off the set. It has happened exactly twice in fifteen years, but it's the kind of story that reputations are made on. "I fight for Brooke and I get bad press.

I don't care what they say about me, because I know that if I've done something wrong, I'm going to pay for it. But if I haven't, I have only God and myself to answer to. So I don't go to bed worrying, 'Oh, this guy is talking about me.' If I did I'd be worrying all day long—and never sleep."

Teri is aware that Brooke is at a particularly vulnerable age: "There are thoughts that confuse her, and there's so much to think about and to adjust to as a human being." Professionally, "things are beginning to happen. People are trying to deal with her when they should be dealing with me—because she's getting older. I remember at the People's Choice Award, where she won the favorite-young-actress trophy, people approached her—right then and there at our dinner table. That's why I'm there to protect her. And people don't like it when anybody gets in their way—especially the mother; that makes it tougher for them, so of course they're going to talk about me."

You frequently hear it said that Teri has used their mother/daughter, manager/client relationship to foster excessive dependence in Brooke. Still, while there's no question that they are exceptionally close, the truth of the matter is that no woman in Teri's position could be more sensitive to the obvious dangers in the situation or take more pains to avoid them. Teri, who was separated from her former husband when Brooke was five months old, has remained friendly with him, and Brooke—with Teri's blessing—is very much part of the life of her father's present family. Equally, she encourages Brooke to "visit with friends and spend time with them. . . . I think ours is closer than any relationship I've ever known, but we do need our separate space. I probably not as much as Brooke. She's growing up, and I want her to develop into an individual . . . independent.

"From thirteen to sixteen is a sensitive time, where you're a little shaky about what you want to do, what you want to be. I've seen her draw closer to me but also resent that she wants to, so

she fights it. But all this proves to me that she's strong and understanding about her feelings, and she's learning to work with them."

It's no secret that until nearly three years ago, Teri had a serious drinking problem; she entered a six-week alcoholism training program at St. Mary's Hospital in Minneapolis, Minnesota, and describes the therapy as "five different people telling you the same things in different ways over and over and over—how bad drinking is for you, what do you really want out of life, and so forth. In a sense it's a brainwashing. But if it works, what's the difference? *I have no desire to drink now* . . . it's like a dream that I ever did. Maybe it was just something I had to go through and come out of, I don't know."

Teri is forty-nine and liking herself better than she has in years. She isn't planning to remarry—and she isn't ruling it out. "If someone came along, I would certainly consider it. . . . That's the way I've always been. I've never anticipated. When I was a child, I never thought, 'What am I going to be when I grow up?' I was—I am—pretty much laid back; what happens will happen. I don't plan that when I'm fifty I'm going to do this, and when I'm sixty I'm going to do that. I never have."

Which isn't the same as not having goals. "I'm working on a regime, because I've neglected myself. The first thing is losing weight. I've lost eighteen pounds, and I'd like to lose another twenty. So I've stopped eating ice cream and sweets. . . . And a new wardrobe. . . . And I'm going to go back to being blond again. I've always been blond—streaked blond—and what's happening now is that gray is slowly growing through my hair, and it looks 'ugh.' So that's on my agenda. And then, maybe—*maybe*—a face lift." Whether she does or not hardly matters. The point is that for Teri right now "everything is in the right direction"; that's what shows in her face—and if you could put it up in jars you'd have the most expensive cosmetic in the whole wide world.

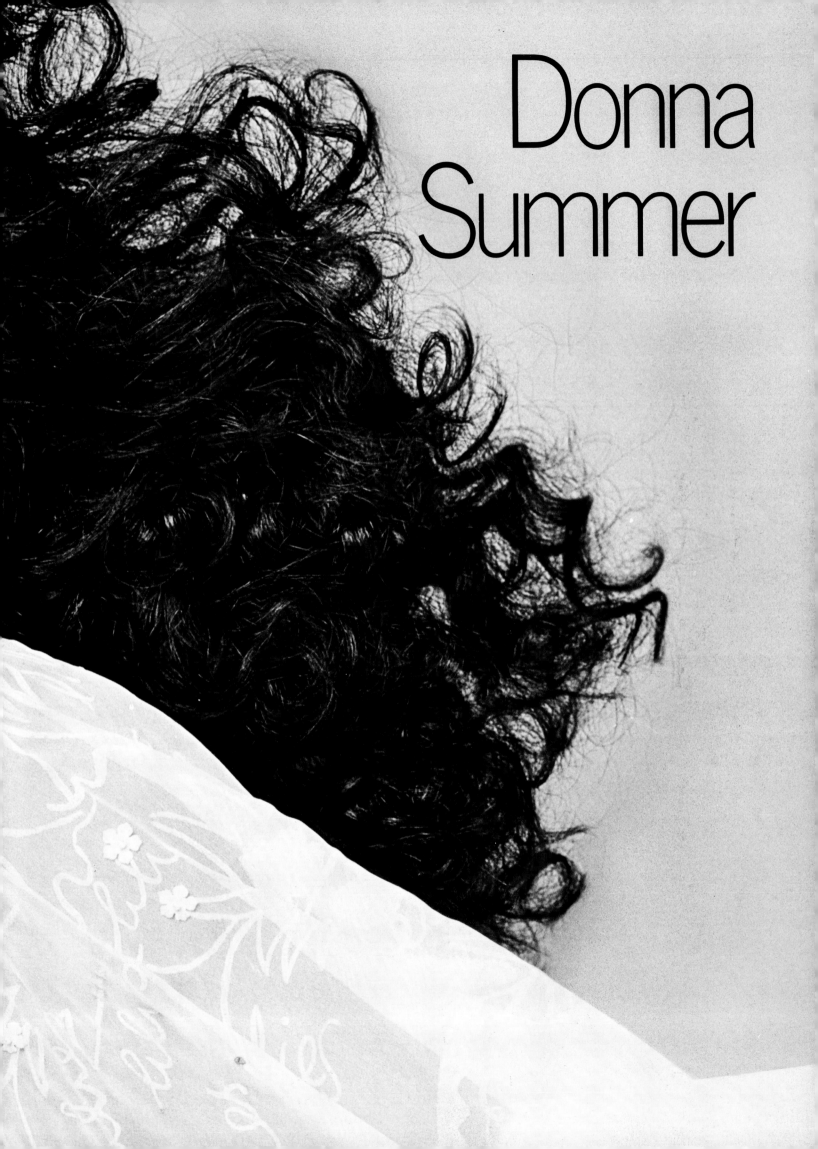

Donna
Summer

Donna
Summer

"Disco is just the ship I happened to come in on. I'm not a disco singer, or a rock-and-roll singer, or a rhythm-and-blues singer, or a classical singer. I am a singer. I will sing anything. It's not in my spirit not to try to use everything I have."

From the moment that Donna Summer walked into my studio for her first album-cover sitting, I knew what I wanted for her was a look that was feminine and at the same time alluring and sensual. The look had to be soft, soft, soft . . . with earthy tones, smudged into each other so there would be no hard lines anywhere. Way Bandy did her makeup divinely and Suga, who is an absolute genius, fashioned her hair just like a fairytale princess (for any woman the secret is this: You have to comb it and comb it and comb it! The result—a head of gorgeous, lustrous hair that looks absolutely great).

Donna loved the way she looked. But it doesn't mean she'll stick with it —or with any other image—any more than she would lock herself into a single image as a singer. To her, it isn't that she stopped doing disco and started doing rock: "Disco is just the ship I happened to come in on. I'm not a disco singer, or a rock-and-roll singer, or a rhythm-and-blues singer, or a classical singer. I am a singer. I will sing anything. It's not in my spirit not to try to use everything I have. I don't look at myself in terms of being

any one thing . . . to be any one thing totally and forever would be complete stagnation. . . . I get very bored with things being the same. I don't even like to eat meals at home most of the time, because the sameness of the food begins to get on my nerves. So, when I go out to eat, I order a lot of different things. I won't eat them all; I just need to taste the variety."

"I get very bored with things being the same."

She is an incredible, galvanizing performer; if you measured the energy in kilowatts, it would cost the earth. Don't think it doesn't cost Donna: "I actually have lumps in my back from the energy I use. I do a lot of moving around onstage, bending over, bending backward, touching my head almost to the floor. . . . If I'm performing outside and the cold air is blowing, I don't feel

it till I come in. Then, I'm as stiff as a board, and my voice is like 'aarrrgh.' I can also get very, very hyper from the continuous flow of energy from performing. I don't take any kind of drugs, but I have to have something to relieve the tension."

What she has is massage: "Massage is my relaxant . . . I get massages every day. My masseuse is a wonderful girl named Jeannie Copeland. She has been coming to me for about five years, and

---

"I think the older you get, the more you have to try to become aware of your body."

---

she's often with me on the road. Within three to five minutes after she starts massaging, I'm out cold. Basically, she uses acupressure. She does my face and she does my feet . . . it's mainly centered in the feet and the hands and in the skull and in the ears. But when she starts doing my feet, I just go 'zzzzzz.' It's fantastic . . . while I was pregnant, it was the best thing that happened to me in the physical world."

Donna and Bruce Sudano, her husband, have a new baby girl named Brooklyn (Bruce, formerly one of the Brooklyn Dreams, comes from you-know-where and will be releasing his solo album this year). Donna's daughter Mimi, the child of her marriage to Helmuth Sommer, an Austrian whom she met in Germany when she was playing in the musical *Hair,* was born in Munich. (In Germany, where Donna lived for eight years, she also did *The Me Nobody Knows, Godspell,* the Vienna Folk Opera's version of *Porgy and Bess,* and began in German clubs to sing the kind of music that, soon after back in the States, zoomed her to fame as the Disco Queen.) Mimi spoke no English when they came here; now she's having to re-learn German: "When you ask her what she is—what nationality—she says, 'I'm a German shepherd.'"

That her mother is also a celebrity isn't a point of conflict for Mimi: "She knows what it's all about. She goes on stage with me a lot—she had her own little number on my TV special. She knows that it's makeup and eyelashes and sparkles. She knows what it takes to make me a star!" Still, the obvious question arises: How does the life of a pop star reconcile with bringing up a child? As Donna found out when Mimi was five, it doesn't. "I wanted to take her everywhere. And yet I knew she really needed to be where she was, in nursery school."

Donna's solution was to take Mimi to her own parents. She says, with a slight edge of justification, "Until I had my second child, I would have to say that my parents raised Mimi. I could never even try to accept the responsibility or the credit. My parents are her parents. I had to do it that way before . . . I was in tears every time I had to leave. It got to the point where I said to myself, You know, grandparents have been raising grandchildren for years. The parents work and bring in the money, and the grandparents stay home and care for the kids . . . it goes down each generation, in all countries.

For a while, she accompanied me on the road, but it was very rough. So I know I shouldn't feel guilty about this; it's what I figured was best for Mimi."

There's no doubt that it is. And the logistics help: Donna's parents live right around the corner, and "Mimi may stay with me for two or three weeks, then at my parents' for two or three weeks, then back. She goes to school from their house, and my

---

"To be any one thing totally and forever would be complete stagnation."

---

mother gets her ready for school and does the things I would normally do; the bottom line is that we are on such different schedules. I can't go to sleep at nine or ten, which I would have to to get up with my daughter . . . so she goes from one to the other. But so far it's worked out well; she feels at home in both places." Mimi's situation will stay as it is for the present. And now that one is affordable, there will be a governess for the new baby.

That she was going to have a baby at all came as a bit of a surprise; tests were negative, her period continued. And the first few months of pregnancy were

---

"I don't take any kind of drugs, but I have to have something to relieve the tension. . . . Massage is my relaxant. . . . I get massages every day."

---

a nightmare: "I was so violently sick, I couldn't eat, I couldn't even smell food. I thought I would never get out of bed; normally, I don't need more than four or six hours sleep. My skin was a mess." When she finally leveled out, she had lost twelve pounds (she gained them back, but it was all she gained) and two lifelong allergies: one to oranges, one to garlic. She eats both now.

P regnancy cut down her exercising to walking, yoga, and a few leg lifts in bed. The non-pregnant Donna is a gung-ho worker-outer—modern jazz, ballet, rollerskating: "I think the older you get, the more you have to try to become aware of your body. You have to say to yourself, 'I've got to take care of this old bod, or I'm not going to have it.' You have to pretend it's like 'the most fine' car you've ever had, and it's the only one you're gonna have for the rest of your life. You're not gonna let anybody drive into it. You're gonna make sure that it gets tuned up. You are not going to blow out the exhaust!"

For Donna Summer, who has accomplished the unprecedented feat of having two Number One albums and two Number One singles on the charts in one year, has earned both an Oscar and a Grammy for her hit song "Last Dance" from the motion picture *Thank God It's Friday,* a film in which she also starred, and has also sold over 20 million albums worldwide, I'd say the chances of the exhaust blowing out simply don't exist. . . . No way.

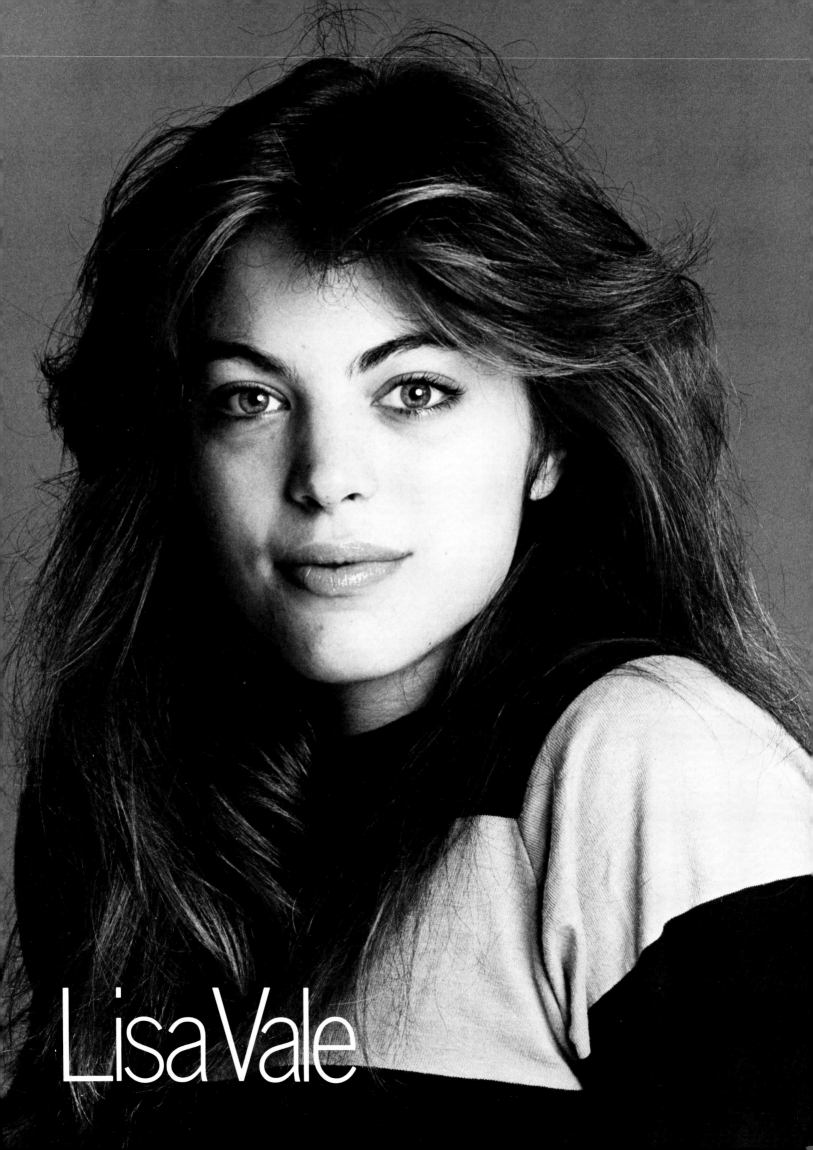

Lisa Vale

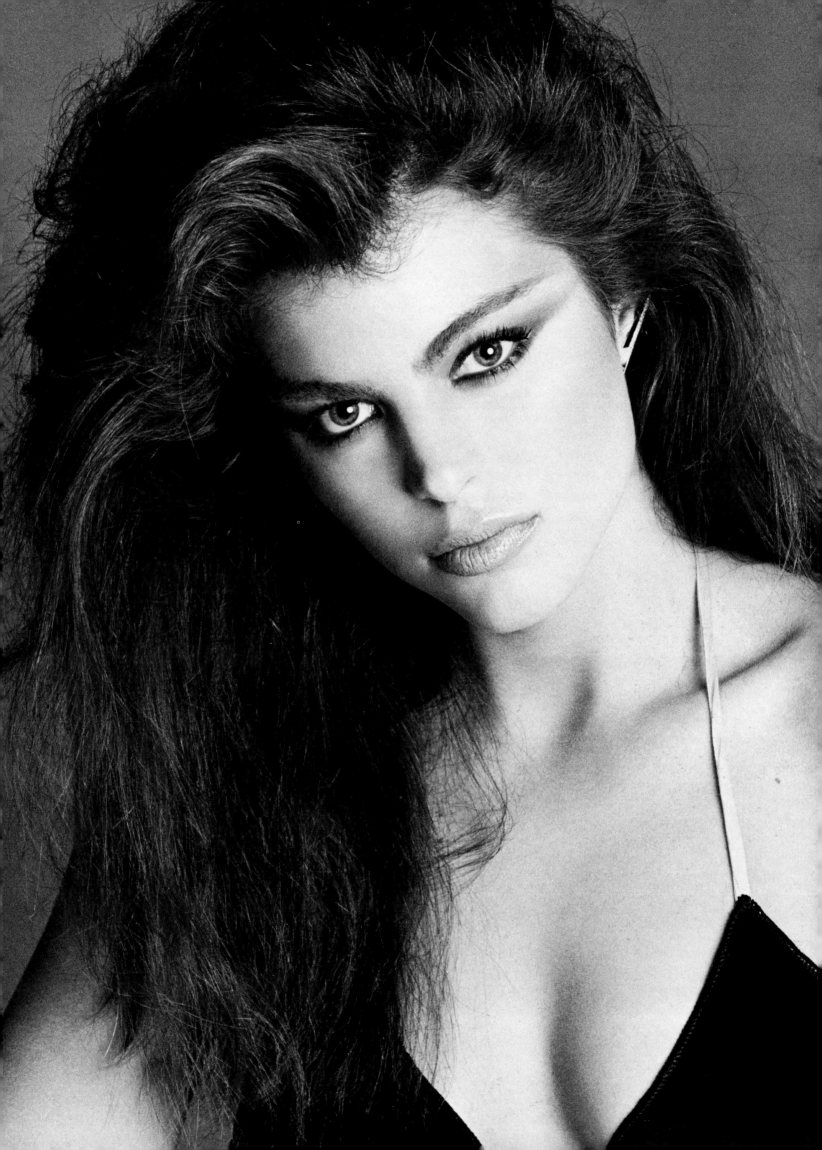

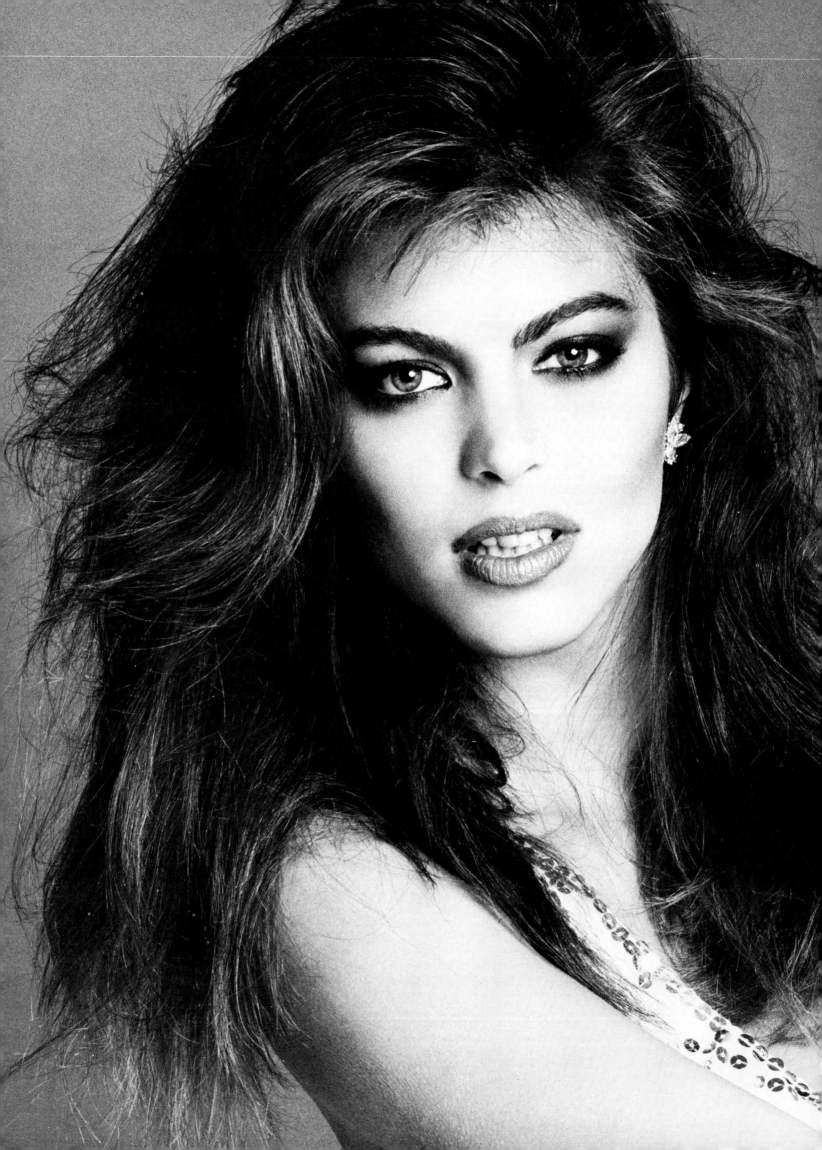

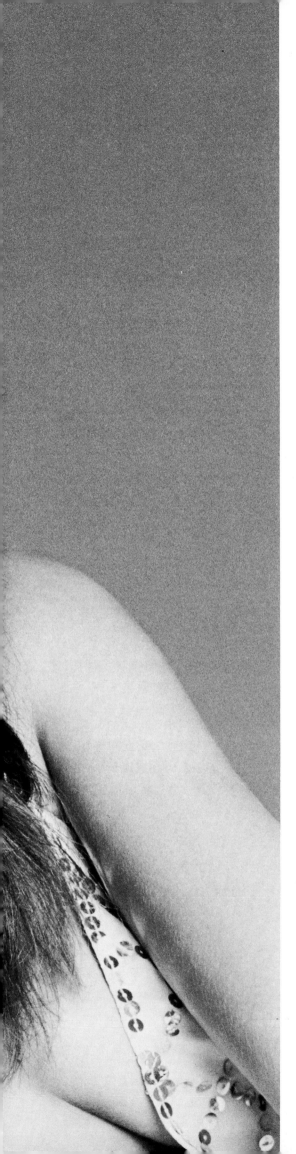

Lisa Vale

Lisa Vale is a beauty. I love her energy and the whole bold brunette look of her. I think I'd faint if she came to the studio in some slickeroo designer creation. What she wears are wonderful, crazy T-shirts and jeans, and her hair is wild and beautiful. And she looks great—sort of rough and tough, as though she might jump on a horse or a bike and blast out of sight. She's modern and exciting, and this is what I think is so fabulous to show in a photograph. But I also realize that not everybody is ready for it (Diana Vreeland once said, "The eye always hates what it hasn't learned to love"); for some people, Lisa is too strong.

So, for some people I soften her. That's the story of the large photograph, for which Way Bandy did the makeup. I told him, "No black. Make everything light . . . make it soft. More round than hard." In the small photograph, left, I had John Richardson do an opposite makeup. This time I wanted to bring out what she has, so there is more of everything: more mascara, more black around the eyes, more contouring on the cheeks, really bringing out those bones. And where in the large picture her eyebrows have been slightly bleached, in this one they've been left as they are, dark and emphatic.

It's how Lisa sees herself; she would rather die than look like the girl next door, though it would probably push her ahead faster. As she is the first to tell you: "I'm not what America is into right now. They're into the blond, blue-eyed, true-blue look. . . . I have a very strong look, a very sexy look. It scares them; it's always going to scare them. And I'm a big girl, which is also hard for them to accept. When I started, I weighed 150 pounds; now I'm about 135; I guess I should be 125. But I'm five-eleven, and I have good proportions. . . . I love the look I have; I wouldn't change it for the world."

There are two kinds of models. There are the girls who will cap their teeth, straighten their noses, straighten their hair, chop it all off, lose thirty pounds in seven days—whatever the agency or the editor or the photographer asks for—and there are the take-me-as-I-am-or-leave-me girls, who hold onto their own image of themselves with both hands. I admire them; they're gutsy ladies, sailing smack against the fashion establishment . . . and often crashing. Lisa crashed: "In the beginning, I was perfectly spontaneous. I loved it . . . just getting out there and working for the camera. It didn't matter which were my good angles and which were bad. Sometimes even your worst angles can be good, because it's really all in the mood, in the dancing of the eyes or whatever, and maybe your face does look fleshy, but the eyes are magnificent and that's what you're going for. . . . Then I started to know the angles. I began playing up this one and playing down that one. And I lost something. It wasn't real or spontaneous anymore. It wasn't me. And I just rebelled against the whole business.

"I wouldn't go on appointments. I would go on bookings with my nails chewed off. I wouldn't lose the weight they wanted me to lose. I wouldn't exercise. I wouldn't keep my body together. . . . I got bitchy. I told off an editor. . . . I was doing drugs, a lot of grass, cocaine. It took me three giant steps back. I was so burnt out, I couldn't talk—I was stuttering—and I couldn't remember things. . . . People in the business knew I was screwing up. I was looking exhausted on shoots. I *was* exhausted."

When you consider the nature of modeling, what happened to Lisa doesn't seem so surprising: Beautiful new models are like beautiful new babies; they are petted and pampered and cooed over. And it's terribly easy—especially at eighteen or nineteen or twenty—to take this sort of thing too seriously. A lot of young women do; they mistake the frills for the whole garment and fail to understand that, as well as sweet and adorable, they are also expected to be grown-up and professional and fully aware of their responsibilities and obligations. When Lisa finally got the message, she got it right: "It's a business; that's the only way to look at it. And it's a good business. I've traveled. I've met people. I've done more fascinating things than I could have in any other job. . . . There is no perfect job, no perfect living conditions, no perfect anything. I couldn't accept that at first, I couldn't handle it. It took me another year and a half to say, 'Hey, do you like yourself this way? No? Then get it together!' . . . I can accept it all now, good and bad, and I'm going for it—all the way!"

Francesco Scavullo uses a Hasselblad camera with a 150-mm Sonar lens and electronic flash. He shoots with Tri-X film and develops with Acufine. The printing is done on Kodak polycontrast F paper. All photo printing for this book was done by Jim Reiher and David Radin.

The text of this book was set in film in a face called *Times Roman,* designed by Stanley Morison for the *Times* (London), and first introduced by that newspaper in 1932. Among typographers and designers of the twentieth century, Stanley Morison has been a strong forming influence, as typographical adviser to the English Monotype Corporation, as a director of two distinguished English publishing houses, and a writer of sensibility, erudition, and keen practical sense.

The book was composed by ComCom, in Allentown, Pennsylvania. It was printed on 80 pound L.O.E. Gloss and bound by the Murray Printing Company, Forge Village, Massachusetts.

FRANCESCO SCAVULLO was born on Staten Island and raised and educated in New York City. He began his career as a professional photographer in 1948. In the past three decades he has photographed nearly every celebrated man and woman in America, as well as many of the most famous men and women in the world. He photographs the fashion collections for major designers in New York, Paris, Rome, and Milan, and the covers for every major magazine, including American *Vogue*, French *Vogue*, Italian *Vogue, Harper's Bazaar, Cosmopolitan, Time, Newsweek, Us, People, Good Housekeeping, Ladies' Home Journal, Essence, Seventeen, Ebony, New York, Interview, Town & Country, Zoom, Playboy, Esquire, Glamour, Life*, and *Redbook*. Generally acknowledged to be the dominant photographic influence on American beauty and fashion, Mr. Scavullo is the author of two previous bestsellers, *Scavullo on Beauty* and *Scavullo Men*, and recently photographed the 1982 souvenir book for the American Ballet Theatre. A series of his portraits of men is in the permanent collection of the Metropolitan Museum of Art in New York City. He photographs many celebrities and artists for record album covers, book covers, and movie posters. Mr. Scavullo also does commissioned portraits for private individuals.